Statins: Understanding Clinical Use

Jawahar L. Mehta, MD, PhD

Professor of Internal Medicine, and Physiology
& Biophysics
Stebbins Chair in Cardiology
Director, Division of Cardiovascular Medicine
University of Arkansas for Medical Sciences
Director, Cardiology Services, Central Arkansas
Veterans Healthcare System
Little Rock, Arkansas

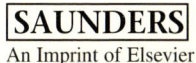

SAUNDERS
An Imprint of Elsevier

SAUNDERS
An Imprint of Elsevier

The Curtis Center
Independence Square West
Philadelphia, Pennsylvania 19106

Library of Congress Cataloging-in-Publication Data

Statins: understanding clinical use / [edited by] J.L. Mehta.–1st ed.
    p. ; cm.
  Includes bibliographical references.
  ISBN 0-7216-0380-7
    1. Statins (Cardiovascular agents) 2. Hypercholesteremia–Chemotherapy.
I. Mehta, Jawahar.
    [DNLM: 1. Hypercholesterolemia–drug therapy. 2. Anticholesteremic
  Agents–therapeutic use. WD 200.5.H8 S797 2004]
  RM666.S714S73 2004
  616.3′997–dc22   2003066883

Acquisitions Editor: Anne Lenehan
Project Manager: Joan Nikelsky
Editorial Assistant: Vera Ginsburgs

Printed in China

Last digit is the print number: 9   8   7   6   5   4   3   2   1

Acknowledgments

I wish to thank my teachers, students and friends for helping me understand science and its application to the well-being of humankind.

I wish to thank my wife, Paulette, for her love and friendship for over a quarter of a century. I thank my children, Asha and Jason, for their support, understanding, and love.

I particularly want to thank Marcy Havelka for her assistance in getting multiple authors to submit manuscripts on time and to compile the different chapters in uniform format, always with a smile.

My thanks to Anne Lenehan, Joan Nikelsky, and Vera Ginsburgs for helping me with the preparation of this book.

Jawahar L. Mehta, MD, PhD

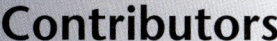

Contributors

Takayuki Asahara, MD, PhD

Professor, Regenerative Medicine Division, Basic Clinical Science Department, Tokai University School of Medicine, Bohseidai Isehara, Kanagawa; Director, Regenerative Medicine and Research Department, Institute of Biomedical Research and Innovation Kobe/RIKEN Kobe Institute Center for Developmental Biology, Kobe, Hyogo, Japan.

Effects of Statins on Endothelial Progenitor Cells: Mobilization, Differentiation, and Contribution to Adult Neovascularization

Gavin J. Blake, MD, MSc, MPH, MRCPI, MRCP

Instructor in Medicine, Harvard Medical School; Associate Physician, Cardiovascular Division, Brigham and Women's Hospital, Boston, Massachusetts.

Statins, Inflammation, and C-Reactive Protein

Raffaele De Caterina, MD, PhD

Associate Professor and Chair, Department of Cardiology, G. D'Annunzio University School of Medicine, Chieti, Italy; Director, Laboratory for Thrombosis and Vascular Research, CNR Institute of Clinical Physiology, Pisa, Italy.

Statins and Reduction of Stroke: Cholesterol-Lowering vs. Pleiotropic Effects

Clarissa Cola, MD

Fellow, Department of Cardiology, University of Tor Vergata School of Medicine, Rome, Italy; Research Fellow, Division of Cardiovascular Medicine, University of Arkansas for Medical Sciences, Little Rock, Arkansas.

New Insights from Trials of Statins in Animal Models of Atherosclerosis

John P. Cooke, MD, PhD

Professor of Medicine, Division of Cardiovascular Medicine; Director, Section of Vascular Medicine, Stanford University School of Medicine; Professor of Medicine, Department of Cardiology/Cardiovascular Medicine, Stanford Hospital, Stanford, California.

Statins and Angiogenesis

Sridevi Devaraj, PhD

Assistant Professor, Department of Pathology, UC Davis
Medical Center, Sacramento, California.
  *Effects of Statins on C-Reactive Protein: Are All Statins
  Similar?*

Pericle Di Napoli, MD

Cardiologist, Department of Cardiology, University of Chieti
School of Medicine; Interventional Cardiologist, Department
of Cardiology, Casa di Cura Villa Pina d'Abruzzo, Chieti, Italy.
  *Statins and Reduction of Stroke: Cholesterol-Lowering
  vs. Pleiotropic Effects*

Louis M. Fink, MD

Professor, Department of Pathology, University of Arkansas
for Medical Sciences; Program Manager, VISN 16 Diagnostic
Services, Central Arkansas Veterans Healthcare System, Little
Rock, Arkansas.
  Anticoagulant Effects of Statins

I. Ross Garrett, PhD

Assistant Professor, Department of Structural and Cellular
Biology, School of Medicine, University of Texas Health
Science Center at San Antonio; Scientific Director,
OsteoScreen, San Antonio, Texas.
  Statins and Bone

Martin Hauer-Jensen, MD, PhD

Professor, Department of Surgery and Pathology, University
of Arkansas for Medical Sciences; Staff Surgeon, Department
of Surgery, Central Arkansas Veterans Healthcare System,
Little Rock, Arkansas.
  Anticoagulant Effects of Statins

Ishwarlal Jialal, MD, PhD

Professor of Pathology and Internal Medicine, and Vice-Chair
for Research, Department of Pathology, University of
California, Davis; Robert E. Stowell Endowed Chair in
Experimental Pathology, and Director, Laboratory for
Atherosclerosis and Metabolic Research, Department of
Pathology, UC Davis Medical Center, Sacramento, California.
  *Effects of Statins on C-Reactive Protein: Are All Statins
  Similar?*

John Kjekshus, MD, PhD

Professor and Head, Department Group of Clinical Medicine, University of Oslo School of Medicine; Senior Consultant, Department of Cardiology, Rikshospitalet, Oslo, Norway.
  Secondary Prevention of Atherosclerosis and Related Events by Statins

Dayuan Li, MD, PhD

Research Assistant Professor, Department of Internal Medicine, University of Arkansas for Medical Sciences, Little Rock, Arkansas.
  Actions of Statins on Ox-LDL–Mediated Signaling and Inflammation

James K. Liao, MD

Associate Professor of Medicine, Harvard Medical School; Director, Vascular Medicine Research, Department of Medicine, Brigham and Women's Hospital, Boston, Massachusetts.
  The Pleiotropic Effects of Statins: Relevance to Their Salutary Effects

Douglas W. Losordo, MD

Associate Professor of Medicine, Tufts University School of Medicine; Chief of Cardiovascular Research, Caritas St. Elizabeth's Medical Center, Boston, Massachusetts.
  Effects of Statins on Endothelial Progenitor Cells: Mobilization, Differentiation, and Contribution to Adult Neovascularization

Ali J. Marian, MD

Associate Professor of Medicine, Baylor College of Medicine, Houston, Texas.
  Statins and the Modulation of Cardiac Hypertrophy and Fibrosis: Implications in the Therapy of Heart Failure

Jawahar L. Mehta, MD, PhD

Professor of Internal Medicine, and Physiology & Biophysics; Stebbins Chair in Cardiology; Director, Division of Cardiovascular Medicine, University of Akansas for Medical Sciences; Director, Cardiology Services, Central Arkansas Veterans Healthcare System, Little Rock, Arkansas
  New Insights from Trials of Statins in Animal Models of Atherosclerosis; Statins in the Primary Prevention of Atherosclerosis-Related Events; Actions of Statins on Ox-LDL–Mediated Signaling and Inflammation;

Anticoagulant Effects of Statins; Statins and Inhibition of Atherosclerosis: Human Studies

Kamal D. Mehta, MPhil, PhD
Associate Professor, Department of Molecular and Cellular Biochemistry, Ohio State University College of Medicine; Investigator, Dorothy M. Davis Heart and Lung Research Institute, Columbus, Ohio.
History and Biochemistry of Statins

Vachaspati Mishra, PhD
Research Associate, Department of Molecular and Cellular Biochemistry, Ohio State University College of Medicine, Columbus, Ohio.
History and Biochemistry of Statins

Gregory R. Mundy, MD, PhD
Professor, Department of Structural and Cellular Biology, Graduate School of Biomedical Sciences, University of Texas Health Science Center at San Antonio, San Antonio, Texas.
Statins and Bone

Francesco Palma, MD
Chair of Cardiology, Clinical Sciences and Bioimaging Department, G. D'Annunzio University School of Medicine; Medical Doctor, Cardiology and Cardiosurgery Department, S. Camillo De Lellis Hospital, Chieti, Italy.
Statins and Reduction of Stroke: Cholesterol-Lowering vs. Pleiotropic Effects

Paul M. Ridker, MD, MPH, FACC, FAHA
Eugene Braunwald Professor of Medicine, Harvard Medical School; Director, Center for Cardiovacular Disease Prevention, Division of Cardiovascular Diseases and Preventive Medicine, Brigham and Women's Hospital, Boston, Massachusetts.
Statins, Inflammation, and C-Reactive Protein

Francesco Romeo, MD
Professor and Chairman, Department of Cardiology, University of Rome Tor Vergata School of Medicine, Rome, Italy.
New Insights from Trials of Statins in Animal Models of Atherosclerosis

Balkrishna M. Singh, MD, FACC
Assistant Professor of Medicine, Division of Cardiovascular
Medicine, University of Arkansas for Medical Sciences; Staff
Cardiologist, Divison of Cardiology, Veterans Affairs Hospital,
Little Rock, Arkansas.
> *Statins and Inhibition of Atherosclerosis: Human
> Studies; Statins in the Primary Prevention of
> Atherosclerosis-Related Events*

Anjan K. Sinha, MD
Assistant Professor of Medicine; Director, Non-Invasive
Laboratories, Division of Cardiovascular Medicine, University
of Arkansas for Medical Sciences, Little Rock, Arkansas.
> *Statins and Inhibition of Atherosclerosis: Human
> Studies; Statins in the Primary Prevention of
> Atherosclerosis-Related Events*

Dirk H. Walter, MD
Fellow in Cardiology, Department of Internal Medicine IV,
Division of Cardiology, University of Frankfurt, Frankfurt,
Germany.
> *Effects of Statins on Endothelial Progenitor Cells:
> Mobilization, Differentiation, and Contribution to
> Adult Neovascularization*

Junru Wang, MD, PhD
Assistant Professor, Department of Surgery, University of
Arkansas for Medical Sciences, Little Rock, Arkansas.
> *Anticoagulant Effects of Statins*

Michael Weis, MD
Head, Working Group Atherosclerosis and Endothelial
Dysfunction, Medizinische Klinik and Poliklinik I, University
Hospital Munich-Grosshadern/Ludwig-Maximilians University
of Munich, Munich, Germany.
> *Statins and Angiogenesis*

Gabriele Weitz-Schmidt, PhD
Head, Research Program, Preclinical Research, Novartis
Pharma AG, Basel, Switzerland.
> *Effects of Statins on Lymphocyte Function–Associated
> Antigen-1*

Sebastian Wolfrum, MD
Research Fellow, Vascular Medicine Research Unit, Brigham and Women's Hospital, Boston, Massachusetts.
   The Pleiotropic Effects of Statins: Relevance to Their Salutary Effects

Preface

Major advances in elucidation of the pathogenesis of atherosclerosis-related diseases and in their diagnosis and treatment have occurred in the last 50 years or so. Understanding of the pathogenesis of atherosclerosis has been greatly enhanced by recognition of the critical role of elevated total cholesterol and low-density lipoprotein (LDL)-cholesterol levels in plasma, although recent observations suggest that oxidatively modified LDL-cholesterol may be even more important than native LDL in atherogenesis. Another major advance has been the recognition that thrombosis is an important part of the process of atherogenesis. Rupture or hemorrhage into a vulnerable atherosclerotic plaque is followed by formation of an occlusive thrombus. Persistence of an occlusive thrombus in the narrowed coronary artery is now believed to be the basis of acute myocardial infarction, whereas an unstable thrombus leads to unstable angina. Similarly, thrombosis occurring in the cerebral circulation is now thought to be a major cause of many cerebrovascular accidents. Information on the causative role of inflammation in atherogenesis is evolving. Although inflammation is seen in all stages of atherosclerosis, there is a predominance of inflammatory cells in the "shoulder" region of vulnerable plaque. In addition, studies in experimental animal models indicate that interference with the pathways of inflammation can limit atherosclerosis.

These concepts in the pathogenesis of atherosclerosis and acute coronary syndromes have led to novel catheter-based, surgical, and pharmaceutical approaches in the management of patients with coronary artery disease (CAD). Among the pharmacologic therapies that have altered the natural history of atherosclerosis and related events are the antiplatelet drugs, such as aspirin, and LDL-cholesterol–lowering agents. Although earlier cholesterol-lowering agents, such as bile acid sequestrants, lowered total cholesterol and LDL-cholesterol, the reduction was modest and the side effects were significant. This resulted in poor acceptance of these agents by patients and physicians alike in the treatment of hypercholesterolemia. The discovery of hydroxymethylglutaryl–coenzyme A reductase inhibitors, commonly known as statins, led to a new era in which we saw a marked 40% to 60% reduction in LDL-cholesterol levels in association with a dramatic reduction in CAD-related events with use of these agents. The reduction in cardiovascular events was observed in both primary and secondary prevention trials. This efficacy of statins has been shown in a wide spectrum of patients with almost any combination and permutation of risk factors for atherosclerosis.

Recent clinical trials show the efficacy of statins in reducing CAD-related events in patients with diabetes, hypertension, and other cardiovascular risk factors regardless of the baseline LDL-cholesterol values, which raises two very important questions. First, should all patients with previous cardiovascular disease and others with coronary risk factors be given statins no matter what the baseline LDL-cholesterol levels? Second, can one attribute all of the benefits of treatment with statins to reduction in LDL-cholesterol, or might there be other effects of statins, unrelated to LDL-cholesterol lowering, that result in the dramatic decrease in cardiovascular events? These latter effects, which have often been called pleiotropic, may well relate to the overall efficacy of statins in patients with atherosclerosis.

A recent search on PubMed with the keyword "statins" revealed 7517 refereed publications. Of course, only a small number of the studies cited relate to the clinical efficacy of these drugs. Most studies relate to the effects of these agents on a number of biochemical pathways, mechanisms of cell injury, and surrogate markers of cardiovascular disease. This book is a compilation of several of these studies by noted experts and different areas of statin research.

There will no doubt be more trials of statins in diverse patient populations, as well as novel mechanistic insights to define the mechanism of the benefit of this group of drugs. For example, a recent study from Japan provided the first visual evidence of stabilization of unstable plaque in patients with acute coronary syndrome with use of atorvastatin. Other studies show reduction in atherosclerosis in the coronary arteries with this agent. We now have newer and more potent statins, such as rosuvastatin, which cause a dramatic reduction in LDL-cholesterol level. With the initial starting dose of rosuvastatin, LDL-cholesterol levels as recommended in ATPIII Guidelines are achieved in 60% of patients. We shall learn to use combinations of these agents with other lifesaving strategies, such as blood pressure–lowering agents and antiplatelet therapies. Along with the evolution of newer statins, we may also encounter unexpected benefits and adverse effects.

All of the new diagnostic and therapeutic strategies have resulted in a significant reduction in mortality from acute myocardial infarction, particularly in the United States, where use of evidence-based therapy is more common. It may be hoped that the developing nations, which have recently seen a surge of new cases with CAD, also will have access to these marvels of modern science.

Better therapies for CAD in other atherosclerosis-related diseases no doubt are yet to come. In the arena of dyslipidemia, these therapies will be directed at raising low levels of HDL-cholesterol and lowering elevated levels of triglycerides, which are components of the metabolic syndrome and often associated with early-onset cardiovascular disease. In addition, we may see evolution of potent antioxidants and insulin-sensitizing agents for use in therapy for atherosclerosis.

However, there is continued concern about the cost of drugs, which affects the national resources, especially when patients think of pills as a substitute for lifestyle modification such as exercise and weight loss. Further, the newer statins aggressively lower cholesterol and we do not really know the lower limit for cholesterol levels.

I hope that this book will be useful to clinicians, investigators, and other healthcare providers alike in understanding the use of statins.

Jawahar L. Mehta, MD, PhD
Little Rock, Arkansas

Contents

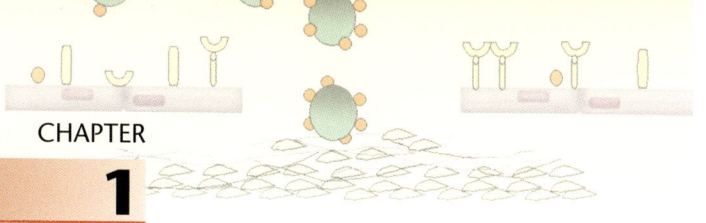

CHAPTER

1

History and Biochemistry of Statins

Vachaspati Mishra and Kamal D. Mehta

Cardiovascular disease (CVD) has been the leading cause of death in the United States since 1900, excluding the 1918 flu epidemic. Every year, more than 1 million deaths occur among 13 million Americans affected with CVD. It causes more deaths than the next six causes of death combined. Contrary to the stereotype that CVD is a man's disease, statistics reveal that more women (503,000) than men (455,000) die each year from this disease as per the American Heart Association website. Among women, CVD is responsible for more deaths than the next 17 causes of death combined. The economic impact of CVD on the U.S. economy each year is staggering: the cost of CVD in 2003 will approach approximately $300 billion.

Of all known risk factors that promote CVD, a high plasma low-density-lipoprotein (LDL) cholesterol level is a major factor. Its role in the pathogenesis of atherosclerotic CVD is well established, being supported by metabolic and pathologic studies in humans and selected animal models as well as by primary and secondary atherosclerosis prevention trials. Now there is evidence that this disease can be arrested and that coronary atherosclerosis can be significantly reversed in patients via drug-induced decrease of plasma LDL cholesterol levels.

Cholesterol can be either derived from the intestinal absorption of dietary cholesterol (approximately 300 to 500 mg/day) or synthesized by a de novo pathway that occurs in most cells of the body but to a greater extent in cells of the liver and intestine (approximately 700 to 900 mg/day). Because the majority of cholesterol is of endogenous origin, it seemed reasonable to lower plasma cholesterol levels by inhibiting its biosynthesis with dietary changes. Because 3-hydroxy-3-methylglutaryl coenzyme A (HMG-CoA) reductase catalyzes a major rate-limiting step in the cholesterol synthetic pathway, it has been the prime target for pharmacologic intervention for several decades. The discovery of statins, inhibitors of HMG-CoA reductase, introduced a new era of cholesterol-lowering therapy. Clinical trials have overwhelmingly established statin therapy as the most effective approach for lipid lowering and the best available choice for

CVD prevention. We will briefly discuss the history and mechanism of the biochemical action of statins in this chapter.

DISCOVERY OF STATINS

By 1960, the role of plasma cholesterol in the development of CVD was quite clear. Several lipid-lowering drugs, such as nicotinic acid, cholestyramine, and clofibrate, were reported and found to reduce the plasma LDL cholesterol level moderately. However, none of these drugs alone was very effective in reducing plasma LDL cholesterol levels to the desired levels for most individuals. As a result, there was a need to introduce a drug that could potentially be more effective with minimal toxicity. The first breakthrough in efforts to find such a drug occurred in 1976 when Endo and colleagues reported the discovery of compactin (ML-236A, ML-236B, ML-236C, renamed mevastatin), a highly functionalized fungal metabolite first isolated from a mold, *Penicillium citrinum*.[1] This compound, a competitive inhibitor of HMG-CoA reductase, was also isolated independently at about the same time from *Penicillium brevicompactum* by researchers at Beecham Laboratories as part of their attempt to discover antifungal agents.[2] Subsequent studies established that mevastatin was an unusually potent inhibitor of HMG-CoA reductase and of cholesterol biosynthesis in various animal studies.[3-9] These studies suggested that mevastatin would be very effective in humans and led to human trials on a few patients in Japan, with great success in reducing their plasma LDL cholesterol levels.[10,11]

Further efforts were made to isolate more natural HMG-CoA reductase inhibitors, which led to the discovery of lovastatin, produced by *Aspergillus terreus* (ATCC20542), in 1979.[12] Merck scientists isolated lovastatin (formerly known as mevinolin), which was found to be more potent than mevastatin in inhibiting HMG-CoA reductase and in lowering plasma cholesterol in experimental animals.[13] Clinical trials of lovastatin began in 1980 on patients with severe hypercholesterolemia in the United States. As expected, lovastatin reduced, in a dose-dependent manner, both total and LDL cholesterol concentrations in patients with heterozygous familial hypercholesterolemia (FH). LDL cholesterol levels were reduced by 24% to 33% at a daily dose of 40 mg and by 38% to 42% at 80 mg, whereas HDL cholesterol was increased by up to 11%.[13] More clinical trials of lovastatin were started in 1984, and the data on more than 1200 patients with severe hypercholesterolemia showed that lovastatin was safe and very effective.[14-16] This drug was approved by the U.S. Food and Drug Administration and first marketed in the United States in 1987. Later, lovastatin was found to be highly effective in treating hyperlipoproteinemias other than FH, including primary moderate and severe hypercholesterolemia, type 3 hyperlipoproteinemia, familial dysbetalipoproteinemia, diabetic dyslipidemia, and nephrotic hyperlipidemia.[17-20]

Since the approval of lovastatin, five other statins have been approved. These include pravastatin, simvastatin, fluvastatin, cerivastatin (withdrawn from the market), atorvastatin, and rosuvastatin. Two of these, pravastatin and simvastatin, are chemically modified derivatives of lovastatin. On the other hand, more recently approved statins—atorvastatin, fluvastatin, and rosuvastatin—are synthetic compounds. More statins are under development, such as crilvastatin (Pan Medica) and nisvastatin (Nissan-Kowa).

Several large, well-controlled clinical trials have documented the efficacy and safety of simvastatin, pravastatin, and lovastatin in reducing CVD.[21-25] It was found that pravastatin (in the WOSCOPS, CARE, and LIPID studies), lovastatin (in the AFCAPS study), and simvastatin (in the 4S study) were very effective in reducing lipid profiles. The results of these trials of statins are remarkable in terms of their size, the consistency of the benefits of treatment, and the lack of serious side effects. A low rate of discontinuations resulting from adverse events was reported in all major statin trials, and there was no suggestion of an imbalance in the placebo versus active drug groups. In general, these statins provoke few serious adverse events. Minor asymptomatic rises in serum transaminases are commonly observed shortly after initiating statin treatment, but they do not normally require discontinuation of the drug. Myopathy and myalgia can occur but are relatively infrequent. Overall, the lack of an adverse influence on noncardiovascular death rates by the statins that have been tested means that substantial clinical benefits from CVD prevention can be obtained against a benign background. Cerivastatin was noted to cause rhabdomyolysis, and the manufacturer chose to withdraw it from the market.

All the known statins share a number of common structural features (Fig. 1-1). First, a portion of the molecule is composed of the substrate analogue, which is present either in the open-chain form (in pravastatin and atorvastatin) or in the closed-ring lactone form (in the other compounds). In vivo, these prodrugs are enzymatically hydrolyzed to their active hydroxy acid form.[26] Second, a complex hydrophobic ring structure is present, which permits tight binding to the reductase enzyme. Third, important structural differences exist between statins in their side groups on the rings. They define the solubility properties of the drugs and hence many of their pharmacokinetic properties and clinical importance. For example, because lovastatin and simvastatin are lactones, they are less soluble in water than are other statins. On the other hand, pravastatin (an acid in the active form), fluvastatin and cerivastatin (sodium salts), and atorvastatin (a calcium salt) are all administered in the active, open-ring form.

BIOCHEMISTRY OF STATINS

The precursor for cholesterol synthesis is acetyl CoA, which is produced from glucose, fatty acids, or amino acids. Two molecules

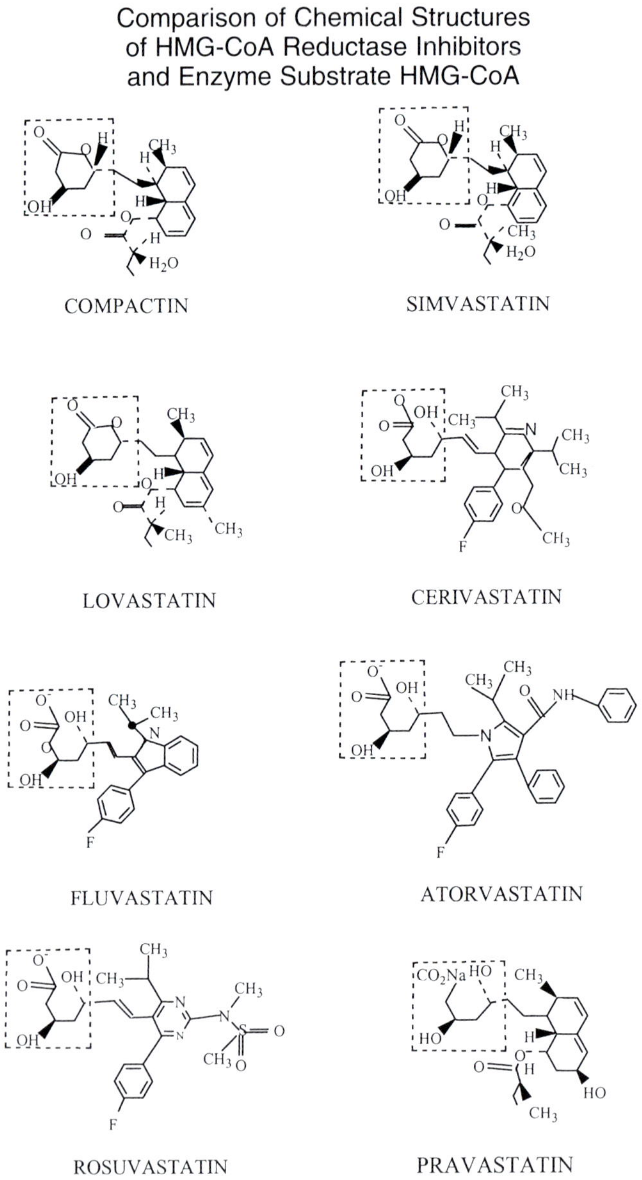

Comparison of Chemical Structures of HMG-CoA Reductase Inhibitors and Enzyme Substrate HMG-CoA

COMPACTIN

SIMVASTATIN

LOVASTATIN

CERIVASTATIN

FLUVASTATIN

ATORVASTATIN

ROSUVASTATIN

PRAVASTATIN

Figure 1-1 Comparison of chemical structures of 3-hydroxy-3-methyl-glutaryl coenzyme A (HMG-CoA) reductase inhibitors and enzyme substrate HMG-CoA with their IC_{50} and Km values. The portion of the statin molecule that resembles natural substrate HMG-CoA is boxed.

of acetyl CoA form acetoacetyl CoA, which condenses with another molecule of acetyl CoA to form HMG-CoA. Reduction of HMG-CoA produces mevalonate. This reaction, catalyzed by HMG-CoA reductase, is the four-electron reductive deacetylation of HMG-CoA to CoA and mevalonate (Fig. 1-2). Mevalonate produces isoprene units that condense, eventually forming squalene. Cyclization of squalene produces the steroid ring system, and a number of consequent reactions generate cholesterol.

All the known statins have structural similarities, and from these structures a mechanism of action is immediately apparent, that of competitive inhibition of HMG-CoA reductase through mimicry of this enzyme's substrate (see Fig. 1-2). As a result of their structural similarity to HMG-CoA, statins are reversible competitive inhibitors of the enzyme's natural substrate, HMG-CoA.[27] They block cholesterol synthesis by inhibiting HMG-CoA reductase, with an inhibition constant (Ki) in the 1-nM range, except cerivastatin, which has a Ki of 0.01 nM.[28] This compares to a Michaelis constant of approximately 4 µM for HMG-CoA.[12] The dissociation constant of HMG-CoA is three orders of magnitude higher than this value. Thus the affinity of HMG-CoA reductase for each statin is approximately 10,000 times higher than its affinity for the natural substrate HMG-CoA. As a result, statins are competitive inhibitors of HMG-CoA reductase with respect to binding of the substrate HMG-CoA, but not with respect to binding of nicotinamide adenine dinucleotide phosphate, reduced (NADPH). They preferentially bind to the active site of the enzyme, which sterically prevents the substrate from binding to the active site.

Early kinetic analysis of the statin inhibition of HMG-CoA reductase suggested that the lactone portion of the mevastatin molecule is bound to the HMG binding site of the reductase molecule.[4] Studies on structure-activity relationships indicated that both the 3- and the 5-hydroxyl groups of the mevastatin molecule (open acid form) played a crucial role in the inhibition process, because inhibitory activity was abolished by the conversion of either of the hydroxyl groups into the methyl ester. Recently, structures of the catalytic portion of human HMG-CoA reductase in complex with either natural substrate HMG or each of the six different statins have been reported.[29] These studies revealed that the HMG-CoA-binding pocket contains a loop spanning residues 682 to 694 (referred to as the *cis* loop). The bulky hydrophobic compounds of statins occupied the HMG-binding pocket, resulting in several polar interactions between the HMG moiety and residues that are located in the *cis* loop (Ser684, Asp690, Lys691, and Lys692). In addition, hydrophobic groups of statins interact with the hydrophobic pocket on the protein involving residues Leu562, Val683, Leu853, Ala856, and Leu857. Despite the structural diversity of statins, their hydrophobic ring structures and surface complementarity between the reductase hydrophobic pocket are prevalent in all enzyme-inhibitor complexes. It has been proposed

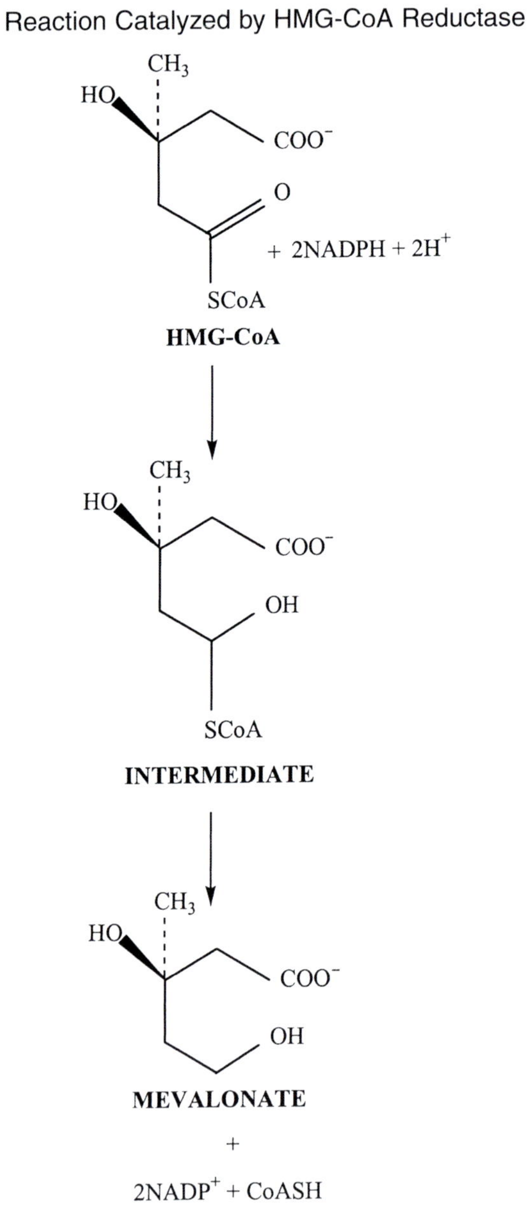

Reaction Catalyzed by HMG-CoA Reductase

Figure 1-2 Reaction catalyzed by 3-hydroxy-3-methylglutaryl co-enzyme A (HMG-CoA) reductase. $NADP^+$ is the oxidized nicotinamide adenine dinucleotide, NADPH is the reduced form of $NADP^+$, and CoASH is the reduced form of CoA.

that these hydrophobic interactions are predominantly responsible for the nanomolar Ki values of statins. The covalent attachment of a nicotinamide-like moiety to statins appears to improve their potency. It is likely that the subtle differences in their modes of binding accounts for the marked differences in cholesterol-lowering efficacy and the wide interindividual variation in response to the same dose of a statin.

MECHANISMS OF LOWERING LDL CHOLESTEROL

The elegant work by Brown and Goldstein, and their collaborators have increased our understanding of the regulation of LDL metabolism and provided an explanation for the actions of a number of cholesterol-lowering drugs, including statins.[30] These authors first showed that circulating LDL cholesterol is cleared largely through LDL receptors in the liver, and the number of hepatic LDL receptors is an important determinant of LDL clearance from the peripheral circulation. Subsequently, in collaboration with David Bilheimer, they showed that cholesterol lowering by lovastatin was primarily a result of enhanced LDL receptor–mediated catabolism in patients with heterozygous FH.[31] When the patients were homozygous for FH, with no capacity to synthesize LDL receptors, treatment with lovastatin even at very high doses was found to cause no decrease in LDL cholesterol levels, or an increase in the turnover rate of LDL.[32] Studies with experimental animals showed that lovastatin increased messenger RNA for LDL receptors in the liver and enhanced the number of LDL receptors expressed on the surface of liver cells.[33,34]

This same group of researchers has identified a family of transcription factors, known as sterol response element binding proteins (SREBPs), which control transcription of the LDL receptor and at least six other key enzymatic steps in the cholesterol biosynthetic pathway, in response to the cellular sterol level.[35] SREBPs are transcription factors that are bound to the endoplasmic reticulum (ER). Immediately after their synthesis on ER membranes, SREBPs bind to SREBP cleavage–activating protein (SCAP), a polytopic membrane protein that serves both an escort function and a sterol-sensing function.[36] A fall in the intracellular cholesterol concentration leads to the proteolysis of the precursor form and the release of mature SREBP from the ER. This 68-kDa protein then travels to the nucleus, where it binds to the sterol response element in the promoter of the LDL receptor gene and activates its transcription, which in turn transports blood LDL into the liver, thus reducing plasma levels of LDL. Although transcription of HMG-CoA reductase is also up-regulated, the increase in its transcription level is not significant enough to overcome the drug effect because the amount of inhibitor present is greater than the amount of enzyme produced. In summary, inhibition of HMG-CoA reductase in the liver suppresses endogenous hepatic cholesterol synthesis and leads to increased transport of SCAP-SREBP complex to the Golgi complex and thus greater transport of active SREBP to the nucleus, resulting in the up-regulation of LDL receptor expression (Fig. 1-3).

In addition to increasing clearance of LDL by LDL receptors, statins exert their effects by enhancing the removal of LDL precursors (very-low-density lipoproteins [VLDLs] and intermediate-density lipoproteins [IDLs]) and by decreasing hepatic VLDL production.[37,38] Because VLDL remnants and IDLs are enriched in apolipoprotein E (apoE), and LDL receptors recognize both apoB-100 and apoE, induction of this receptor by statins has been shown to enhance the clearance of LDL precursors.[39] The reduction in hepatic VLDL production induced by statins is possibly mediated by reduced cholesterol synthesis, an essential component for the VLDL synthesis.[40] This mechanism can also account for the triglyceride-lowering effect of statins.[41]

There is growing evidence to support that statins provide cardiovascular benefit by a range of processes that go beyond their cholesterol-lowering capability.[42,43] On the basis of in vitro and ex vivo data, a multitude of potentially cardioprotective effects are being ascribed to these drugs. Interestingly, statins have been shown to impact endothelial function, plaque stabilization, cellular immunity and inflammation, lipoprotein oxidation, and rheology and blood coagulation. Over the years, a number of tantalizing studies have been published that suggest that statins may have a direct influence on cell growth that is possibly linked to suppression of the production of isoprenoids in the cholesterol synthetic pathway (see Fig. 1-3). Animal and cell culture studies both suggest that cell division and migration are inhibited by the drugs, offering an imaginative but speculative explanation for the suppressive effect that high-dose statin therapy seems to exert on intimal proliferation following vascular injury.[44,45] Among the debatable effects, statin's modulation of the cellularity of arterial walls by inhibiting proliferation of smooth muscle cells and enhancing apoptotic cell death are of greater clinical relevance. Statin administration in rabbits inhibited monocyte infiltration into arterial walls and also inhibited macrophage secretion of matrix metalloproteases.[46,47] These proteases degrade extracellular matrix components and can weaken the fibrous cap of athero-sclerotic plaques. Finally, statins have been suggested to have an anti-inflammatory role.[48] Ridker and colleagues have demonstrated that the C-reactive protein concentration was a marker for high CVD risk and that statin therapy decreased baseline C-reactive protein levels and risk for CVD independently of cholesterol lowering.[49] It remains to be seen whether these potential pleiotropic effects represent a class action effect, differ among statins, or are biologically relevant. If these pleiotropic effects of statins turn out to be of significance in preventing CVD and there are marked differences in effectiveness of statins, then it will be important to discover which part of the molecule governs the additional beneficial effect.

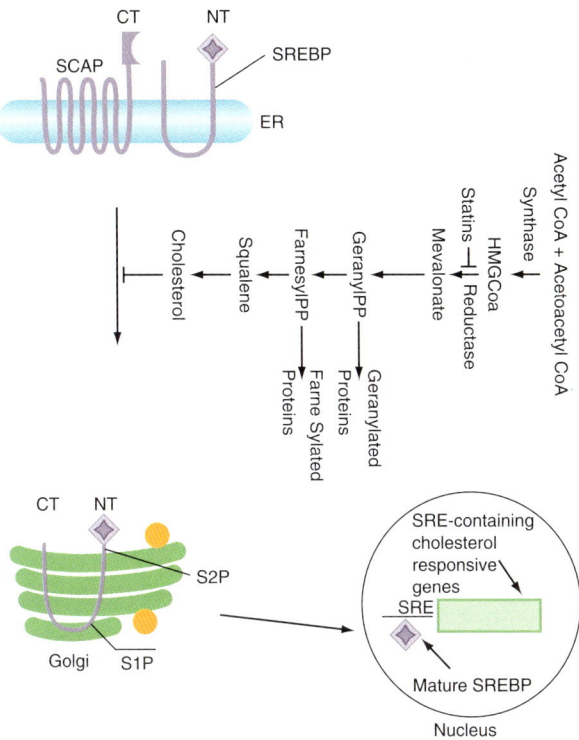

Figure 1-3 **Regulation of cholesterol biosynthesis and low-density-lipoprotein (LDL) receptor in the liver cells.** The expression of the LDL receptor and the genes of the cholesterol biosynthetic pathway is regulated by cellular cholesterol levels. The promoter of known sterol-responsive genes contains sterol response element (SRE), including LDL receptor and 3-hydroxy-3-methylglutaryl coenzyme A (HMG-CoA) reductase. Two SRE binding proteins, SREBP-1 and -2, are localized in the endoplasmic reticulum (ER). When cellular levels of cholesterol are low, SREBP cleavage-activating protein (SCAP) transports the precursor SREBPs from the ER to the Golgi, where two proteases, S1P and S2P, sequentially cleave the SREBPs. As a result, mature SREBP proteins are liberated from the membrane, allowing them to enter the nucleus and bind to the SREs of target genes to induce their transcription. The inhibition of HMG-CoA reductase by statins reduces levels of cellular cholesterol. Cholesterol depletion activates the translocation of the SCAP-SREBP complex and results in the generation of mature SREBPs and up-regulation of SRE-1 containing the LDL receptor gene. Interestingly, the pathway of cholesterol production that statins inhibit is also the route of generation of other molecules critical for cellular processes, including geranyl and farnesyl derivatives that are key components in cell growth. Increased risk of cancer can be a concern and has to be addressed for statin therapy because such a fundamental cellular pathway is being perturbed. CT, carboxy-terminal; NT, amino-terminal.

References

1. Endo A, Kuroda M, Tsujita Y: ML-236A, ML-236B, and ML-236C: New inhibitors of cholesterogenesis produced by *Penicillium citrinum*. J Antibiot (Tokyo) 29:1346-1348, 1976.
2. Brown AG, Smale TC, King J, et al: Crystal and molecular structure of compactin, a new antifungal metabolite from *Penicillium brevicompactum*. J Chem Soc [Perkin 1] 11:1165-1170, 1976.
3. Endo A, Kuroda M, Tanzawa K, et al: Competitive inhibition of HMG CoA reductase by ML-236A and ML-236B fungal metabolites, having hypercholesterolemic activity. FEBS Lett 72:323-326, 1976.
4. Tanzawa K, Endo A: Kinetic analysis of the reaction catalyzed by 3-hydroxy-3-methylglutaryl coenzyme A reductase using two specific inhibitors. Eur J Biochem 98:195-201, 1979.
5. Kanecko I, Hazama-Shimada Y, Endo A: Effects of ML-236B, a competitive inhibitor of 3-hydroxy-3-methylglutaryl coenzyme A reductase, on the lipid metabolism in culture cells. Eur J Biochem 87:313-321, 1978.
6. Doi O, Endo A: Specific inhibition of desmosterol synthesis by ML-236B in mouse LM cells grown in suspension in a liquid-free medium. Jpn J Med Sci Biol 31:225-233, 1978.
7. Endo A, Tsujita Y, Kuroda M, Tanazawa K: Inhibition of cholesterol synthesis in vitro and in vivo by ML-236A and ML-236B, competitive inhibitors of 3-hydroxy-3-methylglutaryl coenzyme A reductase. Eur J Biochem 77:31-36, 1977.
8. Fears R, Richards DH, Ferres H: The effect of compactin, a potent inhibitor of 3-hydroxy-3-methylglutaryl coenzymeA reductase activity, on cholesterogenesis and serum cholesterol levels in rats and chicks. Atherosclerosis 35:439-449, 1978.
9. Tsuijta Y, Kuroda M, Tanzawa K, et al: Hypolipidemic effects in dogs of ML-236B, a competitive inhibitor of 3-hydroxy-3-methylglutaryl coenzyme A reductase. Lipids 14:585-589, 1979.
10. Yamamota A, Sudo H, Endo A: Therapeutic effects of ML-236B in primary hypercholesterolemia. Atherosclerosis 35:259-266, 1980.
11. Mabuchi H, Haba T, Tatami R, et al: Effects of an inhibitor of 3-hydroxy-3-methylglutaryl coenzyme A reductase on serum lipoproteins and ubiquinone-10 levels in patients with familial hypercholesterolemia. N Engl J Med 305:478-482, 1981.
12. Alberts AW, Chen J, Kuron G, et al: A highly-potent competitive inhibitor of hydroxymethylglutaryl-coenzyme A reductase and a cholesterol-lowering agent. Proc Natl Acad Sci USA 77:3957-3961, 1980.
13. Alberts AW: Discovery, biochemistry and biology of lovastatin. Am J Cardiol 62:10J-15J, 1988.
14. Illingworth DR, Sexton GJ: Hypocholesterolemic effects of mevinolin in patients with heterozygous familial hypercholesterolemia. J Clin Invest 74:1972-1978, 1984.
15. Havel RJ, Hunninghake DB, Illingworth DR, et al: Lovastatin (mevinolin) in the treatment of heterozygous familial hypercholesterolemia: A multicenter study. Ann Intern Med 107:609-615, 1987.
16. The Lovastatin Study Group II: Therapeutic response to lovastatin (mevinolin) in nonfamilial hypercholesterolemia: A multicenter study. JAMA 256:2829-2834, 1986.

17. East CA, Grundy SM, Bilheimer DW: Preliminary report: Treatment of type 3 hyperlipoproteinemia with mevinolin. Metabolism 35:97-98, 1986.

18. Vega GL, East CA, Grundy SM: Lovastatin therapy in familial dysbetalipoproteinemia: Effect on kinetics of apoprotein B. Atherosclerosis 70:131-143, 1988.

19. Garg A, Grundy SM: Lovastatin for lowering cholesterol levels in noninsulin-dependent diabetes mellitus. N Engl J Med 314:81-86, 1988.

20. Vega GL, Grundy SM: Lovastatin therapy in nephrotic hyperlipidemia: Effects on lipoprotein metabolism. Kidney Int 33:339-343, 1985.

21. Shepherd J, Cobbe SM, Ford I, et al: Prevention of coronary heart disease with pravastatin in men with hypercholesterolemia. N Engl J Med 333:1301-1307, 1995.

22. Sacks FM, Pfeffer, MA, Moye LA, et al: The effect of pravastatin on coronary events after myocardial infarction in patients with average cholesterol levels. N Engl J Med 335:1001-1009, 1996.

23. LIPID Study Group: Prevention of cardiovascular events and death with pravastatin in patients with coronary heart disease and a broad range of cholesterol levels. N Engl J Med 339:1349-1357, 1998.

24. Downs JR, Clearfield M, Weis S, et al: Primary prevention of acute coronary events with lovastatin in men and women with average cholesterol levels: Results of AFCAPS/TEXCAPS Research Group. JAMA 279:1615-1622, 1998.

25. Scandinavian Simvastatin Survival Study Group: Randomised trial of cholesterol lowering in 4444 patients with coronary heart disease: The Scandinavian Simvastatin Survival Study (4S). Lancet 344:1383-1389, 1994.

26. Corsini A, Maggi FM, Catapano AL: Pharmacology of competitive inhibitors of HMG-CoA reductase. Pharmacol Res 31:9-27, 1995.

27. Endo A: Compactin (ML-236B) and related compounds as potential cholesterol-lowering agents that inhibit HMG-CoA reductase. J Med Chem 28:401-405, 1985.

28. Bischoff H, Angerbauer R, Bender J, et al: Cerivastatin: Pharmacology of a novel synthetic and highly active HMG-CoA reductase inhibitor. Atherosclerosis 135:119-130, 1997.

29. Istavan ES, Deisenhofer J: Structural mechanism for statin inhibition of HMG-CoA reductase. Science 292:1160-1164, 2001.

30. Goldstein JL, Brown MS: Regulation of the mevalonate pathway. Nature 343:425-430, 1990.

31. Bilheimer DW, Grundy SM, Brown MS, Goldstein JL: Mevinolin and colestipol stimulate receptor-mediated clearance of low density lipoprotein from plasma in familial hypercholesterolemia heterozygotes. Proc Natl Acad Sci USA 80:4124-4128, 1983.

32. Uauy R, Vega GL, Grundy SM, Bilheimer DW: Lovastatin therapy in receptor-negative homozygous familial hypercholesterolemia: Lack of effect on low density lipoprotein concentration or turnover. J Pediatr 113:383-392, 1988.

33. Ma PT, Gil G, Sudhof TC, et al: Mevinolin, an inhibitor of cholesterol synthesis, induces mRNA for low density lipoprotein receptor in livers of hamster and rabbits. Proc Natl Acad Sci USA 83:8370-8374, 1986.

34. Kovanen PT, Bilheimer DW, Goldstein JL, et al: Regulatory role for hepatic low density lipoproteins in vivo in the dog. Proc Natl Acad Sci USA 78:1194-1198, 1981.

35. Brown MS, Goldstein JL: A proteolytic pathway that controls the

cholesterol content of membranes, cells, and blood. Proc Natl Acad Sci USA 96:11041-11048, 1999.

36. Korn BS, Shimomura I, Bashmakov Y, et al: Blunted feedback suppression of SREBP processing by dietary cholesterol in transgenic mice expressing sterol-resistant SCAP (D443N). J Clin Invest 102:2050-2060, 1998.

37. Aguilar-Salinas CA, Barrett H, Schonfeld G: Metabolic modes of action of the statins in the hyperlipoproteinemias. Atherosclerosis 141:203-207, 1998.

38. Grundy SM, Vega GL: Influence of mavinolin on metabolism of low density lipoproteins in primary moderate hypercholesterolemia. J Lipid Res 26:1464-1475, 1985.

39. Gaw A, Packard CJ, Murray EF, et al: Effects of simvastatin on apoB metabolism and LDL subfraction distribution. Arterioscler Thromb 13:170-189, 1993.

40. Thompson GR, Naoumova RP, Watts GF: Role of cholesterol in regulating apolipoprotein B secretion by the liver. J Lipid Res 37:439-447, 1996

41. Ginsberg HN: Effects of statins on triglyceride metabolism. Am J Cardiol 81:32B-35B, 1998.

42. Thompson GR, Barter PJ: Clinical lipidology at the end of the millennium. Curr Opin Lipidol 10:521-526, 1999.

43. Davignon J, Laaksonen R: Low-density lipoprotein-independent effects of statins. Curr Opin Lipidol 10:543-559, 1999.

44. Soma MR, Donetti E, Parolini C, et al: HMGCoA reductase inhibitors. In vivo effects on carotid intimal thickening in normocholesterolemic rabbits. Arterioscler Thromb 13:571-578, 1993.

45. Corsini A, Raiteri M, Soma MR, et al: Simvastatin but not pravastatin inhibits the proliferation of rat aorta myocytes. Pharmacol Res 23:173-180, 1991.

46. Bustos C, Hernandez-Presa MA, Ortego M, et al: HMG-CoA reductase inhibition by atorvastatin reduces neointimal inflammation in a rabbit model of atherosclerosis. J Am Coll Cardiol 82:74U-81U, 1998.

47. Bellosta S, Mahley RW, Sanan RW, et al: Macrophage-specific expression of human apolipoprotein E reduces atherosclerosis in hypercholesterolemic apolipoprotein E-null mice. J Clin Invest 96:2170-2179, 1995.

48. Rossen RD: HMG-CoA reductase inhibitors: A new class of anti-inflammatory drugs? J Am Coll Cardiol 30:1218-1229, 1997.

49. Ridker PM, Rifai N, Pfeffer MA, et al: Inflammation, pravastatin, and the risk of coronary events after myocardial infarction in patients with average cholesterol levels: Cholesterol and Recurrent Events (CARE) Investigators. Circulation 98:839-844, 1998.

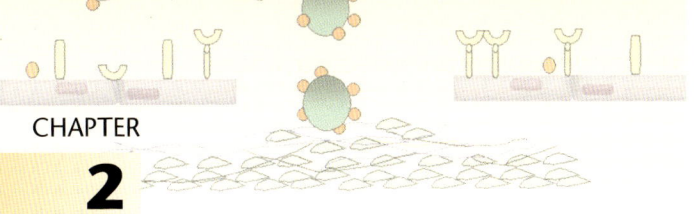

New Insights from Trials of Statins in Animal Models of Atherosclerosis

Clarissa Cola, Francesco Romeo, and Jawahar L. Mehta

An elevated plasma level of cholesterol, especially the low-density-lipoprotein cholesterol (LDL cholesterol), is one of the most important risk factors in atherosclerosis. Certain animals, when fed a diet rich in cholesterol, develop atherosclerosis. Other animal species develop atherosclerosis spontaneously because they have an inability to metabolize cholesterol. The 3-hydroxy-3-methyl-glutaryl coenzyme A (HMG-CoA) reductase inhibitors, or statins, are potent inhibitors of cholesterol biosynthesis. These agents block the production of isoprenoid intermediates. These isoprenoid intermediates activate a number of cell-signaling proteins through prenylation. In particular, members of the G-protein families, such as Rho, Ras, and Rab, are important in cell proliferation, endothelial function, and fibrinolytic balance.[1] The "pleiotropic" effects of statins are supposed to affect the prenylation (Fig. 2-1).

A high cellular cholesterol concentration could provoke a shift in this pathway toward pyrophosphate formation, whereas a decrease in cholesterol concentration could restore the balance; however, this has not been well defined. We do know that a reduction in the lipid pool of the cell raises LDL receptor expression on the cell surface, which then reduces the circulating cholesterol level.

Hepatic cholesterol production, the amount of cholesterol in cells, and circulating cholesterol levels are strictly interrelated. Lipophilic and hydrophilic statins appear to affect these relationships similarly, even though they do not have the same tissue penetration.

Hypercholesterolemia causes injury to the arterial wall, and cholesterol lowering with statins reduces injury to the vessel wall and stabilizes the atherosclerotic plaques.[2] Statins reduce the size of the atherosclerotic lesion by lowering the circulating LDL cholesterol concentration. In addition, these agents influence vascular biology in a number of ways, and affect the size of the atherosclerotic region. Importantly, these agents have an anti-

2

Pathway of Cholesterol Synthesis

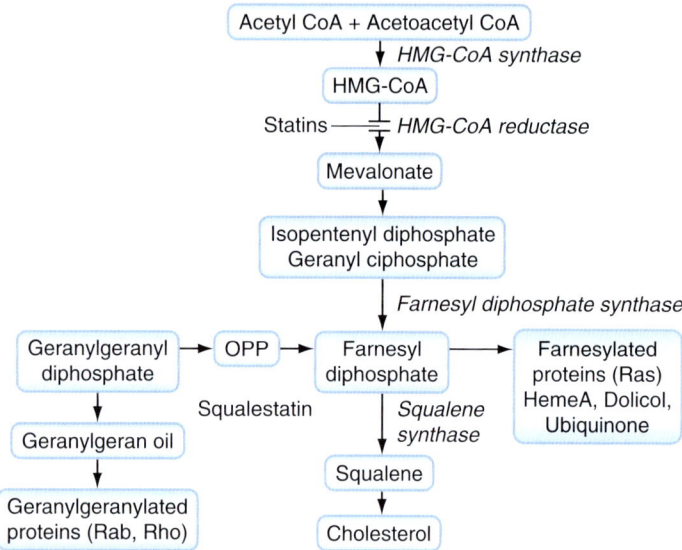

Figure 2-1 **Cholesterol biosynthetic pathway.** Sites of action of 3-hydroxy-3-methylglutaryl coenzyme A (HMG-CoA) reductase inhibitor (statins) and squalene synthetase inhibitor (squalestatin) are shown.

inflammatory effect, decrease plaque calcification, and affect angiogenesis.[3] These effects have been clearly demonstrated in animal models.

Animal models answer certain questions about the pathogenesis of atherosclerosis, but they do not precisely reflect the atherogenesis that occurs in humans and evolves over decades; thus, animal models have major limitations. Furthermore, the doses of statins used in animal models are several-fold higher than those used in humans. Some animals, such as mice, do not develop atherosclerosis without genetic manipulation and have a different lipid physiology. Rats are generally resistant to atherosclerosis, so they require genetic manipulations as well. Monkeys, baboons, and pigs seem to be the best animal models, because they develop atherosclerosis that resembles the pathologic process in humans, but these animals are expensive, their maintenance is difficult, and some species are protected from experimental use by state, federal, and international agencies.[4]

Although the animal models have provided us with a substantial amount of information on the steps involved in atherogenesis and the effects of statins, the mechanism of atherogenesis and our knowledge regarding the action of statins is far from conclusive. Thus, this information must be regarded as preliminary and requires verification in humans. In this chapter, we present evidence for reduction of atherosclerosis with statins and focus on four aspects of atherosclerosis: inflammation, calcification, collagen deposition/degradation, and angiogenesis.

STATINS AND REDUCTION IN THE EXTENT OF ATHEROSCLEROSIS

Atherosclerotic lesion size depends on the accumulation of cholesterol and on the number of intimal macrophages and smooth muscle cells (SMCs) in the arterial wall. Statins have been shown to reduce lesion size and the extent of atherosclerosis in a variety of animal species.[5] Most studies with statins have been done in apoE$^{-/-}$ mice, or in rabbits, monkeys, or pigs fed a high-cholesterol diet. The studies discussed here are by no means a complete listing of the large body of work in this area but have been chosen to represent some salient features of statin therapy.

ApoE$^{-/-}$ mice develop spontaneous hypercholesterolemia and atherosclerotic lesions that increase in size throughout the life span of the animals. In an interesting study conducted in this animal model, simvastatin (100 mg/kg/day) was shown to decrease aortic cholesterol accumulation even though the mice were dosed for only 25% of their lifetime.[6] In association with a decrease in serum LDL cholesterol levels, simvastatin dramatically attenuated the increase in lesion size during the 6-week dosing period.

Chen and colleagues, using a hypercholesterolemic rabbit model, showed reduction in the extent of atherosclerosis, despite an insignificant effect on the plasma levels of LDL cholesterol, by administration of lovastatin.[7] They attributed the potent antiathero-sclerotic effect to the antioxidant properties of lovastatin. The causative role of increased cholesterol level and lipid peroxidation in the development of atherosclerosis has been well documented.[8,9] The activated endothelium in response to oxidized LDL (ox-LDL) is an early target for leukocyte adherence. Activation of leukocytes can damage the vascular tissues by release of free radicals and proteolytic enzymes. Superoxide radicals from activated leuko-cytes adherent to the blood vessels may be a factor in initiating the oxidation of LDL cholesterol. Oxidation of LDL cholesterol is evident during atherogenesis, especially in the early stages.[10] In the study by Chen and co-workers, rabbits treated with lovastatin and fed a high-cholesterol diet had preserved plasma superoxide dismutase (SOD) activity, whereas it was lower in the untreated animals.[7] The lovastatin molecule, per se, does not contain an antioxidant center. However, by inhibiting the isoprenoid reaction during the activation of reduced nicotinamide adenine dinucleotide phosphate (NADPH) oxidase, lovastatin affects the generation of oxygen radicals. Indeed, lovastatin and a related compound, simvastatin, have been reported to inhibit LDL oxidation induced by activated macrophages via reduction of superoxide production.[11] In a study in guinea pigs, Conde and colleagues showed that atorvastatin and simvastatin (10 and 20 mg/kg/day, respectively) both decreased the susceptibility of LDL particles to undergo oxidation by 95%.[12]

Bustos and colleagues showed in rabbits that a 4-week treatment period with atorvastatin (5 mg/kg/day) reduced the extent of atherosclerotic lesions induced by endothelial damage to femoral arteries while the animals were continued on an atherogenic diet.[13] Here, parameters used were maximal stenosis of the femoral artery, intima-to-media ratio, and percentage of the luminal area occupied by the lesion. Other authors who studied the cell composition of lesions in the same animal model found a reduction of macrophages and SMC proliferation with the use of fluvastatin.[14,15]

Alfon and colleagues studied the effects of atorvastatin and simvastatin on lesion composition and expression of genes involved in lesion development in a diet-induced atherosclerotic rabbit model.[16] Both HMG-CoA reductase inhibitors were administered at identical doses of 2.5 mg/kg per day with the hyperlipidemic diet for 10 weeks. Both statins significantly prevented diet-induced increase in LDL cholesterol levels. Relative lesion contents of fibrinogen, macrophages, and SMCs were unaltered by the treatment although the lesion size was reduced; therefore, both statins reduced the overall amount of fibrinogen, macrophages, and SMCs in the vessel wall. Inducible nitric oxide synthase (NOS II or iNOS) gene expression was positively and significantly correlated with the lesion size and inversely correlated with plasma high-density-lipoprotein (HDL) cholesterol levels. The expression of iNOS was markedly down-regulated in simvastatin-treated animals. This study suggested that HMG-CoA reductase inhibition interferes with atherosclerotic lesion development by reducing intimal thickening and the expression of the cytotoxic iNOS.

Effects of cerivastatin and pravastatin on intimal thickening have been studied in rabbits with carotid artery endothelial denudation by a balloon catheter.[17] Rabbits were divided into four groups: control, pravastatin (20 mg/kg/day), and two cerivastatin dose groups (10 or 20 mg/kg/day). Two weeks after balloon catheter injury, the areas of intima and media of the injured carotid arteries were determined, and the intima-to-media ratio was calculated as an index of intimal thickening. Cerivastatin reduced the intima-to-media ratio in the injured artery to approximately half, but pravastatin failed to suppress the intimal thickening. In an in vitro study, SMCs from rabbit aortas were explanted and then cultured, and the effects of cerivastatin on SMC migration and proliferation were examined. Cerivastatin inhibited in a dose-dependent fashion SMC migration and proliferation. The same conclusions were reached by Fukumoto and co-workers, who compared pravastatin to fluvastatin.[18] Thus, it appears that cell-permeating statins have a direct inhibitory effect on SMC proliferation.

In contrast, in a hamster model, pravastatin (34 mg/kg/day for 8 weeks) reduced macrophage foam cell size and fatty streak area by 21% and 31%, respectively.[19] This hydrophilic compound did not show any direct effect on SMC proliferation, but it still reduced lesion size by acting on other plaque components, such as LDL cholesterol and inflammatory cells.

Differences in hydrophilic and lipophilic HMG-CoA reductase inhibitors are important. Pathologic intimal thickening is related to SMC migration and proliferation. On the other hand, collagen production and deposition lead to the formation of a fibrous cap, which makes the atherosclerotic lesion less prone to erosion and rupture.

Masashi and colleagues examined lesion composition and its relation to the stability of coronary plaques in 12-month-old Watanabe heritable hyperlipidemic (WHHL) rabbits.[20] The animals were given pravastatin (50 mg/kg/day) or fluvastatin (20 mg/kg/day) for 1 year. Both statins decreased plasma LDL cholesterol levels by about 25%, but the suppressive effects on the degree of coronary plaque were mild. Macrophage content in fibromuscular cap regions was decreased by pravastatin, and SMC content was decreased by fluvastatin. The plaque vulnerability index was low in macrophage-poor plaques but high in SMC-poor plaques. These results suggest that reduction in the number of macrophages in the fibromuscular cap is related to plaque stabilization, and that reduction in accumulation of SMC in the fibromuscular cap is related to plaque destabilization.

We do not yet know if the direct cellular effects of statins are observed in humans given clinical doses, but we do know that hypercholesterolemia causes injury to the arterial wall, starting with oxidation of LDL cholesterol, and that lipid lowering is good for plaque stability.

STATINS AND INFLAMMATION IN RELATION TO ATHEROGENESIS

Hypercholesterolemia impairs endothelial function, and endothelial dysfunction is one of the early manifestations of atherosclerosis. An important characteristic of endothelial dysfunction is the impaired synthesis, release, and activity of endothelium-derived nitric oxide (NO). Endothelial NO has been shown to inhibit several components of the atherogenic process. For example, endothelium-derived NO mediates vascular relaxation and inhibits platelet aggregation, SMC proliferation, and inflammation.[5] As is well known, atherosclerosis is a complex inflammatory process that is characterized by the presence of monocytes/macrophages and T lymphocytes on the endothelial surface and later in the atheroma itself. Inflammatory cytokines secreted by these macrophages and T lymphocytes can induce SMC migration and proliferation, collagen degradation, and thrombosis.

Endothelium, once activated by pro-atherosclerotic stimuli, such as ox-LDL, angiotensin II, tumor necrosis factor α (TNF-α), or shear stress, expresses adhesion molecules, such as selectins, integrins, and immunoglobulin superfamily members, such as P-selectin and vascular cell adhesion molecule-1 (VCAM-1), which bind monocytes and T lymphocytes. Once adherent to the endothelium, the leukocytes penetrate the intima. Recent studies have identified chemoattractant molecules responsible for this transmigration. For example, monocyte chemoattractant protein-1 (MCP-1) appears responsible for the direct migration of monocytes into the intima at sites of lesion formation. A family of T-cell chemo-attractants may likewise attract lymphocytes into the intima. Once resident in the arterial wall, the blood-derived inflammatory cells participate in the initiation and perpetuation of a local inflammatory response. The macrophages express scavenger receptors for modified lipoproteins, permitting them to ingest lipid and become foam cells. In addition to MCP-1, macrophage colony-stimulating factor (M-CSF) contributes to the differentiation of blood monocytes into macrophage foam cells. T cells likewise encounter signals that cause them to elaborate inflammatory cytokines, such as interferon-γ and TNF-β, which in turn can stimulate macrophages as well as vascular endothelial cells and SMCs. In response to these inflammatory cytokines, SMCs express the inducible enzyme cytochrome C oxidase (COX-2), responsible for the synthesis of pro-inflammatory prostaglandins, such as PGE$_2$, a chemoattractant for leukocytes. Inflammatory processes not only promote initiation and evolution of atheroma but also contribute decisively to precipitation of acute thrombotic complications of atheroma. The activated macrophages abundant in atheroma also produce proteolytic enzymes, such as matrix metallo-proteinases (MMPs), capable of degrading the collagen that lends strength to the plaque's protective fibrous cap, rendering the cap thin, weak, and susceptible to rupture. Macrophages also produce tissue factor, the major procoagulant and trigger for thrombosis (Fig. 2-2).[21-23]

Experimental studies suggest that statins possess anti-inflammatory properties. The precise mechanism of the anti-inflammatory effect, however, has yet to be fully elucidated. Animal models give us some information about the mechanism. Nonhuman primates are a good model because tissues can be obtained from them that have many of the important characteristics of human atherosclerosis. In recent studies, Sukhova and co-workers examined anti-inflammatory properties of different statins in cynomolgus monkeys.[24] The monkeys were fed a high-cholesterol diet for 3 months and then received statins (simvastatin 20 mg/

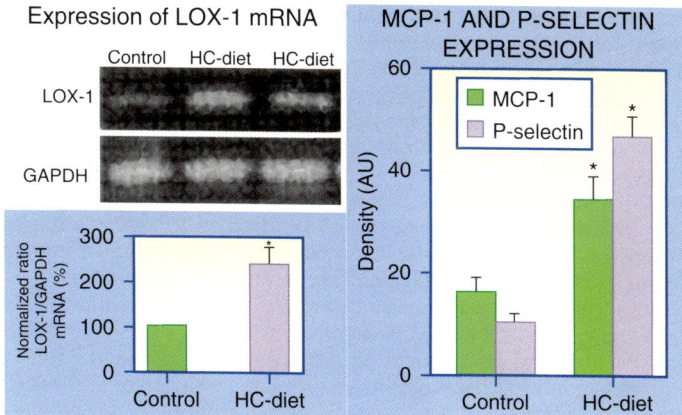

Figure 2-2 *Left*, Expression of oxidized low-density-lipoprotein receptor LOX-1 mRNA in aortic tissue from rabbits fed a high-cholesterol (HC) diet compared with controls. Note that there was only modest amounts of LOX-1 mRNA in the control group. LOX-1 mRNA expression markedly increased in the aortas of rabbits in the HC diet group. *Right*, MCP-1 and P-selectin expression in aortas from rabbits fed HC diet, compared with controls. Both MCP-1 and P-selectin were markedly increased in aortas of rabbits in the HC diet group compared with the control group. (*Right*, Adapted from Chen H, Li DY, Phillips MI, Mehta JL: Attenuation of P-selectin and MCP-1 expression and intimal proliferation by AT1 receptor blockade in hyperlipidemic rabbits. Biochem Biophys Res Commun 282:474-479, 2001; and Chen H, Li DY, Savamura T, et al: Upregulation of LOX-1 expression in aorta of hyper-cholesterolemic rabbits: Modulation by losartan. Biochem Biophys Res Commun 276:1100-1104, 2000.)

kg/day or pravastatin 40 mg/kg/day) with the same diet for an additional 15 months. These authors found that both statins decreased VCAM-1, interleukin-1 beta (IL-1β), tissue factor, and macrophages in atherosclerotic lesions. These were considered lipid-lowering independent effects because the plasma levels of LDL cholesterol were not appreciably lowered. However, statins work primarily on endogenously produced cholesterol, whereas in cholesterol-fed monkeys, lipid in plasma was derived primarily from exogenous sources. It is noteworthy that simvastatin is lipophilic and pravastatin is hydrophilic, yet both compounds had similar effects.

As primates, pigs are also a very good model to study athero-genesis, especially because they develop atherosclerosis even on a normal diet. When fed a cholesterol-rich diet, they develop elevated plasma levels of LDL cholesterol and atherosclerotic lesions very similar to those seen in humans. Anti-inflammatory properties of statins have been reported in these animals. Martínez-González and co-workers fed pigs a high-cholesterol diet for 50 days and found that vascular MCP-1 expression was down-regulated in the early lesions either by atorvastatin (3 mg/kg/day) or pravastatin (3 mg/kg/day).[25] Vascular MCP-1 inhibition by statins could be linked to the modulation of nuclear factor kappa B (NF-κB); this factor plays a pivotal role in vascular cell activation and induction of a wide spectrum of genes linked to the inflammatory response, including MCP-1. In this context, the modulation of gene expression by HMG-CoA reductase inhibitors seems to be derived from depletion of nonsteroidal isoprenoids in the cells. Isoprenoids participate in signal transduction through small G proteins. Again, this effect was not restricted to atorvastatin (lipophilic) and it was shared by pravastatin (hydrophilic), in agreement with results of earlier studies showing the ability of pravastatin to attenuate MCP-1 expression induced by $N(\omega)$nitro-L-arginine methylester (L-NAME) in rat coronary arteries.[26] L-NAME is an inhibitor of endothelial NO synthase (eNOS or NOS III), and it induces early vascular inflammation as well as subsequent arteriosclerosis in rats. In this model, cerivastatin and pravastatin decreased inflammatory features (e.g., there was reduction of MCP-1 and transforming growth factor-β [TGF-β] expression and a subsequent decrease in monocyte infiltration) and restored NO synthesis in endothelial cells (Fig. 2-3).

Several other studies have been conducted in rats, despite their resistance to atherosclerosis and different lipid metabolism. The endothelium-protective action of statins has been demonstrated in normocholesterolemic rats.[27] In this study, simvastatin was shown to down-regulate P-selectin expression and reduce leukocyte–endothelial cell interactions in the mesenteric artery after induction of inflammation by superfusion with L-NAME or thrombin. The endothelial fibrinolytic system also seems to be affected by statins. In one study,[28] aortas isolated from rats treated for 2 days with lovastatin (4 mg/kg/day) showed a threefold increase in tissue plasminogen activator (tPA) activity. Leukocyte–endothelial cell adhesion was significantly attenuated by fluvastatin in a hyper-cholesterolemic rat model, whereas blood lipid levels were not affected.[15] These anti-inflammatory actions of statins in rats were thought to be related to depletion of isoprenoids, particularly since these animals are known to be tolerant to the lipid-lowering effects of HMG-CoA reductase inhibitors.

Rabbits fed large amounts of cholesterol develop lipid-rich arterial lesions with some of the features of human atherosclerosis. Indeed, it was in cholesterol-fed rabbits that aortic cholesterol accumulation was first noted by Anitschkow in St. Petersburg 90 years ago.[29] Anti-inflammatory actions of statins have also been studied in this animal model. Hernandez-Presa and co-workers[30] demonstrated that atorvastatin decreases COX-2 mRNA expression and NF-κB activity in atherosclerotic lesions of hypercholesterolemic New Zealand male rabbits. Tissue factor expression and

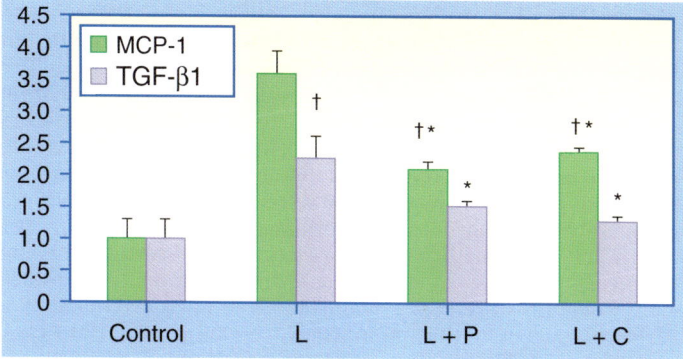

Effects of Statins on Cardiac MCP-1 and TGF-β1

Figure 2-3 Effect of statin treatment on rat cardiac monocyte chemo-attractant protein-1 (MCP-1) and transforming growth factor-β (TGF-β1) gene expression: summary of densitometric analysis of data. Data are expressed as ratio of MCP-1 and TGF-β1 mRNA to reduced glyceraldehyde-phosphate dehydrogenase (GAPDH) mRNA relative to control, which was assigned an arbitrary value of 1. L, group receiving L-NAME alone; L+P, group receiving L-NAME and pravastatin; L+C, group receiving L-NAME and cerivastatin; *, $P < .05$ versus L group; †, $P < .05$ versus control group. Each bar represents a sample size of five or six animals. (Adapted from Ni W, Egashira K, Kataoka C, et al: Anti-inflammatory and antiarteriosclerotic actions of HMG-CoA reductase inhibitors in a rat model of chronic inhibition of nitric oxide synthesis. Circ Res 89:415-421, 2001.)

macrophage accumulation were both reduced by fluvastatin (5 mg/kg/day) in the intimal lesions of WHHL rabbits, and this effect was independent of lipid lowering in another study.[31] Fluvastatin (3 mg/kg/day) was shown to protect LDL from oxidative modification in rabbits fed a high-cholesterol diet.[32] In another study in the rabbit model, arterial macrophage infiltration was abolished by atorvastatin treatment, MCP-1 was significantly diminished in the neointima and media of the femoral artery, and NF-κB activity and plasma lipid levels were reduced.[13] In this study, atherosclerosis was induced in the femoral arteries of rabbits by endothelial damage and by feeding an atherogenic diet for 4 weeks. NF-κB activity was found to be greater in the aorta and liver of high-cholesterol diet animals. Importantly, NF-κB activity was increased in tissues exposed only to hypercholesterolemia without local injury, suggesting a role for circulating cholesterol as a pro-inflammatory factor. Lipid lowering with statins in these animals decreased expression of VCAM-1, MCP-1, and iNOS expression.[33]

Further studies are needed to clarify the contribution and importance of direct cellular anti-inflammatory effects of statins. A broad knowledge base concerning atherosclerosis has recently emerged from genetically modified mouse models of athero-sclerosis. The role of HMG-CoA reductase inhibitors has been extensively studied in these animals. However, it is important to recall the fundamental limitations of the mouse model. Mice do not develop atherosclerosis without genetic manipulation. The physiology of lipid metabolism is radically different in mice from that in humans, because most of the cholesterol is transported in HDL-like particles. The mouse model demonstrates the central role of MCP-1 in the development of atherosclerotic lesions, because mice lacking MCP-1 or its receptor (CC-chemokine receptor-2) are considerably resistant to plaque formation. In wild-type mice, the in vivo anti-inflammatory effect of statins was investigated using the mouse airpouch model of local inflammation.[34] Lovastatin and pravastatin were orally administered to mice according to a treatment schedule that significantly inhibited the HMG-CoA reductase activity without affecting total blood cholesterol. At a dose of 10 mg/kg, lovastatin and pravastatin reduced by approximately 50% the lipopolysaccharide-induced leukocyte recruitment and MCP-1 production. These effects of statins were believed be a result of nonsterol mevalonate products and inde-pendent of circulating lipid lowering, in agreement with another study conducted in mice, where squalestatin, a selective inhibitor of sterol synthesis, was compared to lovastatin.[35] Squalestatin alone did not have any anti-inflammatory effect, whereas lovastatin (10 mg/kg/day) did. It is worth noticing that the short treatment schedule used in the case of lovastatin did not reduce the levels of circulating cholesterol but caused a significant drop in hepatic HMG-CoA reductase activity. Under the same experimental conditions, squalestatin, unlike lovastatin, caused a rapid drop in circulating cholesterol levels. Through the negative feedback mechanism controlling cholesterol synthesis, squalestatin induced hepatic HMG-CoA reductase activity. In this model, it is impossible to deduce the effect of these therapies through alterations in tissue cholesterol, in particular the concentration of lipid in the cell membrane.

In an elegant study by Sparrow and colleagues, anti-inflam-matory actions of simvastatin were confirmed by using a classic model of inflammation: carrageenan-induced foot pad edema.[36] Simvastatin administered orally to mice 1 hour before carrageenan injection significantly reduced the extent of edema. Simvastatin was comparable to indomethacin in this model. To determine whether the anti-inflammatory activity of simvastatin might affect atherogenesis, simvastatin was tested in apoE$^{-/-}$ mice. The mice were dosed daily for 6 weeks with simvastatin (100 mg/kg/day). Simvastatin did not alter plasma lipids. Atherosclerosis was quan-tified by measurement of aortic cholesterol content. Simvastatin significantly decreased the accumulation of free cholesterol and cholesteryl ester in the aorta without any effect on plasma cholesterol levels. These data suggest a reduction in tissue cholesterol in concert with anti-inflammatory actions when statins are given.

Every animal model gives us some useful information, but each comes with some limitation, such as the need for high doses to manifest the effect. It is too soon to say if any of these actions of statins are really independent of lipid lowering, particularly in doses used in humans.

STATINS AND REDUCTION IN ARTERIAL CALCIFICATION

Calcification of atherosclerotic lesions is an organized, regulated process similar to bone formation. Nonhepatic Gla-containing proteins (e.g., osteocalcin), which are actively involved in the transport of calcium out of vessel walls, are suspected to have key roles in the pathogenesis of arterial calcification. Osteopontin, as well as core-binding factor alfa-1, which are known to be involved in bone mineralization, have been identified in calcified atherosclerotic lesions. Calcified human atherosclerotic plaque also contains mRNA for bone morphogenetic protein-2, a potent factor for osteoblastic differentiation, matrix Gla protein, a potent inhibitor, and cells that are capable of osteoblastic differentiation.[37] Cells that are capable of osteoblastic differentiation, when exposed to oxidatively modified lipoproteins and inflammatory cytokines, may be derived from SMC and pericytes. These and other recent findings indicate that calcification is an active process and not simply a passive precipitation of calcium phosphate crystals, as once thought. Although calcification is found more frequently in advanced lesions, it may also occur in small amounts in earlier lesions that appear in the second and third decades of life.[38] Acute coronary syndromes generally result from less extensive coronary atherosclerosis. This explains why calcium is frequently observed in patients with acute coronary syndromes, although calcium cannot be used to identify unstable plaques. Rather, a calcium-rich fibrous cap is supposed to be resistant to erosion and less prone to rupture.[39] Calcium is associated less frequently with plaque erosion, and the most extensively calcified plaques are healed ruptures.[40]

HMG-CoA reductase inhibitors decrease mineralization in the atherosclerotic plaques. Whether this effect is good or bad has yet to be determined. Decreased mineralization can be considered good at the beginning of the atherosclerosis process; however, when the lesion is already established (late-stage atherosclerosis), calcification with collagen in the fibrous cap may be considered beneficial. Some studies have indeed addressed this subject. Williams and co-workers analyzed the effects of pravastatin on plaque characteristics in a monkey model.[41] Cynomolgus monkeys were fed an atherogenic diet for 2 years (progression phase) and then fed a lipid-lowering diet, either with or without pravastatin for an additional 2 years (treatment phase). As per design, plasma total and HDL cholesterol concentrations did not differ between the groups at the beginning of or during the treatment phase of the experiment. Histochemical analysis of the atherosclerotic lesions indicated that arteries from pravastatin-treated monkeys had significantly fewer macrophages in the intima as well as the media, less calcification, and less neovascularization in the intima. These effects of pravastatin occurred independently of plasma lipoprotein concentrations and despite similar changes in plaque size between the groups. Again, we do not know the cholesterol concentration in the tissue during the treatment phase.

In another interesting study, simvastatin (50 mg/kg/day) was given to apoE$^{-/-}$ mice, and changes in plaque size and composition were evaluated over 24 weeks of treatment.[42] In the untreated animals, there was a continuous increase in the frequency of calcified lesions, whereas the simvastatin-treated animals exhibited reduction in the frequency of calcification during the entire study. This effect of a statin was independent of lipid lowering, because HMG-CoA reductase inhibitors in general did not reduce plasma lipid levels (Fig. 2-4). On the other hand, van de Poll and co-workers studied atherosclerotic plaque formation in apoE*3 Leiden mice that were fed a high-cholesterol diet.[43] These mice, which carry the dysfunctional apoE variant from patients with a dominantly inherited form of familial dysbetalipoproteinemia, develop severe hyperlipidemia that results in rapid atherosclerotic plaque formation when they are fed a diet enriched with saturated fats and cholesterol. The authors treated these mice with atorvastatin (15 mg/kg/day) and compared their lesions in the aortic arch to those

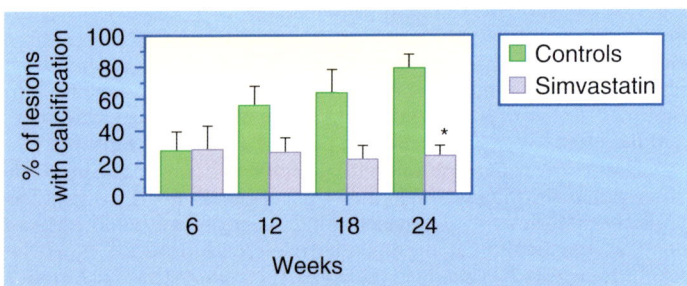

Effects of Simvastatin on Plaque Calcification

Figure 2-4 **Frequency of calcified lesions in the innominate artery of simvastatin-treated and control apoE$^{-/-}$ mice.** Values are mean ± standard error. *, $P < .01$ versus control. (Adapted from Bea F, Blessing E, Bennett B, et al: Simvastatin promotes atherosclerotic plaque stability in apoE-deficient mice independently of lipid lowering. Arterioscler Thromb Vasc Biol 22:1832-1837, 2002.)

in the control group without treatment. Raman spectroscopy[44] was used to evaluate changes in atherosclerotic plaque extent and composition as a function of cholesterol exposure and treatment with the lipid-lowering atorvastatin. They found significant reduction in plasma LDL concentration, average plaque surface, and calcification in the treated animals compared to controls.

Despite these studies, it is difficult to pinpoint the mechanism by which statins reduce plaque calcification. Nonetheless, the relationship between arterial mineralization and plaque vulnerability deserves additional investigation, particularly with regard to the clinical utility of statins.

STATINS AND ANGIOGENESIS

Angiogenesis has different roles in atherosclerosis. It can be considered to have a salutary effect when neovascularization occurs in ischemic tissues; on the other hand, it may be hazardous if microvascularization occurs inside the atherosclerotic plaque. Increased vascularization is a major feature during plaque development.[41] Neovascularization is an important process that is required for the progression of atherosclerosis.[45] Its pathogenic role includes the supply of nutrients and oxygen and facilitation of the accumulation of blood monocytes.[46] However, angiogenesis could also be involved in destabilization of the plaque, leading to hemorrhage and rupture.[47] By examining plaque from patients with ischemic events, Jeziorska and Woolley concluded that local hemorrhages as a result of rupture of microvasculature within the atherosclerotic plaque contribute to the acute complications of atherosclerosis by favoring plaque destabilization.[48] McCarthy and colleagues also reported that there was significantly more neovascularization in plaques and fibrous caps in symptomatic compared with asymptomatic plaques.[49]

Possible stimuli for plaque angiogenesis include local hypoxia and leukocyte-derived cytokines, such as vascular endothelial growth factor (VEGF) and basic fibroblast growth factor (bFGF).[50] Oncostatin M (OSM), secreted by activated monocytes and largely overexpressed in atherosclerotic plaque, has also been characterized as an angiogenic factor.[51] The same stimuli, such as hypoxia and VEGF in ischemic tissues, can promote endothelial cell survival,[52] NO synthesis,[53] and migration[54]; these cellular responses contribute to new blood vessel growth and stabilization of the vascular network.

Statins exert a biphasic dose-dependent action on angiogenesis. High doses of statins inhibit angiogenesis, whereas low doses can promote neovascularization. Relevant studies that have elucidated this effect are reviewed here. Vincent and colleagues evaluated the effect of cerivastatin on angiogenesis in the Matrigel model in mice.[55] Mice that received Matrigel containing 1 µg of bFGF and 100 µg of cerivastatin developed a limited number of discontinuous vessel spots around the Matrigel plugs. In contrast, mice that received Matrigel containing only bFGF exhibited an abundant and continuous vascular network in the connective tissue around the Matrigel plugs. To explore the mechanism of action, the authors conducted an in vitro study and demonstrated that cerivastatin (10 to 25 ng/mL) inhibited microvascular endothelial cell proliferation induced by growth factors, whereas it had no effect on unstimulated cells. This growth arrest occurred at the G_1/S phase and was related to the increase of the cyclin-dependent kinase inhibitor $p21^{Waf1/Cip1}$. These effects were reversed by geranylgeranyl pyrophosphate (GGPP), suggesting that the inhibitory effect of cerivastatin is related to RhoA inactivation. This mechanism was confirmed by RhoA delocalization from cell membrane to cytoplasm and actin fiber depolymerization, which are also prevented by GGPP. Vincent and associates[55] also found that RhoA-dependent inhibition of cell proliferation is mediated by the inhibition of focal adhesion kinase and protein kinase B (PKB)/Akt activation. The PKB/Akt serves as a multifunctional regulator of cell survival, growth, and glucose metabolism. With respect to its cardiovascular function, Akt acts downstream of the angiogenic growth factors VEGF and angiopoietin[56] to confer endothelial cell survival and ensure proper blood vessel development.[57] In addition to its cytoprotective role, Akt functions as an activator of endothelial cell NO production in response to VEGF; it is also essential for direct endothelial cell migration toward VEGF, mediating, therefore, the response of the endothelium to angiogenic stimuli.

In another study in pigs, simvastatin attenuated the increase in coronary vasa vasorum in the absence of lipid lowering, suggesting attenuation of the compensatory neovascularization by a direct non–lipid-lowering effect.[58] Previous studies have demonstrated a correlation between the extent of vasa vasorum neovascularization and severity of coronary atherosclerosis.[59] One potential mechanism of the relationship between neovascularization and atherosclerosis might be endothelial dysfunction of the vasa vasorum at an early stage, which leads to a reduction in oxygen supply to the coronary artery wall with subsequent activation of hypoxia-inducible factor (HIF), a transcription factor that regulates the expression of pro-angiogenic factors, such as VEGF.[60] It may also be postulated that simvastatin attenuates hypoxia in the coronary artery wall and hence reduces neovascularization in experimental hypercholesterolemia, despite an absence of change in plasma lipids. It is noteworthy that in all studies mentioned thus far, animals were given high doses of statins.

Pro-angiogenic effects of statins have also been demonstrated in animal models given statins in low doses. Kureishi and co-workers studied normocholesterolemic rabbits; these animals underwent unilateral resection of the femoral artery and its main branches, resulting in a marked decrease in hind-limb perfusion.[61]

To test the effects of simvastatin on limb revascularization, a dose of 0.1 mg/kg/day was administered by intraperitoneal injection after femoral artery resection. Animals receiving statin treatment displayed more detectable collateral vessels with characteristic corkscrew morphology than the untreated control group at 40 days after femoral resection. Simvastatin administration also promoted capillary formation in the ischemic limb. To explore the mechanism, the authors conducted an in vitro study on human umbilical vein endothelial cells and found that simvastatin (1 μM) increased Akt activity during the first 30 minutes of incubation; Akt activity fell thereafter but remained higher than in the untreated cells.

These apparently inconsistent and contradictory results depend on the dose of statin and the incubation time used. It appears that low-dose statin may enhance angiogenesis by activation of endothelial NO synthase via the PKB/Akt pathway. In contrast, high-dose statins may decrease angiogenesis via a reduction in GGPP and/or MCP-1 and MMPs.

Weis and co-workers have studied the effects of different doses of statins in inflammation-induced angiogenesis in mice.[62] They observed that low doses of cerivastatin or atorvastatin (0.5 mg/kg/day) enhanced, whereas higher doses inhibited, angiogenesis. Plasma concentrations in humans closely mimic the low doses used in animals. These authors also showed pro-angiogenic effects at concentrations between 0.005 and 0.05 μmol/L (low- to mid-range concentrations observed in humans), and angiostatic effects at greater than 0.05 μmol/L of cerivastatin or atorvastatin (high-dose concentrations observed in humans). These in vitro and in vivo studies are concordant with the concept of a biphasic effect of statins on angiogenesis (Fig. 2-5).

STATINS AND PLAQUE COLLAGEN CONTENT

The proliferation of vascular SMCs is a central event in the pathogenesis of vascular lesions. SMCs synthesize the interstitial collagens, major constituents of the arterial extracellular matrix responsible for resistance to rupture of atherosclerotic plaques. The balance between collagen production and degradation is a key determinant of plaque disruption, the trigger of most acute coronary events. An atherosclerotic lesion contains highly thrombogenic materials in the lipid core that are separated from the bloodstream by the fibrous cap. Collagen is the main component of the fibrous cap and is responsible for its tensile strength. Because macrophages are capable of degrading the collagen-containing fibrous cap, they play an important role in the development and subsequent stability of atherosclerotic plaques.[63] Indeed, degradation of the plaque matrix appears to be most active in macrophage-rich regions. Secretion of proteolytic enzymes, such as MMPs, by activated macrophages weakens the fibrous cap, particularly at

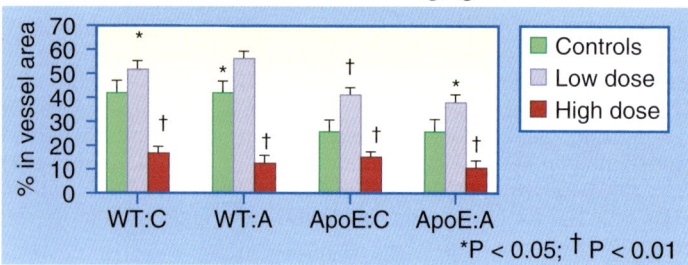

Figure 2-5 **Inflammation-induced angiogenesis was enhanced with low-dose statins but diminished with high doses. Angiogenesis was impaired in hyperlipidemic apoE$^{-/-}$ mice compared with wild-type (WT) mice.** High-dose statins further impaired angiogenesis in these mice. A, atorvastatin; C, cerivastatin. (Adapted from Weis M, Heeschen C, Glassford AJ, Cooke JP: Statins have biphasic effects on angiogenesis. Circulation 105:739-745, 2002.)

the "vulnerable" shoulder region, where the fibrous cap joins the arterial wall.

Macrophages in atheroma overexpress MMP-1 (collagenase-1), MMP-3 (stromelysin-1), and MMP-9 (gelatinase-β). Matrix remodeling by MMPs liberates SMCs from their pericellular matrix cage and permits their migration during response to injury. Pathologic studies have shown that MMPs colocalize with morphologic and mechanical determinants of plaque rupture. Inflammatory mediators, such as interleukin-1 (IL-1), CD40 ligand, and TNF-α, up-regulate MMP activity in vascular cells. Tissue inhibitors of metalloproteinases (TIMPs) inhibit MMP activity, and hence they reduce matrix remodeling.[64]

Lipid lowering by statins may contribute to plaque stability by reducing plaque size or by modifying the physiochemical properties of the lipid core. The clinical benefits from lipid lowering are probably the result of a decrease in macrophage accumulation in atherosclerotic lesions and inhibition of production of MMPs by activated macrophages. Indeed, statins inhibit the expression of MMPs and tissue factor. As such, the plaque-stabilizing properties of statins are mediated through a combined reduction in lipids, macrophages, and MMPs. Many animal studies have been reported that address this issue

In a study in monkeys, sections of normal abdominal aortas showed that medial SMCs contained immunoreactive MMP-2 and its selective inhibitor TIMP-2, but no MMP-3 or MMP-9.[24] However, these segments consistently displayed expression of TIMP-1, indicating that the inhibitors of MMPs prevail in normal arteries. Fatty streak–like atherosclerotic lesions, on the other hand,

MMP-1 Immunohistochemistry

Control   HC-diet

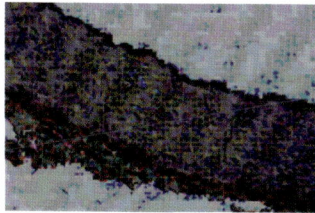 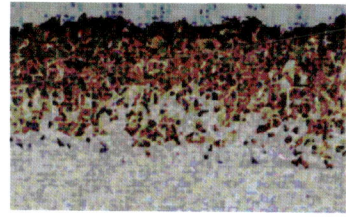

Figure 2-6 MMP-1 immunohistochemistry in aortic tissues of rabbits fed a high-cholesterol (HC) diet or control diet. Note that the HC diet increased the expression of MMP-1 in the neointima and media. (Adapted from Chen H, Li DY, Mehta JL: Mutation of matrix metalloproteinase-1, its tissue inhibition and nuclear factor-κB by losartan in hypercholesterolemic rabbits. J Cardiovasc Pharmacol 39:332-339, 2002.)

generally exhibited higher levels of MMPs than did uninvolved arteries, particularly in neointimal foam cells. Conversely, the expression of MMP inhibitors was much more prominent in the underlying media than in the expanded intima. This pattern increased in advanced atheroma, wherein the intimal SMCs and macrophages frequently colocalized with immunoreactive MMPs but little TIMP-1; the medial SMCs contained much fewer immuno-reactive MMPs but more TIMPs. Intimal macrophage-derived foam cells produce cytokines such as IL-1β that can augment MMP expression. Interestingly, treatment of a group of monkeys with atherosclerosis with pravastatin (40 mg/kg/day) and simvastatin (20 mg/kg/day) reduced immunostaining for IL-1β.

In a study from our laboratory, Chen and colleagues showed markedly increased MMP-1 expression in proliferating intima in hypercholesterolemic rabbits (Fig. 2-6).[65] Aikawa and co-workers studied WHHL rabbits for 32 weeks and measured macrophage accumulation and expression of MMPs in aortic atheroma.[66] Cerivastatin (0.6 mg/kg/day) diminished the enhanced accumulation of macrophages in aortic atheroma. Macrophage expression of MMP-1, MMP-3, and MMP-9 also decreased with cerivastatin treatment. Cerivastatin reduced the number of macrophages expressing mRNA, a sensitive marker of cell proliferation, but did not alter macrophages undergoing apoptosis (Fig. 2-7). These findings suggest that statins can decrease the number of macrophages in the lesion by inhibiting their proliferation, but not by induction of cell death. More interestingly, Luan and co-workers studied secretion of MMPs and TIMPs from SMCs and macrophages in cholesterol-fed rabbits.[67] Cerivastatin, simvastatin, and lovastatin inhibited inducible MMP-1, -3, and -9 and constitutive MMP-2 secretion, but not TIMP-1 or -2 secretion, which implies that statins

2

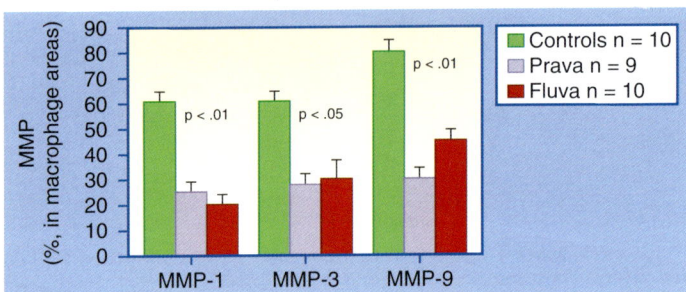

Figure 2-7 Quantitative analysis of matrix metalloproteinase-1 (MMP-1), MMP-3, or MMP-9 expression by macrophages in atheroma of WHHL rabbits. Data are reported as percentage of MMP-1-, MMP-3-, or MMP-9–positive area within macrophage-containing regions by computer analysis. MMP-1 expression by macrophages was significantly reduced in the fluvastatin group compared with the control group. MMP-3 and MMP-9 expression by macrophages were significantly reduced in the pravastatin and fluvastatin groups compared with the control group. (Adapted from Aikawa M, Rabkin E, Sugiyama S, et al: An HMG-CoA reductase inhibitor, cerivastatin, suppresses growth of macrophages expressing matrix metalloproteinases and tissue factor in vivo and in vitro. Circulation 103:276-283, 2001.)

shift the MMP/TIMP balance toward TIMPs. Importantly, all these statins similarly decreased collagenolytic, caseinolytic, and gelatinolytic activity. Mevalonate and geranylgeranyl pyrophosphate, but not squalene, reversed the effects of statins, suggesting dependence on isoprenoids, not on plasma cholesterol–lowering effect.

By inhibiting secretion of MMPs, statins can limit collagen degradation in plaque, but statins also reduce total collagen content of plaque by inhibiting SMC proliferation and intimal migration.[16,17] SMCs are collagen producers. In a previously mentioned study, Fukumoto and colleagues administered pravastatin (50 mg/kg/day), fluvastatin (20 mg/kg/day), or placebo to WHHL rabbits.[18] Immunohistochemistry revealed that MMP-1, -3, and -9 expression by macrophages in the intima was less in both the pravastatin and fluvastatin groups than in the placebo group, without any difference in macrophage numbers. Numbers of intimal SMCs and expression of type I procollagen mRNA, however, were significantly higher in the pravastatin group than in the fluvastatin group. Treatment with pravastatin, but not fluvastatin, preserved interstitial collagen content in vivo. The authors concluded that although both statins reduced expression of MMPs, only the cell-permeant fluvastatin decreases SMC number and collagen gene expression in vivo.

Reduction of SMCs and collagen is associated with plaque instability. On the other hand, reduction of macrophages and MMPs is related to plaque stability. In a study in rabbits, atherosclerosis was induced with balloon injury and an atherogenic diet for 4 months; then the rabbits were continued on a hyperlipemic or a lipid-lowering diet for the next 8 or 16 months.[68] At baseline, atherosclerotic lesions expressed high levels of MMP-1 and contained many macrophages. These features of plaque instability persisted in rabbits continued on the hyperlipemic diet. However, the lipid-lowering diet resulted in a progressive reduction in both macrophage content and MMP-1 immunoreactivity over time. Aortic interstitial collagen content increased in the lipid-lowering diet group compared with the hyperlipemic group, indicating that lipid lowering reinforced the fibrous skeleton of the atheroma.

These studies are just a small example of the large amount of work that has been done in several laboratories. However, we do not yet know if lipophilic statins are superior and whether isoprenoid-dependent actions are significant in patients given clinically used doses, but we do know that lipid lowering itself can stabilize plaques by reducing proteolytic activity.

CONCLUSIONS

It is well recognized that plaque characteristics and anatomo-pathology are related to clinical syndromes; for example, unstable lipid- and macrophage-rich plaques are responsible for acute coronary syndromes, whereas stable plaques with low lipid content are the basis of chronic ischemia. Ideally, one would like to convert unstable to stable plaque. The animal data on the effect of statins have been mixed. Particularly problematic is the effect of different statins on plaque content and collagen-forming and collagen-depositing enzymes. Similarly, the effect of statins on angiogenesis in the clinical setting needs to be examined. Likewise, the relative differences between lipophilicity and hydrophilicity have not been translated into differences in clinical outcomes of patients.

It must be recognized that animal models have several limitations, such as use of high doses, differences in lipid metabolism (from humans), and lack of tissue cholesterol measurement. Nevertheless, studies in animal models provide clues about the mechanisms of disease and potential therapeutic targets.

References

1. Palinski W, Napoli C: Unraveling pleiotropic effects of statins on plaque rupture. Arterioscler Thromb Vasc Biol 22:1745-1750, 2002.
2. Liao JK: Beyond lipid lowering: The role of statins in vascular protection. Int J Cardiol 86: 5-18, 2002.
3. Libby P, Aikawa M: Mechanisms of plaque stabilization with statins. Am J Cardiol 91:4B-5B, 2003.

4. Cullen P, Baetta R, Bellosta S, et al: Rupture of the atherosclerotic plaque: Does a good animal model exist? Arterioscler Thromb Vasc Biol 23:535-542, 2003.

5. Takemoto M, Liao JK: Pleiotropic effects of 3-hydroxy-3-methylglutaryl coenzyme A reductase inhibitors. Arterioscler Thromb Vasc Biol 21:1712-1719, 2001.

6. Wright SD, Burton C, Hernandez M, et al: Infectious agents are not necessary for murine atherogenesis. J Exp Med 191:1437-1442, 2000.

7. Chen L, Haught H, Yang B, et al: Preservation of endogenous antioxidant activity and inhibition of lipid peroxidation as common mechanisms of antiatherosclerotic effects of vitamin E, lovastatin and amlodipine. J Am Coll Cardiol 30:569-575, 1997.

8. Polette A, Blache D: Effect of vitamin E on acute iron load-potentiated aggregation, secretion, calcium uptake and thromboxane biosynthesis in rat platelets. Atherosclerosis 96:171-179, 1992.

9. Grundy SM: HMG-CoA reductase inhibitors for the treatment of hypercholesterolemia. N Engl J Med 319:24-33, 1988.

10. Carpenter KLH, Taylor SE, van der Veen C, et al: Lipids and oxidized lipids in human atherosclerotic lesions at different stages of development. Biochim Biophys Acta 1256:141-150, 1995.

11. Aviram M, Dankner G, Cogan U, et al: Lovastatin inhibits low-density lipoprotein oxidation and alters its fluidity and uptake by macrophages: In vitro and in vivo studies. Metabolism 41:229-235, 1992.

12. Conde K, Pineda G, Newton RS, Fernandez ML: Hypocholesterolemic effects of 3-hydroxy-3-methylglutaryl coenzyme A (HMG-CoA) reductase inhibitors in the guinea pig: Atorvastatin versus simvastatin. Biochem Pharmacol 58:1209-1219, 1999.

13. Bustos C, Hernandez-Presa MA, Ortego M, et al: HMG-CoA reductase inhibition by atorvastatin reduces neointimal inflammation in a rabbit model of atherosclerosis. J Am Coll Cardiol 32:2057-2064, 1998.

14. Igarashi M, Takeda I, Mori S, et al: Suppression of neointimal thickening by a newly developed HMG-CoA reductase inhibitor, BAYw6228, and its inhibitory effect on vascular smooth muscle cell growth. Br J Pharmacol 120:1172-1178, 1997.

15. Kimura M, Kurose I, Russell J, Granger N: Effects of fluvastatin on leukocyte-endothelial cell adhesion in hypercholesterolemic rats. Arterioscler Thromb Vasc Biol 17:1521-1526, 1997.

16. Alfon J, Guasch JF, Berrozpe M, Badimon L: Nitric oxide synthase II (NOS II) gene expression correlates with atherosclerotic intimal thickening: Preventive effects of HMG-CoA reductase inhibitors. Atherosclerosis 145:325-331, 1999.

17. Komukai M, Wajima YS, Tashiro J, et al: Carvastatin suppresses intimal thickening of rabbit carotid artery after balloon catheter injury probably through the inhibition of vascular smooth muscle cell proliferation and migration. Scand J Clin Lab Invest 59:159-166, 1999.

18. Fukumoto Y, Libby P, Rabkin E, et al: Statins alter smooth muscle cell accumulation and collagen content in established atheroma of Watanabe heritable hyperlipidemic rabbits. Circulation 103:993-999, 2001.

19. Kowala MC, Valentine M, Recce R, et al: Enhanced reduction of atherosclerosis in hamsters treated with pravastatin and captopril: ACE in atheromas provides cellular targets for captopril. J Cardiovasc Pharmacol 32:29-38, 1998.

20. Masashi S, Takashi I, Yasuhiko H, Makoto E: Stability of atheromatous plaque affected by lesional composition: Study of WHHL rabbits treated with statins. Ann N Y Acad Sci 947:419-423, 2001.
21. Libby P, Ridker PM, Maseri A: Inflammation and atherosclerosis. Circulation 105:1135-1143, 2002.
22. Chen H, Li DY, Phillips MI, Mehta JL: Attenuation of P-selectin and MCP-1 expression and intimal proliferation by AT1 receptor blockade in hyperlipidemic rabbits. Biochem Biophys Res Commun 282:474-479, 2001.
23. Chen H, Li DY, Savamura T, et al: Upregulation of LOX-1 expression in aorta of hypercholesterolemic rabbits: Modulation by losartan. Biochem Biophys Res Commun 276:1100-1104, 2000.
24. Sukhova GK, Williams JK, Libby P: Statins reduce inflammation in atheroma of nonhuman primates independent of effects on serum cholesterol. Arterioscler Thromb Vasc Biol 22:1452-1458, 2002.
25. Martínez-González J, Alfon J, Berrozpe M, Badimon L: HMG-CoA reductase inhibitors reduce vascular monocyte chemotactic protein-1 expression in early lesions from hypercholesterolemic swine independently of their effect on plasma cholesterol. Atherosclerosis 159:27-33, 2001.
26. Ni W, Egashira K, Kataoka C, et al: Antiinflammatory and antiarteriosclerotic actions of HMG-CoA reductase inhibitors in a rat model of chronic inhibition of nitric oxide synthesis. Circ Res 89:415-421, 2001.
27. Pruefer D, Scalia R, Lefer AM: Simvastatin inhibits leukocyte-endothelial cell interactions and protects against inflammatory processes in normocholesterolemic rats. Arterioscler Thromb Vasc Biol 19:2894-2900, 1999.
28. Essig M, Nguyen G, Prié D, et al: 3-Hydroxy-3-methylglutaryl coenzyme A reductase inhibitors increase fibrinolytic activity in rat aortic endothelial cells. Circ Res 83:683-690, 1998.
29. Anitschkow N: Über die veränderungen der kaninchenaorta bei experimenteller cholesterinsteatose. Beitr Pathol Anat Allg Pathol 56:379:404, 1913.
30. Hernandez-Presa MA, Martin-Ventura JL, Ortego M, et al: Atorvastatin reduces the expression of cyclooxygenase-2 in a rabbit model of atherosclerosis and cultured vascular smooth muscles cells. Atherosclerosis 160:49-58, 2002.
31. Baetta R, Camera M, Comparato C, et al: Fluvastatin reduces tissue factor expression and macrophage accumulation in carotid lesions of cholesterol fed rabbits in the absence of lipid lowering. Arterioscler Thromb Vasc Biol 22:692-698, 2002.
32. Yasuhara M, Suzumura K, Tanaka K, et al: Fluvastatin, an HMG-CoA reductase inhibitor, protects LDL from oxidative modification in hypercholesterolemic rabbits. Biol Pharm Bull 23:570-574, 2000.
33. Aikawa M, Sugiyama S, Hill CC, et al: Lipid lowering reduces oxidative stress and endothelial cell activation in rabbit atheroma. Circulation 106:1390-1396, 2002.
34. Romano M, Diomede L, Sironi M, et al: Inhibition of monocyte chemotactic protein-1 synthesis by statins. Lab Invest 80:1095-1100, 2000.
35. Diomede L, Albani D, Sottocorno M, et al: In vivo anti-inflammatory effect of statins is mediated by nonsterol mevalonate products. Arterioscler Thromb Vasc Biol 21:1327-1332, 2001.

36. Sparrow CP, Burton CA, Hernandez M, et al: Simvastatin has anti-inflammatory and antiatherosclerotic activities independent of plasma cholesterol lowering. Arterioscler Thromb Vasc Biol 21:115-121, 2001.
37. Proudfoot D, Davies JD, Skepper JN, et al: Acetylated low-density lipoprotein stimulates human vascular smooth muscle cell calcification by promoting osteoblastic differentiation and inhibiting phagocytosis. Circulation 106: 3044-3050, 2002.
38. Wexler L, Brundage B, Crouse L, et al: Coronary artery calcification: Pathophysiology, epidemiology, imaging methods, and clinical implications: A statement for health professionals from the American Heart Association. Circulation 94:1175-1192, 1996.
39. Schmermund A, Erbel R: Unstable coronary plaque and its relation to coronary calcium. Circulation 104:1682-1687, 2001.
40. Taylor AJ, Burke AP, O'Malley PG, et al: A comparison of the Framingham risk index, coronary artery calcification, and culprit plaque morphology in sudden cardiac death. Circulation 101:1243-1248, 2000.
41. Williams JK, Sukhova GK, Herrington DM, Libby P: Pravastatin has cholesterol-lowering independent effects on the artery wall of atherosclerotic monkeys. J Am Coll Cardiol 31:684-691, 1998.
42. Bea F, Blessing E, Bennett B, et al: Simvastatin promotes atherosclerotic plaque stability in apoE-deficient mice independently of lipid lowering. Arterioscler Thromb Vasc Biol 22:1832-1837, 2002.
43. van de Poll SW, Römer TJ, Volger OL, et al: Raman spectroscopic evaluation of the effects of diet and lipid-lowering therapy on atherosclerotic plaque development in mice. Arterioscler Thromb Vasc Biol 21:1630-1635, 2001.
44. Brennan JF III, Römer TJ, Lees RS, et al: Determination of human coronary artery composition by Raman spectroscopy. Circulation 96:99-105, 1997.
45. Battegay EG: Angiogenesis: Mechanistic insights, neovascular diseases, and therapeutic prospects. J Mol Med 73:333-346, 1995.
46. Zhang Y, Cliff WJ, Schoefl GI, Higgins G: Immunohistochemical study of intimal microvessels in coronary atherosclerosis. Am J Pathol 143:164-172, 1993.
47. Lee RT, Libby P: The unstable atheroma. Arterioscler Thromb Vasc Biol 17:1859-1867, 1997.
48. Jeziorska M, Woolley DE: Local neovascularization and cellular composition within vulnerable regions of atherosclerotic plaques of human carotid arteries. J Pathol 188:189-196, 1999.
49. McCarthy MJ, Loftus IM, Thompson MM, et al: Angiogenesis and the atherosclerotic carotid plaque: An association between symptomatology and plaque morphology. J Vasc Surg 30:261-268, 1999.
50. Shweiki D, Itin A, Soffer D, Keshet E: Vascular endothelial growth factor induced by hypoxia may mediated hypoxia-initiated angiogenesis. Nature 359:843-845, 1992.
51. Vasse M, Pourtau J, Trochon V, et al: Oncostatin M induces angiogenesis in vitro and in vivo. Arterioscler Thromb Vasc Biol 19:1835-1842, 1999.
52. Gerber HP, McMurtrey A, Kowalski J, et al: Vascular endothelial growth factor regulates endothelial cell survival through the phosphatidylinositol 3′-kinase/Akt signal transduction pathway: Requirement for Flk-1/KDR activation. J Biol Chem 273:30336-30343, 1998.

53. Fulton D, Gratton JP, McCabe TJ, et al: Regulation of endothelium-derived nitric oxide production by the protein kinase Akt. Nature 399:597-601, 1999.

54. Morales-Ruiz M, Fulton D, Sowa G, et al: Vascular endothelial growth factor-stimulated actin reorganization and migration of endothelial cells is regulated via the serine/threonine kinase Akt. Circ Res 86:892-896, 2000.

55. Vincent L, Soria C, Mirshahi F, et al: Cerivastatin, an inhibitor of 3-hydroxy-3-methylglutaryl coenzyme A reductase, inhibits endothelial cell proliferation induced by angiogenic factors in vitro and angiogenesis in in vivo models. Arterioscler Thromb Vasc Biol 22:623-629, 2002.

56. Kim I, Kim HG, So JN, et al: Angiopoietin-1 regulates endothelial cell survival through the phosphatidylinositol 3′-kinase/Akt signal transduction pathway. Circ Res 86:24-29, 2000.

57. Carmeliet P, Lampugnani MG, Moons L, et al: Targeted deficiency or cytosolic truncation of the *VE-cadherin* gene in mice impairs VEGF-mediated endothelial survival and angiogenesis. Cell 98:147-157, 1999.

58. Wilson SH, Herrmann J, Lerman LO, et al: Simvastatin preserves the structure of coronary adventitial vasa vasorum in experimental hypercholesterolemia independent of lipid lowering. Circulation 105:415-418, 2002.

59. Kumamoto M, Nakashima Y, Sueishi K: Intimal neovascularization in human coronary atherosclerosis: Its origin and pathophysiological significance. Hum Pathol 2:450-456, 1995.

60. Kwon HM, Sangiorgi G, Ritman EL: Enhanced coronary vasa vasorum neovascularization in experimental hypercholesterolemia. J Clin Invest 101:1551-1556, 1998.

61. Kureishi Y, Luo Z, Shiojima I, et al: The HMG-CoA inhibitor simvastatin activates the protein kinase Akt and promotes angiogenesis in normocholesterolemic animals. Nat Med 6:1004-1010, 2000.

62. Weis M, Heeschen C, Glassford AJ, Cooke JP: Statins have biphasic effects on angiogenesis. Circulation 105:739-745, 2002.

63. Moreno PR, Falk E, Palacios IF, et al: Macrophage infiltration in acute coronary syndromes: Implications for plaque rupture. Circulation 90:775-778, 1994.

64. Galis ZS, Khatri JJ: Matrix metalloproteinases in vascular remodeling and atherogenesis: The good, the bad, and the ugly. Circ Res 90:251-262, 2002.

65. Chen H, Li DY, Mehta JL: Mutation of matrix metalloproteinase-1, its tissue inhibition and nuclear factor-κB by losartan in hypercholesterolemic rabbits. J Cardiovasc Pharmacol 39:332-339, 2002.

66. Aikawa M, Rabkin E, Sugiyama S, et al: An HMG-CoA reductase inhibitor, cerivastatin, suppresses growth of macrophages expressing matrix metalloproteinases and tissue factor in vivo and in vitro. Circulation 103:276-283, 2001.

67. Luan Z, Chase AJ, Newby AC: Statins inhibit secretion of metalloproteinases-1, -2, -3, and -9 from vascular smooth muscle cells and macrophages. Arterioscler Thromb Vasc Biol 23:769-775, 2003.

68. Aikawa M, Rabkin E, Okada Y, et al: Lipid lowering by diet reduces matrix metalloproteinase activity and increases collagen content of rabbit atheroma: A potential mechanism of lesion stabilization. Circulation 97:2433-2444, 1998.

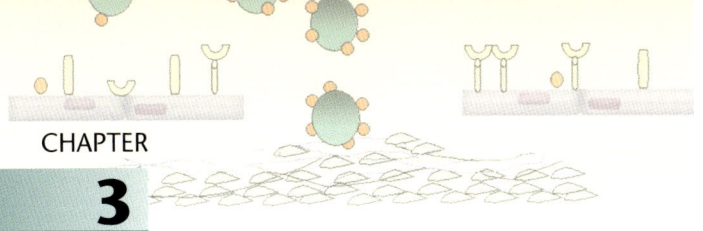

CHAPTER

3

Statins and Inhibition of Atherosclerosis: Human Studies

Anjan K. Sinha, Balkrishna M. Singh, and
Jawahar L. Mehta

3

HISTORICAL PERSPECTIVE

Hypercholesterolemia is associated with coronary atherosclerosis. Its initial description included dominant co-segregation of high levels of cholesterol, xanthomas, and early coronary heart disease in multiple kindred, which later became known as familial hypercholesterolemia.[1] Duguid and Aberd first suggested that lipids came from degenerate thrombus.[2] This concept was later proven to be wrong but it gave an insight into new pathophysiology. Gofman and colleagues, in their seminal publication "The Role of Lipids and Lipoproteins in Atherosclerosis," showed an association between lipoprotein fractions and risk for atherosclerosis.[3] Chandler and Hand subsequently provided the first mechanistic support for the view that atherosclerosis is associated with thrombosis (appropriately called atherothrombosis).[4,5] Equally important, this occurred at a time when the prevailing opinion held that cholesterol was the principal (if not sole) determinant of plaque formation. Their first report demonstrated that macrophages could phagocytose platelets and thereby evolve into foam cells.[4] Their second report indicated that autologous, fragmented blood clots injected into the pulmonary circulation of normal rabbits in amounts that do not increase pulmonary pressures are alone sufficient to induce plaque formation.[5] Although there had been strong evidence for the role of lipids in the pathogenesis of atherosclerosis, there were no experimental models until Vesselinovitch and co-workers created a mice model to study atherosclerosis.[6] Several studies have since utilized molecular biology, biochemistry, integrative physiology, and metabolism to gain insight into the complex processes leading to cardiovascular events, from the initiation of plaque formation to plaque rupture and thrombosis. Recent pathologic studies have shown that the plaques that are likely to cause clinical sequelae have a high content of lipid and foam cells[7] and an eccentric morphology. In addition, angiographic studies have shown that the majority of plaques that cause events are less than totally occlusive.[8]

In 1987, Glagov and co-workers demonstrated in their seminal paper that human coronary arteries enlarge in relation to plaque area and that functionally important luminal stenosis may be delayed until the lesion occupies 40% of the internal elastic laminar area (Fig. 3-1).[9] Because it was evident that atherosclerosis was closely linked to lipids, it was intuitive to evaluate the effect of lipid lowering and assess angiographic progression or regression. Progression of coronary atherosclerosis as measured by coronary angiography has been shown to be predictive of nonfatal myocardial infarction, coronary heart disease mortality, and a need for revascularization procedures. Therapies that decrease the progression of coronary atherosclerosis as assessed by angiography should also decrease clinical events. The evidence accumulated in experimental studies during the past few decades indicates that atherogenesis initially involves the intima, particularly the endothelium, with progression of disease until it affects the entire vessel wall. Recently, several studies have been performed with lipid-lowering strategies in different animal models of atherosclerosis.[10] These strategies result in important biologic changes within the atherosclerotic plaque, especially in areas of high macrophage and lipid content.

Angiographic trials of lipid-lowering therapies were initially called "regression trials" on the basis of the mistaken idea that lipid modification would "regress" the lesions and lead to large anatomic improvements. Multiple angiographic trials with or without statins have reported excellent low-density-lipoprotein (LDL) cholesterol reduction and have convincingly demonstrated that regression is not achieved but that progression is decreased. These results have

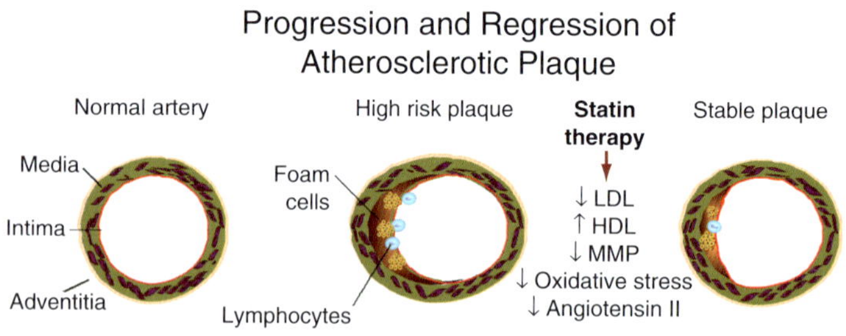

Progression and Regression of Atherosclerotic Plaque

Figure 3-1 **Progression and regression of atherosclerotic plaque.** There is a compensatory enlargement of the vessel wall to accommodate the atherosclerotic plaque. Therefore, despite significant atherosclerotic disease, the lumen is not compromised until very late. Statin therapy does not significantly alter the luminal diameter; however, preliminary investigations have demonstrated significant changes in plaque burden. This may represent a reverse Glagov phenomenon.

led to the concept that lipid-lowering therapy may lead to plaque stabilization. There had been no trials in humans demonstrating the effects of lipid lowering on the rate of progression of arteriosclerosis until recently. The classic 4S (Scandinavian Simvastatin Survival Study) trial[11] of 4444 Scandinavian patients reviewed in Chapter 4 provided the first demonstration of the lifesaving capacity of statins. However, no data showed whether atherosclerosis progression was minimized or, more importantly, whether regression of atherosclerosis occurred.

PROGRESSION AND REGRESSION TRIALS

Smaller angiographic studies have shown that the progression of coronary atherosclerosis can be slowed and, in some cases, atherosclerosis can be reversed by cholesterol-lowering interventions. The anatomic changes in the coronary arteries, however, are small and occur too slowly to account for the clinical benefit, which is evident soon after initiating cholesterol-lowering therapy. Evidence suggests that plaque stabilization is the most important mechanism by which cholesterol-lowering therapy reduces the incidence of adverse cardiac events and affects progression of coronary atherosclerosis. Here we review major trials that show the effect of cholesterol-lowering therapy on coronary atherosclerosis (Table 3-1).

Coronary Artery Disease Trials

PROGRAM ON THE SURGICAL CONTROL OF THE HYPERLIPIDEMIAS

The Program on the Surgical Control of the Hyperlipidemias (POSCH), a randomized clinical trial, was designed to test whether cholesterol lowering induced by the partial ileal bypass operation would favorably affect overall mortality or mortality due to coronary heart disease.[12] The study population consisted of 838 patients (417 in the control group and 421 in the surgery group), both men (90.7%) and women, with an average age of 51 years, who had survived a first myocardial infarction. The mean follow-up period was 9.7 years. When compared with the control group at 5 years, the surgery group had a mean plasma total cholesterol level that was 23.3% lower ($P < .0001$), an LDL cholesterol level 37.7% lower ($P < .0001$), and a high-density-lipoprotein (HDL) cholesterol level 4.3% higher ($P = .02$). A comparison of baseline coronary arteriograms with those obtained at 3, 5, 7, and 10 years subsequently showed less disease progression in the surgery group ($P < .001$). Although this first report was published more than 10 years ago, the surgical group continues to have a lower cardiovascular event rate.

LIFESTYLE HEART TRIAL

The Lifestyle Heart Trial was performed in two tertiary care university hospitals.[13] Forty-eight patients with moderate to severe

Table 3-1

Summary of Major Progression/Regression Coronary Trials with Statins

Trial	Number of Agents	Participants	TG	In Trial LDL	LDL	HDL	Angiographic Outcomes			Cardiovascular Events
							Progression	Regression	No Change	
CCAIT[18]	Lovastatin	146/153	174/188	172/171	120/167	43/42	48/76	14/10	84/67	18/21
MARS[16]	Lovastatin	114/106	121/164	157/157	86/152	45/43	33/42	26/14	57/50	15/20
MAAS[21]	Simvastatin	178/167	149/170	170/173	117/174	46/42	41/54	33/20	104/93	25/33
REGRESS[20]	Pravastatin	314/327	129/152	166/167	125/170	39/36	142/181	54/30	118/116	50/79
FATS[29]	Colestipol, lovastatin	38/46	137/264	190/175	107/162	41/40	17/21	26/5	31/20	5/10
SCOR[30]	Colestipol, niacin, lovastatin	40/32	90/109	283/275	172/243	59/51	8/13	13/4	19/40	0/1
SCRIP[31]	Colestipol, niacin, lovastatin, gemfibrozil, probucol	119/127	126/156	158/156	121/150	52/45	60/63	24/13	35/51	38/47
HARP[17]	Pravastatin, niacin, cholestyramine, gemfibrozil	40/39	130/174	140/135	85/138	44/41	14/15	4/5	22/19	4/4
PLAC[19]	Pravastatin	206/202	166	164	—	41	42/59	22/22	99/76	55/81

HDL, high-density lipoprotein; LDL, low-density lipoprotein; TG, triglyceride; CCAIT, Canadian Coronary Atherosclerosis Intervention Trial; MARS, Monitored Atherosclerosis Regression Study; MAAS, Multicentre Anti-Atheroma Study; REGRESS, Regression Growth Evaluation Statin Study; FATS, Familial Atherosclerosis Treatment Study; SCOR, Specialized Center for Research; SCRIP, The Stanford Coronary Risk Intervention Project; HARP, Harvard Atherosclerosis Reversibility Study; PLAC, Pravastatin Limitation of Atherosclerosis in the Coronary Arteries.

coronary heart disease were randomized to an intensive lifestyle change group or to a usual care control group, and 35 completed the 5-year follow-up quantitative coronary arteriography procedure. Intensive lifestyle changes included a vegetarian diet with 10% of daily intake from fat, aerobic exercise, stress management, smoking cessation, and psychosocial support. Notably, these patients did not receive any lipid-lowering drugs. Changes in coronary artery stenosis and cardiac events were recorded. In the experimental group, 20 of 28 patients completed the 5-year follow-up and maintained comprehensive lifestyle changes throughout the study, whereas the control group (15 of 20 patients completed the 5-year follow-up) made more modest changes. In the experimental group, the coronary artery stenosis decreased by 1.75 absolute percentage points after 1 year (a 4.5% relative improvement) and by 3.1 absolute percentage points after 5 years (a 7.9% relative improvement). In contrast, the coronary artery stenosis in the control group increased by 2.3 percentage points after 1 year (a 5.4% relative worsening) and by 11.8 percentage points after 5 years (a 27.7% relative worsening) (P = .001 between groups). In the 28 patients in the experimental group, 25 cardiac events occurred (versus 45 events in the 20 patients in the control group) during the 5-year follow-up (risk ratio for any event for the control group, 2.47 [95% CI, 1.48-4.20]).

ST. THOMAS' ATHEROSCLEROSIS REGRESSION STUDY

The St. Thomas' Atherosclerosis Regression Study (STARS) in Britain assessed the effect of dietary reduction of plasma cholesterol concentrations on coronary atherosclerosis.[14] It was a randomized, controlled, endpoint-blinded trial based on quantitative image analysis of coronary angiograms in patients with angina or past myocardial infarction. To determine the effect of a greater reduction in circulating cholesterol, the intervention group received diet and cholestyramine. Ninety men with coronary heart disease, who had a mean plasma cholesterol of 7.23 ($\pm$0.77 SD) mmol/L (279 [$\pm$30 SD] mg/dL), were randomized to receive usual care, dietary intervention, or diet plus cholestyramine. Coronary angiography was performed at baseline and at 39 (mean) months. Mean plasma cholesterol levels during the trial were 6.93, 6.17, and 5.56 mmol/L (268, 238, and 215 mg/dL) in the usual care, dietary intervention, and diet plus cholestyramine groups, respectively. The proportion of patients who showed overall progression of coronary atherosclerosis was significantly reduced by both interventions (46%, 15%, 12% in usual care, diet alone, and diet plus cholestyramine, respectively), whereas the proportion that showed an increase in luminal diameter rose significantly (4%, 38%, and 33% in usual care, diet alone, and diet plus cholestyramine, respectively). The absolute width of the coronary segments studied decreased by 0.201 mm (mean) in the usual care group, increased by 0.003 mm in the diet alone group, and increased by 0.103 mm in the diet plus cholestyramine group ($P < .05$), with improvement also seen in the minimum width of segments, percentage of stenosis diameter, and edge irregularity index in both intervention groups. The change in indices of coronary narrowing was independently and significantly correlated with LDL cholesterol concentration and LDL/HDL cholesterol ratio during the trial period. Both interventions significantly reduced the frequency of total cardiovascular events. Dietary change alone reduced overall progression and indeed some regression of coronary atherosclerosis disease, and diet plus cholestyramine had an additive effect with a net increase in coronary luminal diameter.

LIPOPROTEIN AND CORONARY ATHEROSCLEROSIS STUDY

The Lipoprotein and Coronary Atherosclerosis Study (LCAS), a more recent and larger study, included men and women, 35 to 75 years old, with angiographic coronary heart disease and a mean LDL cholesterol of 2.97 to 4.92 mmol/L (115 to 190 mg/dL) despite dietary modification.[15] Patients ($N = 429$; 19% women) were randomized to fluvastatin, 20 mg twice daily, or placebo. One fourth of patients were also assigned open-label adjunctive therapy with cholestyramine (up to 12 g/day) because prerandomization LDL cholesterol had remained at 4.14 mmol/L (160 mg/dL) or higher. The primary endpoint, assessed by quantitative coronary angiography, was a within-patient, per-lesion change in minimum luminal diameter of qualifying lesions. Over 2.5 years of follow-up, the mean LDL cholesterol level fell by 23.9%, from 3.78 to 2.87 mmol/L (146 to 111 mg/dL), in all patients treated with fluvastatin plus cholestyramine, and by 22.5%, from 3.54 to 2.74 mmol/L (137 to 106 mg/dL), in the fluvastatin-only subgroup. Primary analysis in 340 patients showed significantly less lesion progression in all fluvastatin-treated patients than in all placebo-treated patients (change in minimal luminal diameter, –0.028 versus –0.100 mm, respectively, $P < .01$), Patients treated with fluvastatin alone also showed a greater change in luminal diameter than placebo-treated patients (change in minimal luminal diameter, –0.024 versus –0.094 mm, respectively, $P < .02$). Similar benefit was observed with treatment whether baseline LDL cholesterol was above 4.14 or below 3.37 mmol/L (160 or 130 mg/dL). Beneficial effects of lipid lowering were persistent regardless of baseline LDL cholesterol (Fig. 3-2).

MONITORED ATHEROSCLEROSIS REGRESSION STUDY

The Monitored Atherosclerosis Regression Study (MARS) included 270 patients, 37 to 67 years old, with a total cholesterol level ranging from 4.92 to 7.64 mmol/L (190 to 295 mg/dL) and angiographically defined coronary artery disease.[16] This was a randomized, double-blind, placebo-controlled, multicenter coronary angiographic trial performed in community- and university-based centers. The patients were on a cholesterol-lowering diet, and either lovastatin (80 mg/day) or placebo was administered. Change in coronary

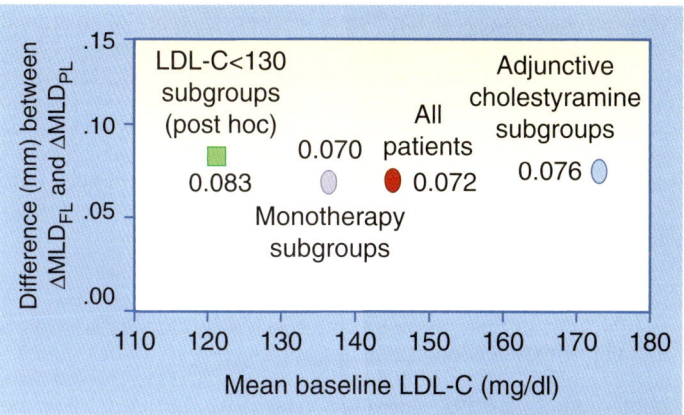

Relation of LDL-Concentrations
and Minimum Luminal Diameter In LCAS

Figure 3-2 Across the range of baseline low-density-lipoprotein cholesterol (LDL-C) concentrations included in the Lipoprotein and Coronary Atherosclerosis Study (LCAS), the difference between minimum luminal diameter (MLD) changes with fluvastatin and with placebo (MLD_{FL} and MLD_{PL}) was consistent. (Adapted from Herd JA, Ballantyne CM, Farmer JA, et al: Effects of fluvastatin on coronary atherosclerosis in patients with mild to moderate cholesterol elevations (Lipoprotein and Coronary Atherosclerosis Study [LCAS]). Am J Cardiol 80:278-286, 1997.)

stenosis by quantitative coronary angiography was the primary endpoint. Global change in coronary atherosclerosis, based on the consensus of blinded expert readers, was the secondary endpoint. The average percentage diameter of the stenosis increased 2.2% in placebo recipients and 1.6% in lovastatin recipients ($P > .20$). For lesions 50% or greater, the average percentage diameter of the stenosis increased 0.9% in placebo recipients and decreased 4.1% in lovastatin recipients ($P = .005$). The mean global change score was +0.9 (indicating progression) in the placebo group and +0.4 in the lovastatin group ($P = .002$); 13 placebo recipients and 28 lovastatin recipients had global change scores indicating regression ($P < .02$). There was no evidence of regression.

Harvard Atherosclerosis Reversibility Project Group

In a study by the Harvard Atherosclerosis Reversibility Project (HARP) group, 79 normocholesterolemic patients with CHD (70 men, 9 women) were studied.[17] Their mean age was 58 years, all were nonsmokers, and their mean total cholesterol concentration was 5.5 mmol/L (212 mg/dL). All patients received dietary advice and were randomly assigned placebo (39) or active treatment (40) with pravastatin, nicotinic acid, cholestyramine, and gemfibrozil stepwise as needed to reach the specified goal (total cholesterol ≤ 4.1 mmol/L [158 mg/dL], ratio of LDL/HDL cholesterol ≤ 2.0). Coronary angiograms at baseline and after 2.5 years of treatment were analyzed by computer-assisted quantitative techniques. There was no significant difference in the extent of coronary atherosclerosis during follow-up between the active treatment and placebo groups; the minimum diameter narrowed significantly but to the same extent in both groups (change from baseline over 2.5 years, 0.14 mm [SD = 0.42] and 0.15 mm [SD = 0.42], respectively, both $P < .001$). Similarly, the change in percentage stenosis did not differ between the groups (2.1 [SD10.6] versus 2.4 [SD10.3]%).

CANADIAN CORONARY ATHEROSCLEROSIS INTERVENTION TRIAL

In the Canadian Coronary Atherosclerosis Intervention Trial, 331 patients with diffuse coronary atherosclerosis documented on a recent arteriogram and with fasting serum cholesterol between 5.7 and 7.7 mmol/L (220 and 300 mg/dL) were enrolled in a randomized, double-blind, placebo-controlled trial.[18] All patients received intensive dietary counseling. Lovastatin or placebo was begun at 20 mg/day and was titrated to 40 and 80 mg during the first 16 weeks to attain a fasting LDL cholesterol of 3.37 mmol/L (130 mg/dL) or less. The mean lovastatin dose was 36 mg/day. Coronary arteriography was repeated after 2 years. In 299 patients (90%), 3858 coronary segments containing 2309 stenoses were measured blindly with an automated computerized quantitative system. Total and LDL cholesterol decreased by 21 ± 11% and 29 ± 11%, respectively, in the lovastatin-treated group but changed by less than 2% in the placebo-treated group. The primary endpoint, coronary artery lumen change, defined as the per-patient mean of the minimum luminal diameter changes (follow-up minus baseline angiogram) for all lesions measured, excluding those less than 25% on both films, worsened by 0.09 ± 0.16 mm in the placebo group and by only 0.05 ± 0.13 mm in the lovastatin group ($P = .01$). The beneficial effect of treatment was most pronounced in the more numerous, milder lesions and in patients whose baseline total or LDL cholesterol levels were above the group median.

PRAVASTATIN LIMITATION OF ATHEROSCLEROSIS IN THE CORONARY ARTERIES

In the Pravastatin Limitation of Atherosclerosis in the Coronary Arteries (PLAC I) study, the 3-hydroxy-3-methylglutaryl coenzyme A (HMG-CoA) reductase inhibitor pravastatin was used to evaluate the effect on progression of coronary atherosclerosis and ischemic events in patients with coronary artery disease (CAD) and mild to moderate hyperlipidemia.[19] In this 3-year study, 408 patients (mean age, 57 years) with CAD and LDL cholesterol 3.37 mmol/L (130 mg/dL) or more, but less than 4.9 mmol/L (190 mg/dL) despite diet, were randomized to receive pravastatin or placebo. Atherosclerosis progression was evaluated by quantitative coronary arteriography.

Baseline mean LDL cholesterol in all the patients was 4.25 mmol/L (164 mg/dL). Pravastatin decreased total and LDL cholesterol and triglyceride levels by 19%, 28%, and 8%, respectively, and increased HDL cholesterol by 7% ($P \leq .001$ versus placebo for all lipid variables). Progression of atherosclerosis was reduced by 40% as assessed by coronary artery diameter ($P = .04$). This relationship was particularly pronounced in lesions with less than 50% stenosis at baseline. There was a consistent although not statistically significant effect on mean diameter and percentage diameter stenosis. There were also fewer new lesions in patients assigned to pravastatin therapy ($P \leq .03$).

REGRESSION GROWTH EVALUATION STATIN STUDY

The Regression Growth Evaluation Statin Study (REGRESS) was a double-blind, placebo-controlled, multicenter study to assess the effects of 2 years of treatment with pravastatin on progression and regression of coronary atherosclerosis in 885 men with a serum total cholesterol level between 4.0 and 8.0 mmol/L (155 and 310 mg/dL) by quantitative coronary arteriography.[20] Primary endpoints were change in coronary artery diameter and minimum obstruction diameter. Clinical events were also analyzed. Of the 885 patients, 778 (88%) had an evaluable final angiogram. Mean coronary artery segment diameter decreased 0.10 mm in the placebo group versus 0.06 mm in the pravastatin group ($P = .019$). The difference in coronary artery diameter between the two treatment groups was 0.04 mm, with a 95% CI of 0.01 to 0.07 mm. The median minimum obstruction diameter decreased 0.09 mm in the placebo group versus 0.03 mm in the pravastatin group ($P = .001$).

MULTICENTRE ANTI-ATHEROMA STUDY

The Multicentre Anti-Atheroma Study (MAAS) was a randomized, double-blind clinical trial in 381 patients with coronary heart disease treated with either placebo or simvastatin, 20 mg daily, for 4 years.[21] Patients who received simvastatin had a 23% reduction in serum cholesterol, a 31% reduction in LDL cholesterol, and a 9% increase in HDL cholesterol compared with placebo. Quantitative coronary angiography done at baseline and after 2 and 4 years showed significant reductions in mean luminal diameter (–0.08 mm) and in minimum luminal diameter (–0.13 mm) in the placebo group. In the simvastatin group, changes in mean luminal diameter and minimum luminal diameter were significantly superior to those in the placebo group ($P = .006$). Patients on placebo had an increase in mean diameter stenosis of 3.6%, whereas in those on simvastatin there was a 2.6% decrease in diameter. On a per-patient basis, angiographic progression occurred less often in the simvastatin group (41 versus 54 patients) and regression was more frequent (33 versus 20 patients). Significantly, more new lesions and new total occlusions developed in the placebo group (48 versus 28, and 18 versus 8, respectively). There was no difference in the clinical outcome. However, more patients in the placebo group underwent coronary angioplasty or revascularization (34 versus 23 on simvastatin).

Peripheral Vascular Disease Trials

Increased carotid intima media thickness (IMT) is a relatively simple, inexpensive, and reproducible noninvasive marker of global atherosclerotic disease. As an experimental tool, it is frequently used in epidemiologic studies to identify and follow vascular disease. Ultrasonographic noninvasive assessment of easily accessible arteries has been advocated as a surrogate marker for less accessible vessels such as those in the coronary and cerebral arterial systems.[22] Numerous clinical trials have shown that treatment of dyslipidemia retards progression of IMT, as quantified by carotid two-dimensional ultrasound.

REGRESS ULTRASOUND STUDY

In the REGRESS ultrasound study, in addition to coronary artery evaluation, carotid and femoral artery walls were imaged at baseline and at 6, 12, 18, and 24 months.[23] Pravastatin treatment effect was defined as the difference in progression of the combined intima and media thicknesses between treatment groups. This substudy included 255 patients out of a total of 885 men. Pravastatin treatment effects were highly significant (combined IMT, $P = .0085$; combined far wall IMT, $P < .0001$; common femoral artery far wall IMT, $P = .004$).

The Asymptomatic Carotid Artery Progression Study randomized asymptomatic individuals with early carotid atherosclerosis and moderately elevated serum LDL cholesterol. In this study, there was significant reduction in the incidence of cardiovascular events in the lovastatin-treated group. After 6 months, although IMT continued to progress in the placebo group, there was a progressive reduction in the lovastatin group.[24] The Kuopio Atherosclerosis Prevention Study showed a similar trend in the pravastatin-treated group during a 3-year follow-up period.[25]

It is clear from a review of the randomized angiographic trials that cholesterol lowering results in a favorable shift in the balance between progression and regression of CAD. Progression and regression are likely to happen with all the statins and are possible with other agents as long as a lipid-lowering effect is achieved (Fig. 3-3). In most of the trials, a significant reduction in mortality occurred within 2 years. Notably, patients treated with statin regimens demonstrated the same degree of CAD progression, albeit at a reduced rate compared with patients in the control group. In the PLAC I study, pravastatin therapy reduced the progression of coronary artery diameter stenosis (0.43%/year), whereas the difference in minimum luminal diameter between pravastatin and placebo-treated patients was only 0.02 mm per year. These changes in coronary atherosclerosis are clearly out of proportion to the

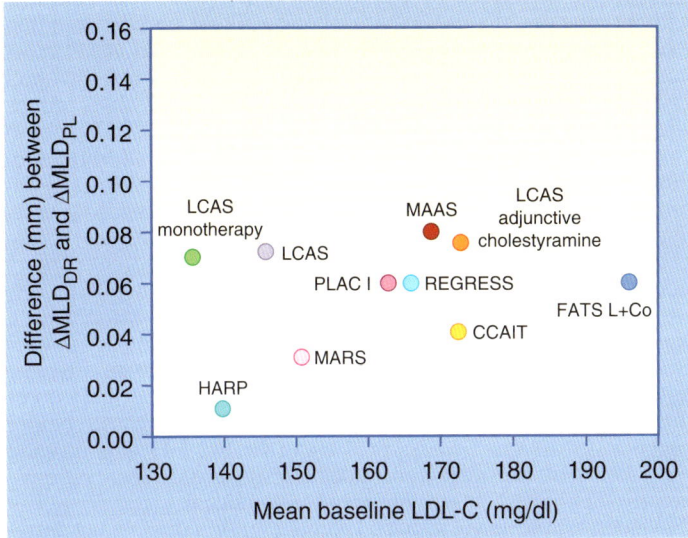

Comparison of MLD Change in Minimal Luminal Diameter in Trials of Statin Therapy

Figure 3-3 Despite marked variation in baseline low-density-lipoprotein cholesterol (LDL-C) in angiographic trials with different statins, the difference in minimum luminal diameter changes with statin and with placebo (MLD_{DR} and MLD_{PL}) was consistent regardless of the statin used. CCAIT, Canadian Coronary Atherosclerosis Intervention Trial; FATS, Familial Atherosclerosis Treatment Study; HARP, Harvard Atherosclerosis Reversibility Study; L+Co, lovastatin and colestipol; LCAS, Lipoprotein and Coronary Atherosclerosis Study; MAAS, Multicentre Anti-Atheroma Study; MARS, Monitored Atherosclerosis Regression Study; PLAC I, Pravastatin Limitation of Atherosclerosis in the Coronary Arteries; REGRESS, Regression Growth Evaluation Statin Study. (Adapted from Herd JA, Ballantyne CM, Farmer JA, et al: Effects of fluvastatin on coronary atherosclerosis in patients with mild to moderate cholesterol elevations (Lipoprotein and Coronary Atherosclerosis Study [LCAS]). Am J Cardiol 80:278-286, 1997.)

marked reduction in clinical events and do not account for the early treatment benefit attributable to statins.

Corti and colleagues recently described beneficial effects of long-term, lipid-lowering therapy by simvastatin on previously established aortic and carotid atherosclerotic lesions.[26] Magnetic resonance imaging of aortic and carotid plaques performed serially demonstrated that simvastatin not only might reduce the vessel wall area (vascular atherosclerotic burden) but, if treatment is maintained, might also increase the arterial luminal area. This observation emphasizes the need for sustained lowering of LDL cholesterol to favorably impact the progression of atherosclerotic disease. The earliest change noted in this study was a regression in plaque size, illustrated by the reduction of the arterial wall area without affecting the luminal area. Longer follow-up indicated that regression of atherosclerotic lesions continues for at least 24 months and that progressive remodeling of the arterial wall produces a significant increase in luminal area. These observations suggest that, at least in the early lesions, plaque shrinkage and vascular remodeling may be achieved earlier than alterations in luminal dimensions. Interestingly, the feature of arterial remodeling, detected as a decrease in the total vessel wall area, may not be sustained after the first 18 months of treatment. These data confirm the original observation by Glagov and co-workers that in the early stages of atherogenesis, lipid deposition is associated with a positive outer remodeling of the arterial wall, whereas at later stages, continuous lipid and cell accumulation start compromising the arterial lumen.[9] On the other hand, an effective lipid-lowering treatment may, by reducing the lipid content of the lesions, affect the remodeling of the vascular wall before significantly affecting the luminal area (see Fig. 3-1). The imaging capabilities of high-resolution magnetic resonance imaging have greatly facilitated these observations. Recent data from the Cleveland Clinic have provided similar information using intravascular ultrasound (unpublished data). Significant atherosclerotic plaque burden regression has been shown without significant difference in luminal diameter of coronary arteries in subjects treated with high-dose pravastatin.

LIMITATIONS AND FUTURE DIRECTIONS

The greatest limitation of all the progression and regression trials has been lack of uniformity. Some trials evaluate minimal luminal diameter, whereas others consider degree of stenosis. Moreover, coronary luminography, which has been the method of choice in all the trials, is a poor technique to assess plaque burden. Degree of remodeling to accommodate plaque is variable, particularly in the setting of diabetes. Some recent ongoing trials are using intravascular ultrasound to accurately measure luminal area and thickness. This is a more accurate way to assess plaque burden,[27] but randomized placebo-controlled trials can no longer be performed because of the known significant survival benefits of statins.

If regression indeed occurs with cholesterol-lowering therapy, then we should expect improvement in stable angina and in perfusion scans related to improvement of blood flow. The number of studies evaluating lipid-lowering therapy with assessment of myocardial perfusion is limited. Thallium-201 scintigraphy and positron emission tomography scanning have been used for semiquantitative evaluation. In these studies, myocardial perfusion defects improved in the actively treated patient groups, without significant changes in coronary anatomy as measured by coronary luminography. In a long-term intense risk factor modification study, the change in dipyridamole positron emission tomography scans of normalized counts worsened in control subjects by 13.5% and improved in the experimental group by 4.2%.[28] Similarly, in the short-term lipid-lowering study with fluvastatin, the improvement of perfusion defects could be observed after about 12 weeks of therapy. The improvement was especially noticeable in the previously ischemic areas. The positive effects of these studies on myocardial perfusion have not yet been elucidated. Suggested mechanisms are improved endothelium-dependent vasodilation, improved collateral circulation, and changes in blood viscosity, but the possibility of plaque regression still exists. Recent meta-analyses have suggested that it is the change in lipid level rather than the prevailing concentration of LDL cholesterol that determines the angiographic therapeutic response, supporting the recommendation that lipid-lowering therapy not be restricted to those with severe hyperlipidemia.

Utilization of intravascular ultrasound in addition to coronary angiography will provide increased sensitivity to assess treatment effects on CAD progression. Other noninvasive methods—such as quantitative assessment of coronary calcium by ultrafast computed tomography, magnetic resonance imaging, and ultrasound—may provide useful means of assessing the benefits of pharmacologic treatment of atherosclerosis. Smaller trials utilizing surrogate endpoints will be useful in determining the beneficial effects of a drug, but larger morbidity and mortality studies will remain a necessity to understand fully the benefits and the risks of any given treatment.

References

1. Müller C: Angina pectoris in hereditary xanthomatosis. Arch Intern Med 64:675-700, 1939.
2. Duguid JB, Aberd MD: Pathogenesis of atherosclerosis. Lancet 257:925-936, 1947.
3. Gofman JW, Lindgren F, Elliott H, et al: The role of lipids and lipoproteins in atherosclerosis. Science 111:166-171, 1950.
4. Chandler AB, Hand RA: Phagocytized platelets: A source of lipids in human thrombi and atherosclerotic plaques. Science 134:946-947, 1961.
5. Hand RA, Chandler AB: Atherosclerotic metamorphosis of autologous pulmonary thromboemboli in the rabbit. Am J Pathol 40:469-486, 1962.
6. Vesselinovitch D, Wissler RW, Doull J: Experimental production of atherosclerosis in mice. 1. Effect of various synthetic diets and radiation on survival time, food consumption and body weight in mice. J Atheroscler Res 8:483-495, 1968.
7. Libby P, Aikawa M: Stabilization of atherosclerotic plaques: New mechanisms and clinical targets. Nat Med 8:1257-1262, 2002.
8. Ambrose JA, Tannenbaum MA, Alexopoulos D, et al: Angiographic progression of coronary artery disease and the development of myocardial infarction. J Am Coll Cardiol 12:56-62, 1988.

9. Glagov S, Weisenberg E, Zarins CK, et al: Compensatory enlargement of human atherosclerotic coronary arteries. N Engl J Med 316:1371-1375, 1987.

10. Aikawa M, Rabkin E, Sugiyama S, et al: An HMG-CoA reductase inhibitor, cerivastatin, suppresses growth of macrophages expressing matrix metalloproteinases and tissue factor in vivo and in vitro. Circulation 103:276-283, 2001.

11. Scandinavian Simvastatin Survival Study Group: Randomised trial of cholesterol lowering in 4444 patients with coronary heart disease: The Scandinavian Simvastatin Survival Study (4S). Lancet 344:1383-1389, 1994.

12. Buchwald H, Varco RL, Matts JP, et al, and the POSCH Group: Effect of partial ileal bypass surgery on mortality and morbidity from coronary heart disease in patients with hypercholesterolaemia: Report of the Program on the Surgical Control of the Hyperlipidemias (POSCH). N Engl J Med 323:946-955, 1990.

13. Ornish D, Brown SE, Scherwitz LW, et al: Can lifestyle changes reverse coronary heart disease? The Lifestyle Heart Study. Lancet 336:129-133, 1990.

14. Watts GF, Lewis B, Brunt JNH, et al: Effects on coronary artery disease of lipid-lowering diet, or diet plus cholestyramine, in the St Thomas' Atherosclerosis Regression Study (STARS). Lancet 339:563-569, 1992.

15. Herd JA, Ballantyne CM, Farmer JA, et al, for the LCAS Investigators: Effects of fluvastatin on coronary atherosclerosis in patients with mild to moderate cholesterol elevations (Lipoprotein and Coronary Atherosclerosis Study [LCAS]). Am J Cardiol 80:278-286, 1997.

16. Blankenhorn DH, Azen SP, Kramsch DM, et al. Coronary angiographic changes with lovastatin therapy: The Monitored Atherosclerosis Regression Study (MARS). Ann Intern Med 119:969-976, 1993.

17. Sacks FM, Pasternak RC, Gibson CM, et al, for the Harvard Atherosclerosis Reversibility Project (HARP) Group: Effect on coronary atherosclerosis of decrease in plasma cholesterol concentrations in normocholesterolaemic patients. Lancet 344:1182-1186, 1994.

18. Waters D, Higginson L, Gladstone P, et al: Effects of monotherapy with an HMG-CoA reductase inhibitor on the progression of coronary atherosclerosis as assessed by serial quantitative arteriography: The Canadian Coronary Atherosclerosis Intervention Trial. Circulation 89:959-968, 1994.

19. Pitt B, Mancini GBJ, Ellis SG, et al, for the PLAC I Investigators: Pravastatin Limitation of Atherosclerosis in the Coronary Arteries (PLAC I): Reduction in atherosclerosis progression and clinical events. J Am Coll Cardiol 26:1133-1139, 1995.

20. Jukema JW, Bruschke AVG, van Boven AJ, et al, on behalf of the REGRESS Study Group: Effects of lipid lowering by pravastatin on progression and regression of coronary artery disease in symptomatic men with normal to moderately elevated serum cholesterol levels: The Regression Growth Evaluation Statin Study (REGRESS). Circulation 91:2528-2540, 1995.

21. MAAS Investigators: Effect of simvastatin on coronary atheroma: The Multicentre Anti-Atheroma Study (MAAS). Lancet 344:633-638, 1994.

22. Sinha AK, Eigenbrodt M, Mehta JL: Does carotid intima media thickness indicate coronary atherosclerosis? Curr Opin Cardiol 17:526-530, 2002.

23. de Groot E, Jukema JW, Montauban van Swijndregt AD, et al: B-mode ultrasound assessment of pravastatin treatment effect on carotid and femoral artery walls and its correlations with coronary arteriographic findings: A report of the Regression Growth Evaluation Statin Study (REGRESS). J Am Coll Cardiol 31:1561-1567, 1998.

24. Furberg CD, Adams HP Jr, Applegate WB, et al: Effect of lovastatin on early carotid atherosclerosis and cardiovascular events: Asymptomatic Carotid Artery Progression Study (ACAPS) Research Group. Circulation 90:1679-1687, 1994.

25. Salonen R, Nyyssonen K, Porkkala E, et al: Kuopio Atherosclerosis Prevention Study (KAPS): A population-based primary preventive trial of the effect of LDL lowering on atherosclerotic progression in carotid and femoral arteries. Circulation 92:1758-1764, 1995.

26. Corti R, Fuster V, Fayad ZA, et al: Lipid lowering by simvastatin induces regression of human atherosclerotic lesions: Two years' follow-up by high-resolution noninvasive magnetic resonance imaging. Circulation 106:2884-2887, 2002.

27. Schartl M, Bocksch W, Koschyk DH, et al: Use of intravascular ultrasound to compare effects of different strategies of lipid-lowering therapy on plaque volume and composition in patients with coronary artery disease. Circulation 104:387-392, 2001.

28. Sdringola S, Nakagawa K, Nakagawa Y, et al: Combined intense lifestyle and pharmacologic lipid treatment further reduce coronary events and myocardial perfusion abnormalities compared with usual-care cholesterol-lowering drugs in coronary artery disease. J Am Coll Cardiol 41:263-272, 2003.

29. Brown G, Albers JJ, Fisher LD, et al: Regression of coronary artery disease as a result of intensive lipid-lowering therapy in men with high levels of apolipoprotein B. N Engl J Med 323:1289-1298, 1990.

30. Kane JP, Malloy MJ, Ports TA, et al: Regression of coronary atherosclerosis during treatment of familial hypercholesterolemia with combined drug regimens. JAMA 264:3007-3012, 1990.

31. Haskell WL, Alderman EL, Fair JM, et al. Effects of intensive multiple risk factor reduction on coronary atherosclerosis and clinical cardiac events in men and women with coronary artery disease: The Stanford Coronary Risk Intervention Project (SCRIP). Circulation 89:975-990, 1994.

3

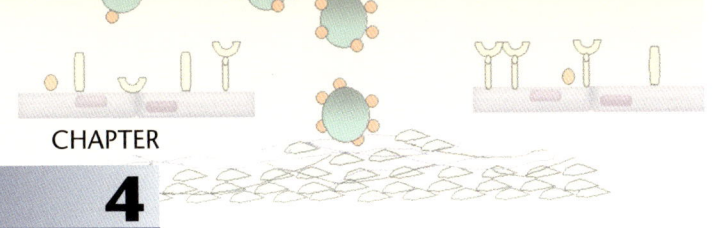

Statins in the Primary Prevention of Atherosclerosis-Related Events

Balkrishna M. Singh, Anjan K. Sinha, and
Jawahar L. Mehta

Atherosclerosis is responsible for almost all cases of coronary heart disease (CHD), and it contributes to a variety of other cardiovascular problems. Atherosclerosis begins with fatty streaks, which are first seen in adolescence; these lesions progress insidiously into plaques in early adulthood, and culminate in thrombotic occlusions and coronary events in middle age and later life. Improved understanding of the natural history of this disease process has led to the concept that thrombosis plays a key role in acute manifestations, and this disease has come to be recognized as atherothrombosis. A variety of factors, often acting in concert, are associated with an increased risk for atherosclerotic plaques in coronary arteries and other arterial beds. Thus, atherosclerosis is currently being seen as a complex disease process. Recognized risk factors of atherosclerosis are increased age, male sex, a family history of premature CHD, hypertension, hyperlipidemia, diabetes mellitus, tobacco smoking, and sedentary lifestyle. Recent studies have led to the identification of additional risk factors, which may have an impact on both prevention and treatment of CHD. The growing list of these risk factors includes the role of inflammation, estrogen deficiency, and obesity, and elevated plasma levels of homocysteine, fibrinogen, and uric acid.

Atherosclerosis tends to be a generalized, diffuse, and progressive disease. Hence, it is not surprising to learn that clinical events are related to multiple organ systems. Some of the clinical events are directly and strongly related to atherosclerosis, whereas others are indirectly and weakly related. On the basis of both laboratory and clinical evidence, 3-hydroxy-3-methylglutaryl coenzyme A (HMG-CoA) reductase inhibitors (statins) are known to have powerful modulatory effects on atherogenesis and are known to reduce major cardiovascular events in both primary and secondary prevention trials. Statins seem to exert important modulating effects on dyslipidemia, with a potent reduction in LDL cholesterol and a modest increase in HDL cholesterol. Although the exact mechanism of benefits in clinical trials remains debatable, many pleiotropic effects of statins (discussed separately in Chapter 8) have also been implicated in reducing major cardiovascular events. The role of statins in the primary prevention of these atherosclerosis-related events is the subject of this review.

CORONARY ARTERY DISEASE–RELATED EVENTS: ANGINA, MYOCARDIAL INFARCTION, REVASCULARIZATION, AND DEATH

Treating hypercholesterolemia in patients who do not have clinical evidence of coronary artery disease (CAD) to prevent clinical events is called primary prevention. The rationale for this approach is based on epidemiologic data documenting a continuous, graded relationship between total plasma cholesterol concentration and CAD events and mortality.[1,2] The causal role of cholesterol in this relationship is suggested by clinical trials that have demonstrated that targeted lowering of LDL cholesterol in patients with hyper-cholesterolemia reduces CAD morbidity.

In earlier studies with cholesterol-lowering agents, the higher death rate from noncardiac causes raised a concern regarding the safety of cholesterol-lowering therapy, particularly in a relatively low-risk population. This concern confounded management guidelines for primary preventive therapy in hypercholesterolemic subjects, until they were addressed in subsequent trials. A meta-analysis of primary prevention trials in which statins were administered showed a 26% reduction in overall mortality that was primarily the result of a 37% reduction in cardiovascular deaths, with no effect on noncardiovascular deaths and no difference in the incidence of fatal or nonfatal cancer.[3] The availability of the statin group of drugs thus can be considered a major breakthrough in the primary prevention of CHD. The data from some of the studies utilizing statins strongly support the use of statins for the prevention of CHD-related events and are summarized here.

The WOSCOPS Trial

The West of Scotland Coronary Prevention Study (WOSCOPS) trial was designed to evaluate the effect of pravastatin (40 mg/day) for 5 years on the rate of nonfatal myocardial infarction (MI) and CHD death in 6595 men with hypercholesterolemia and no prior evidence of MI or cardiac revascularization.[4,5] The study included men aged 45 to 64 years with a total cholesterol level greater than 252 mg/dL (6.5 mmol/L) on initial screening, LDL cholesterol greater than 155 mg/dL (4.0 mmol/L) on visits 2 and 3, and greater than 174 mg/dL (4.5 mmol/L) but less than 232 mg/dL (6.0 mmol/L) on one occasion after dietary therapy for 4 weeks. Reduction in nonfatal myocardial infarction or CHD death from approximately 9.4% to 6.4% was observed over a 6-year follow-up. Thus, the absolute benefit was 3%. The reduction in clinical events began within 6 months after randomization. Another important observation was that, in contrast to results seen in the earlier primary prevention trials, there was no difference in noncardiovascular death (56 in the pravastatin group versus 62 in the placebo group [P = .54]) or incidence of cancers (115 versus 106 in the placebo group [P = .55]). Reduction in major clinical events in the WOSCOPS trial is summarized in Table 4-1.

The AFCAPS/TexCAPS Trial

The Air Force/Texas Coronary Atherosclerosis Prevention Study (AFCAPS/TexCAPS) was a randomized, placebo-controlled trial of lovastatin (20 to 40 mg daily) in 6605 patients without CHD.[6] It differed from WOSCOPS in two major ways: 997 postmenopausal women were also included, and the mean serum total and LDL cholesterol concentrations of the participants were near the average value in the general population (221 mg/dL and 150 mg/dL [5.7 and 3.9 mmol/L], respectively); the mean HDL concentration was somewhat low (36 mg/dL [0.94 mmol/L]).[6] Lovastatin reduced the serum LDL cholesterol concentration by 25% and increased the HDL concentration by 6%.

After a 5.2-year follow-up, an absolute benefit was noted in subjects treated with lovastatin. For every 1000 men and women treated with lovastatin for 5 years, 19 major coronary events, 12 myocardial infarctions, and 17 coronary revascularizations could

4

Table 4–1
Reduction in Clinical Events in the WOSCOPS Trial

Clinical Events	Relative Risk Reduction	Significance
Nonfatal MI or CHD death	31%	P < 0.001
Nonfatal MI	31%	P < 0.001
All CVD deaths	32%	P = 0.033
Total mortality	22%	P = 0.051
Coronary revascularization (CABG, PCI)	31% to 37%	P < 0.01

CABG, coronary artery bypass surgery; CHD, coronary heart disease; CVD, cardiovascular disease death; MI, myocardial infarction; PCI, percutaneous coronary intervention; WOSCOPS, West of Scotland Coronary Prevention Study.

From Shepherd J, Cobbe SM, Ford I, et al: Prevention of coronary heart disease with pravastatin in men with hypercholesterolemia. N Engl J Med 333:1301-1307, 1995; and West of Scotland Coronary Prevention Study Group: Baseline risk factors and their association with outcome in the West of Scotland Coronary Prevention Study. Am J Cardiol 79:756-762, 1997.

be prevented.[6] The total absolute benefit was approximately 2%, such that those 50 patients had to be treated to prevent one event at 5 years. Again, the benefit was independent of the absolute level of LDL cholesterol.

The AFCAPS/TexCAPS trial extended the observations seen in the WOSCOPS study in two ways. First, it demonstrated the efficacy of primary prevention in women, as was noted in the Scandinavian Simvastatin Survival study of secondary prevention[7]; second, it demonstrated the efficacy of primary prevention in patients with "normal" serum cholesterol concentrations. The clinical implications of this study for treating asymptomatic subjects with a statin have led to some major revisions in the National Cholesterol Education Program (NCEP) (Adult Treatment Panel III [ATP III]) guidelines.

The Heart Protection Study

The Medical Research Council/British Heart Foundation (MRC/BHF) Heart Protection Study (HPS) randomly assigned 20,536 subjects to simvastatin (40 mg/day) or placebo; 33% had a baseline LDL cholesterol level of less than 116 mg/dL (<3 mmol/L), 25% had a level of 116 to 135 mg/dL (3 to 3.5 mmol/L), and 42% had a level greater than 135 mg/dL (>3.5 mmol/L). HPS was truly a study of both primary and secondary prevention, because it included patients with known CAD, occlusive arterial disease, and diabetes mellitus. After an average follow-up of 5.5 years, significant benefits with simvastatin were observed (Table 4-2). There was no effect on the incidence of noncardiovascular deaths, and the reduction in

Table 4–2

Reduction in Clinical Events in the Heart Protection Study

Clinical Events	Relative Risk Reduction	Absolute Event Rate in Treated versus Placebo Group
All-cause mortality	12%	12.9% versus 14.7%
CHD death	17%	5.7% versus 6.9%
Major cardiovascular events	24%	20% versus 25.4%
Stroke	27%	4.3% versus 5.7%
MI and stroke in diabetics without CVD	28%	14% versus 18.7%
Nonfatal MI and CHD death	26%	8.7% versus 11.8%

CHD, coronary heart disease, CVD, cardiovascular disease, MI, myocardial infarction.
    From Heart Protection Study Collaborative Group: MRC/BHF Heart Protection Study of cholesterol lowering with simvastatin in 20536 high-risk individuals: A randomized controlled trial. Lancet 360:1623-1630, 2002.

stroke rate was primarily the result of a decrease in ischemic strokes without an increase in hemorrhagic strokes.[8] The benefit of simvastatin treatment extended to patients with low LDL cholesterol, women, and older adults. This interesting observation suggests that patients at high risk for cardiovascular events would benefit from statin therapy regardless of their baseline LDL cholesterol level.

The ASCOT-LLA Trial

The benefits of cholesterol lowering in the primary prevention of CHD in hypertensive patients who are not conventionally deemed dyslipidemic were shown in the recently published Anglo-Scandinavian Cardiac Outcomes Trial—Lipid-Lowering Arm (ASCOT-LLA).[9] Hypertensive patients (sample total, 19,342) between the ages of 40 and 79 years and with at least three other cardiovascular risk factors were randomized to one of two antihypertensive regimens; of this group, 10,305 patients with nonfasting total cholesterol concentrations of 6.5 mmol/L or lower were randomized to atorvastatin, 10 mg, or placebo. Treatment was stopped prematurely after a median follow-up of 3.3 years, when the lipid-lowering arm of ASCOT showed that in hypertensive patients, who on average were at moderate risk for developing cardiovascular events, cholesterol lowering with atorvastatin, 10 mg, conferred a 36% reduction in fatal CHD and nonfatal myocardial infarction compared with the placebo group. Table 4-3 shows the outcomes in major cardiovascular events in the ASCOT trial.

Table 4–3

Reduction in Clinical Events in ASCOT-LLA Trial

Clinical Events	Relative Risk Reduction	Absolute Event Rate in Treated versus Placebo Group
Nonfatal MI plus fatal CHD	36%	1.9% versus 3.0%
Total cardiovascular events and procedures	21%	7.5% versus 9.5%
Total coronary events	29%	3.4% versus 4.8%
All-cause mortality	13%	3.6% versus 4.1% (NS)
Cardiovascular mortality	12%	1.4% versus 1.6% (NS)

ASCOT-LLA, Anglo-Scandinavian Cardiac Outcomes Trial, Lipid-Lowering Arm; CHD, coronary heart disease; MI, myocardial infarction.

From ASCOT-LLA: Prevention of coronary and stroke events with atorvastatin in hypertensive patients who have average or lower-than-average cholesterol concentrations, in the Anglo-Scandinavian Cardiac Outcome Trial—Lipid Lowering Arm (ASCOT-LLA): A multicentre randomized controlled trial. Lancet 361:1149-1158, 2003.

The ALLHAT Study

The Antihypertensive and Lipid-Lowering Treatment to Prevent Heart Attack Trial (ALLHAT) is the only trial other than ASCOT-LLA that has been done specifically among hypertensive patients.[10] In the ALLHAT study, the effects of different antihypertensive drugs on fatal and nonfatal CHD events were compared, and a subgroup of 10,355 patients were also randomly assigned to pravastatin, 40 mg, or usual care. The patients included in the lipid-lowering arm of ALLHAT were a slightly older cohort, 14% had a history of preexisting CHD, and a greater proportion were women and nonwhite patients.

No significant benefits in terms of all-cause mortality or coronary and stroke events were apparent with statin use in the ALLHAT. This is somewhat surprising in view of ASCOT-LLA. The potential benefits of pravastatin in this study may have been compromised by a substantial use of statins in the usual care group, leading to differences in total cholesterol and LDL cholesterol of only 9% and 17%, respectively, between the two groups. Analysis of the hypertensive subgroups in earlier statin trials[6,8,11-13] has shown that the overall benefits of lipid lowering with statins among hypertensive patients could be expected to be at least as large as those noted among normotensive patients.

The PROSPER Study

The efficacy and safety of statins in older adults were the subject of the Prospective Study of Pravastatin in the Elderly at Risk (PROSPER), which included 5804 patients aged 70 to 82 years with a history of, or risk factors for, vascular disease.[14] Again, this was a study that combined both primary and secondary prevention. Patients were randomized to pravastatin, 40 mg, or placebo and followed for an average period of 3.2 years. Primary endpoints, a composite of CHD death, nonfatal MI, and fatal or nonfatal stroke were reduced by 15%, with an absolute reduction of 2.1%. Similarly, the CHD death rate was reduced by 24%. Although the incidence of transient ischemic attacks was reduced, there was no reduction in stroke rate. Of the patients in PROSPER, 56% were free of overt arterial disease (primary prevention group) and there was no significant difference in the outcome compared with patients who had arterial disease at the beginning of the trial.

The Cardiovascular Health Study

In older adult patients, evidence of a benefit of statins in primary prevention, in contrast to secondary prevention, remains scarce.[15] Observational data from the Cardiovascular Heath Study (CHS) showed a similar lowering of risk for cardiovascular events in patients 65 years and older treated with statins.[16] In this study of 1250 women and 664 men (with a mean follow-up of 7.3 years), the hazard ratios for cardiovascular events and all-cause mortality were

0.44 and 0.56, respectively, in the statin-treated group. Notably, patients over the age of 74 years derived similar benefit from statins in this study.

STROKE AND TRANSIENT ISCHEMIC ATTACKS
Link between Cholesterol, Atherosclerosis, and Stroke

Although the association between cholesterol and CHD are well accepted, the association between cholesterol and stroke has been a subject of some confusion. This may partly relate to the heterogeneous nature of stroke types, such as hemorrhagic and nonhemorrhagic strokes. It is usually understood that most nonhemorrhagic ischemic strokes are related to atherosclerotic disease in the cerebral circulation. However, a large number of patients with embolic strokes may also have underlying atherosclerosis.

Hypertension is well recognized as a risk factor for stroke, and controlling blood pressure has been demonstrated to reduce the risk for stroke. When blood pressure is well controlled to greatly reduce hypertensive strokes, dyslipidemia is revealed as a stroke risk factor.[17] In the large population of men screened for the Multiple Risk Factor Intervention Trial (MRFIT), there was a graded increase in the rate of fatal nonhemorrhagic stroke with increasing plasma levels of total cholesterol, whereas that of fatal hemorrhagic stroke was highest in those with the lowest total cholesterol plasma concentration. In the MRFIT trial, the incidence of nonhemorrhagic strokes far outweighed hemorrhagic strokes after myocardial infarction.[17]

In an Israeli study, researchers followed 11,177 patients with documented CHD, but no history of stroke, for 6 to 8 years and identified 941 patients who developed nonhemorrhagic cardiovascular disease.[18] The investigators observed a positive correlation between stroke and transient ischemic attack (TIA) risk and both total cholesterol and LDL cholesterol, as well as an inverse correlation between stroke and TIA risk and HDL cholesterol. Similarly, the Women's Pooling Project, a longitudinal prospective cohort study of 24,343 women with no previous cardiovascular disease, showed that among women younger than 55 years at baseline, those whose total cholesterol levels were in the highest quintile (relative to those whose levels were in the lowest quintile) were 2.13 times more likely to die of a nonhemorrhagic stroke.[19] However, these studies did not include patients who had a prior stroke, and there is limited or no analysis of the relationship between cholesterol levels and specific stroke subtypes.

Some studies suggest that serum cholesterol is not a risk factor for stroke.[20,21] The fact that nonstatin cholesterol-lowering drugs lack beneficial effects on risk for stroke corroborate this finding. Despite some differences in the existing information about the relationship of lipids and stroke, there is growing evidence that statins reduce the risk for stroke. Some of these effects may be related to its lipid-lowering effect, but there is increasing evidence that cholesterol-independent effects may also be important. This may include an anti-inflammatory effect, an antithrombotic effect, an improvement of endothelial function, an effect on platelets, or even a decrease in myocardial infarction and thus a reduction of a cardiac source of the embolus. Because hypertension is an important and known risk factor for stroke, the blood pressure–lowering effect of statins may also be contributory.[22] Some of these ancillary benefits of statins may explain the statin paradox—that benefit from treatment with statins seems to extend to people aged 65 to 75 despite the fact that cohort studies[23] and Framingham studies[24] strongly suggested that cardiovascular mortality is not related to serum cholesterol concentration in the older age group. Similarly, some observational cohort studies, which included about 500,000 people and 13,500 stroke events, did not suggest that elevated serum cholesterol was a risk factor for stroke.[20,25] There was no clear relationship between plasma cholesterol and total (fatal and nonfatal) stroke. There was, however, a weak positive association between cholesterol concentration and the risk for ischemic stroke and a weak negative association with hemorrhagic stroke.[25-27]

The Physicians' Health Study (PHS), which followed 1986 apparently healthy men for 8 years, found that subjects with the highest levels of C-reactive protein (CRP), a marker of inflammation, were twice as likely as those with the lowest CRP levels to have a stroke.[28] This increased risk was independent of other nonlipid and lipid risk factors. Similarly, a prospective study of 137 patients scheduled for carotid endarterectomy showed that CRP concentrations were significantly higher in the subgroup of 125 patients who had cerebrovascular symptoms than they were in the 12 patients who were asymptomatic.[29] Because statins are known to reduce the levels of CRP, it is possible that some of the benefits seen with statin treatment may be related to its anti-inflammatory effect.

Despite weak evidence of the link between serum total cholesterol level and stroke and TIA, it is becoming increasingly apparent that statins reduce the risk for stroke in certain patients.

Clinical Trial Evidence of the Benefit of Statins in Stroke Reduction

The clinical trials of statin use and data on stroke prevention in major statin trials are summarized in Tables 4-4 and 4-5.

The Heart Protection Study

In the HPS study, a 25% reduction in the incidence of a first stroke was observed with the use of statins.[8] This outcome was a secondary endpoint in the study. The benefit was mainly in the form of a reduction in ischemic stroke; simvastatin treatment did not affect the rate of hemorrhagic stroke. Also, simvastatin use significantly reduced TIA risk by about 17%.

Table 4-4		
Stroke Reduction in Major Statin Trials		
Trial	Reference	Relative Risk Reduction (%)
4S	7	30
WOSCOPS	4	11 (NS)
CARE	33	31
LIPID	12	19
HPS	8	30
ASCOT-LLA	9	27
PROSPER	14	25 for TIA, but no reduction in stroke
GREACE	13	47

4S, Scandinavian Simvastatin Survival Study; ASCOT-LLA, Anglo-Scandinavian Cardiac Outcome Trial-Lipid Lowering Arm; CARE, Cholesterol and Recurrent Events; GREACE, Greek Atorvastatin and Coronary Heart Disease Evaluation study; HPS, Heart Protection Study; LIPID, Long-term Intervention with Pravastatin in Ischemic Disease; PROSPER, Pravastatin in elderly individuals at risk of vascular disease; WOSCOPS, West Of Scotland Coronary Prevention Study.

4

THE MIRACL STUDY

Statin therapy was linked to a significant (51%) reduction in fatal and nonfatal stroke, although wide confidence intervals were noted in a subanalysis of this study.[30] In the Myocardial Ischemia Reduction with Aggressive Cholesterol Lowering (MIRACL) study, 3086 patients with unstable angina or non–Q-wave myocardial infarction and a total cholesterol level of 270 mg/dL (6.9 mmol/L) or lower were randomized to receive atorvastatin, 80 mg daily, or placebo. Treatment was begun 24 to 96 hours after hospital admission and continued for 16 weeks. In the atorvastatin group, LDL cholesterol was reduced by 40% from baseline to a mean of 72 mg/dL. Most strokes were ischemic. The absolute number of cerebrovascular events was small (12 in the atorvastatin group and 24 in the placebo group) and hence should be interpreted with caution.

OTHER TRIALS

Data from three major secondary prevention statin trials (Scandinavian Simvastatin Survival Study [4S], Cholesterol and Recurrent Events [CARE], and Long-term Intervention with Pravastatin in Ischemic Disease [LIPID]) show a 19% to 29% reduction in the incidence of stroke, with no increase in the risk for a hemorrhagic event.[31] This is consistent with the results of the Prospective Pravastatin Pooling (PPP) Project,[32] in which combined CARE and LIPID data revealed a significant (22%) reduction in the incidence of total stroke and a 23% decrease in risk for nonhemorrhagic stroke with pravastatin therapy.[32,33]

Table 4-5

Meta-Analysis of Statin Trials in the Prevention of Stroke

Author (Reference No.)	Year of Publication	Drugs Used	Number of Trials Included	Total Number of Patients	Stroke Reduction	Comments
Hebert et al[34] Crouse et al[35]	1997 1997	Statins Statins	16 12	29,000	29% 27%	Mortality reduced by 22%, CV death by 28% 15% stroke reduction in primary prevention trials and 32% reduction in secondary prevention trials
Bucher et al[36]	1998	Any LLT	28	>100,000	24%	24% reduction is only for the statin-treated group; no stroke reduction in other forms of lipid-lowering treatment
Warshafsky et al[37]	1999	Statins	13	19,921	29%	OR for nonfatal stroke 0.64, and OR for fatal stroke 1.25
Di Mascio et al[38]	2000	Any LLT	41	80,000	23%	23% RRR is only for statin-treated group; 16% RRR for the total group
Byington et al[39]	2001	Pravastatin	3	19,768	22%	Most benefits seen in the secondary prevention group, with 25% reduction in nonfatal and 23% reduction in nonhemorrhagic stroke
Sirol et al[40]	2001	Statins	13	>32,0000	24%	RRR of 25% in the secondary prevention and 15% in the primary prevention studies
Glorioso et al[41]	2003	Any LLT	38	83,161	26%	26% RRR is for statin-treated group only, RRR of 17% for the overall group; stroke reduction more evident when TC lowered to values less than 232 mg/dL

CV, cardiovascular; LLT, lipid-lowering treatment; OR, odds ratio; RRR, relative risk reduction; TC, total cholesterol.

Importantly, the major benefits in stroke reduction have been noted in patients with known CHD or with CHD risk equivalents. An 11% reduction in stroke was observed in WOSCOPS during the 5-year follow-up that did not reach statistical significance.

Evidence from Meta-Analyses

The use of statins for stroke reduction has been the subject of intense debate. There are no published clinical trials that have examined the effects of statin on stroke reduction as the primary endpoint. Most of the information comes from the use of statins in several primary and secondary cardiac event prevention trials in which stroke has been analyzed as a secondary endpoint. On the basis of published data, most of the positive benefit of stroke reduction has been seen in middle-aged patients with a known history of prior CHD. Older adults, who have higher stroke risk, have been excluded from most studies. Results of the meta-analyses are tabulated in Table 4-5.[34-41] There appears to be consistent benefit in terms of stroke risk reduction of about 15% to 29% in different trials. The benefit is more striking in trials of secondary prevention of CHD, and the use of statins appears most impressive compared with other forms of lipid-lowering treatment.

Ongoing Studies

It is important to keep in mind that until the publication of the HPS study, the clinical benefit of statins for stroke prevention in patients without CAD was not proven. The reduction in stroke risk, seen in HPS patients both with and without CHD and even in older adults, suggests that the benefit appears to be uniform across a spectrum of patient populations. The ongoing Stroke Prevention by Aggressive Reduction of Cholesterol Levels (SPARCL) trial has been designed to prospectively evaluate the benefits of aggressive lipid-lowering therapy (atorvastatin, 80 mg daily) on cerebrovascular events in patients who have had a previous stroke or a TIA but who have no prior history of coronary artery disease.[42]

An ongoing trial of primary stroke prevention with statins in older patients is RESPECT; a similar trial, FAME, was discontinued for commercial reasons. The Cholesterol Treatment Trialists Collaboration carried out a meta-analysis of all randomized trials of cholesterol reduction that were of more than 2 years' duration and included more than 1000 people.[43] The first cycle of analyses, when combined with the MRC/BHF-HPS, included data from 57,000 patients and 2200 strokes.

Potential Benefit of Statins in Neuroprotection

Cognitive impairment in older adults, once called senile dementia, is now known to be a heterogeneous condition that in most cases has pathologic features consistent with Alzheimer's disease.[44] Another, less common cause of cognitive impairment is vascular dementia, whose definition and distinction remain ill defined. Mixed dementia has features of both Alzheimer's dementia and vascular dementia. Although a small number of early-onset, dominantly inherited cases of familial Alzheimer's disease are caused by genetic mutations, the cause of most sporadic cases of dementia is presently unknown. There is evidence that even one or two small strokes increase the risk for Alzheimer's disease by 20-fold.[45] Dementia is a heterogeneous disorder and cannot be considered a purely atherosclerotic disease. The use of statins for the prevention of dementia has been prompted by some observations, such as associations of an apolipoprotein allele (apoE=ε4) with Alzheimer's disease, degradation of amyloid precursor protein by cholesterol in cell culture, the abnormal appearance of microvascular endothelial cells in affected brain areas in Alzheimer's disease, and a possible role of LDL receptor-related protein in Alzheimer's disease.[46]

Treatment of hypercholesterolemia and other vascular risk factors may have major implications in the prevention of Alzheimer's disease. For example, sterol metabolism in the brain is an active process, well controlled and regulated by 24-hydroxylase, an enzyme that is uniquely expressed in the brain. In animal models of ischemic stroke, statins have been shown to reduce infarct size, possibly through up-regulation of endothelial nitric oxide synthase (eNOS), thus preserving blood flow to regions exposed to an ischemic insult. Moreover, putative anti-inflammatory and antioxidant properties of statins may confer additional neuroprotection.

Statins inhibit small GTPases Rho and Ras, which require isoprenoids (intermediates of the cholesterol biosynthesis pathway) for activation. Inhibition of Rho attenuates infarct size in a rat model of brain ischemia via the elevation of eNOS expression and suppresses vascular smooth muscle proliferation through up-regulation of cyclin-dependent kinase inhibitor p27kip1.[47]

Several case-control studies have suggested a beneficial effect of statins in reducing the occurrence of Alzheimer's disease and dementia. Wolozin and colleagues described the prevalence of probable Alzheimer's disease in the cohort taking statins to be 65% to 73% lower than in the total patient population or in patients taking other medications typically used in the treatment of hypertension or cardiovascular disease but not statins.[48] In another case-control study, Jick and co-workers described a substantially lowered risk for developing dementia in individuals 50 years or older who were prescribed statins.[46] These findings were independent of the presence or absence of untreated hyperlipidemia or exposure to nonstatin lipid-lowering agents. Although the benefits of statins in reduction of dementia have been shown in other studies as well,[46,48] some recent studies[8] and PROSPER[14] did not report changes in cognitive impairment with the use of simvastatin or pravastatin. Although causative mechanisms cannot be inferred on the basis of these data, these studies suggest an interesting association of statin use and development of dementia.

PERIPHERAL ARTERIAL DISEASE

Evidence of Benefit of Statin Use

Lower extremity peripheral arterial disease (PAD) with claudication and gangrene is one of the significant atherosclerosis-related events with tremendous impact on quality of life. Men and women with lower extremity PAD have impaired functioning compared with those without PAD. Greater PAD severity, as measured by the ankle brachial index (ABI), is associated with more extensive functional impairment. There are limited data on the relationship between statins and PAD outcome. The Scandinavian Simvastatin Survival Study demonstrated that subjects randomized to simvastatin had a 38% reduction in new or worsening claudication compared with subjects randomized to placebo over a median follow-up of 5.4 years ($P = .008$).[49] Mayer and Hromadka have made similar observations in the prolongation of claudication interval with the use of statins in patients with arterial occlusive disease of the lower extremities.[50]

A recent study on statin use and leg functioning in patients with and without lower extremity PAD supports the beneficial role of statins in PAD.[51] This study included 392 men and women with an ABI of less than 0.9, and 249 with an ABI of 0.9 to 1.5. Adjusting for age, sex, ABI, comorbidities, education level, medical insurance status, cholesterol, and other confounders, participants taking statins had better 6-minute walk performance, faster walking velocity, and a higher summary performance score than participants not taking statins. No significant association was found between lower extremity functioning and aspirin, angiotensin-converting enzyme (ACE) inhibitors, vasodilators, or beta blockers. The favorable association between statin use and functioning observed in participants with an ABI between 0.90 and 1.49 may relate to the beneficial influence of statins in subclinical lower extremity atherosclerosis. The superior leg functioning with the use of statin was independent of cholesterol levels, suggesting that non-cholesterol-lowering properties of statins may be important.

Mechanisms of Benefit for PAD

Potential mechanisms of the benefit of statins have been extensively discussed in separate chapters in this book. A large body of literature has established that statins have favorable actions on atherosclerosis and vascular properties in addition to those attributed to cholesterol lowering.[52-59] Statins increase production of nitric oxide in the endothelium, which has local vasodilatory properties in addition to antithrombogenic, antiproliferative, and leukocyte-adhesion inhibiting effects. Other mechanisms by which statins favorably influence atherosclerosis include enhancement of endothelium-dependent relaxation, inhibition of platelet function, and inhibition of endothelin-1, a potent vasoconstrictor and mitogen. Statin-associated reduction of inflammatory cytokines may play a role in improvement of blood flow, regression of atherosclerosis, and improvement of end-organ function.

AORTIC VALVE SCLEROSIS AND AORTIC STENOSIS

Similarity between Atherosclerosis and Aortic Valve Sclerosis and Stenosis

Aortic valvular sclerosis, defined as a thickening and calcification of a trileaflet aortic valve without obstruction to the left ventricular outflow, is a common disease in older adults and frequently leads to calcific aortic valve stenosis, which is the most common reason for aortic valve replacement. Calcific aortic stenosis is usually seen in patients over the age of 65 years, and as the population continues to grow older, the number of patients with aortic stenosis is almost certain to rise. For many years, the progression of calcific aortic stenosis was considered a wear-and-tear phenomenon—a consequence of aging coupled with increased hydrodynamic stresses on the aortic valve. This mechanical stress theory emphasizes that wear and tear of the valve disrupts collagen and leads to calcification. On the other hand, the petrification theory suggests that cell aging and death, with petrification of cellular degradation products, causes dystrophic calcification of valve leaflets.

Some studies have indicated that valve calcification is not a passive process but involves inflammation similar to that seen in atherosclerosis of central and peripheral arteries. Roberts has suggested that aortic cuspal calcium is a form of atherosclerosis.[60] The link between calcific aortic stenosis and atherosclerosis is based on data from both histochemical studies and epidemiologic data. The calcified lesions of arteries and valves both contain lipid and inflammatory cells. Edwards showed that primary changes in calcific aortic valves included an "alteration of valvular collagen with extra-cellular droplets of a neutral fat occurring in bundles," an alteration presumably followed by calcification.[61] There is substantial evidence of a link between lipids and tissue calcification. Histochemical stains reveal an intimate relationship between the calcium-containing mineral of atherosclerotic plaques and cholesterol at the ultrastructural level. Cholesterol is contained in the center of calcified granules of coronary artery atherosclerotic plaques, which suggests that lipids are involved in the precipitation of calcium and mineral crystals.[62] Also, 25-hydroxycholesterol, a product of cholesterol oxidation found in coronary artery atherosclerotic lesions, accelerates in vitro vascular and valvular calcification.[63,64] Thus, the calcified regions of cardiac valves have features generally associated with arterial atherosclerotic plaques, such as inflammatory changes and lipid content. Not only inflammatory cells, such as macrophages and lymphocytes, but also bone cells, such as osteoblasts and osteoclasts, have been found in ossified areas of stenotic calcified valves.[65] As in calcified atherosclerotic lesions, neoangiogenesis has also been identified in calcified valve tissue.

Epidemiologic data suggest a close association between atherosclerosis and aortic stenosis. Not only are both conditions more prevalent with increasing age but both disorders also demonstrate associations with sex, hyperlipidemia, hypertension, diabetes, and smoking. The classic risk factors for atherosclerosis have also been reported to affect the progression of calcific aortic stenosis and have been summarized by Mohler.[66] Despite some studies demonstrating only a weak or absent association between serum cholesterol and calcific aortic stenosis,[67-71] the overwhelming body of evidence seems to suggest a positive association between hyperlipidemia and calcific aortic stenosis.[72-77] In a prospective trial, the presence of aortic sclerosis was associated with an approximately 50% increase in CHD mortality and myocardial infarction, even after correction for age, sex, known CAD, and clinical factors associated with aortic sclerosis.[78]

Evidence for a Benefit of Statins in the Prevention of Aortic Valve Sclerosis and Stenosis

There is no medical treatment for aortic valve calcification. On the basis of (1) evidence that aortic valve calcification is an inflammatory process fueled by atherosclerotic risk factors and (2) the demonstrated benefit of statins in reducing atherosclerotic cardiovascular events, statins are now being investigated to see if they stabilize the lesions of atherosclerotic cardiac valves, retard calcification, and thus prevent the progression of calcific aortic stenosis.

Electron beam computed tomography (EBCT), which has been used to quantify coronary artery calcification, is also a highly reproducible method of quantifying aortic valve calcification. Using EBCT, Pohle and colleagues observed a strong influence of LDL cholesterol level on the progression of aortic valve calcium and coronary calcium accumulation, suggesting that lipid-lowering therapy may decrease the progression of aortic valve calcification.[79] In a retrospective study, Shavelle and co-workers studied the effect of statins on aortic valve calcium.[80] In this retrospective study, they identified 65 patients who had undergone two EBCT scans at a mean interval of 2.5 years; 43% of them were receiving statins. Those who were treated with statins had a 62% to 63% lower median rate of aortic valve calcium accumulation ($P = .006$), and 44% to 49% fewer statin patients had definite aortic valve calcium progression ($P = .043$). Despite this study's several limitations, it suggests that a pharmacologic intervention, such as statin therapy, may favorably alter the natural history of calcific aortic valvular disease.

Aronow and colleagues studied the association of coronary risk factors and the use of statins for progression of mild valvular aortic stenosis in older persons.[72] The data from this study showed that independent significant predictors of the progression of aortic stenosis were male sex, cigarette smoking, systemic hypertension, diabetes mellitus, a serum LDL cholesterol of 125 mg/dL or higher at follow-up, a HDL cholesterol level of 35 mg/dL or lower at follow-up, and the use of statins (inverse association). In this study, the rate of progression of aortic stenosis as noted by an increase in peak systolic pressure gradient across aortic valve was 6.3 mm Hg/year for patients with an initial LDL cholesterol level of 125 mg/dL or greater not treated with statin, versus 3.4 mm Hg/year for patients with an initial LDL cholesterol level of 125 mg/dL or higher treated with statins ($P < .0001$). This was a retrospective analysis of all patients over 60 years of age with mild valvular aortic stenosis (peak systolic gradient across the aortic valve of 10 to 25 mm Hg) who had follow-up Doppler echocardiograms at 2 years or longer to detect progression of aortic stenosis.

Novaro and co-workers studied the effect of statins on the progression of calcific aortic stenosis. In this retrospective study of 174 patients with mild to moderate stenosis, 57 patients (33%) received treatment with statins and the remaining 117 (67%) did not.[81] The statin group was older and had a higher prevalence of hypertension, diabetes mellitus, and CAD. During the mean follow-up of 21 months, patients treated with statin had a smaller increase in peak and mean gradients and a smaller decrease in aortic valve area. When annualized, the decrease in aortic valve area for the nonstatin group was 0.11 ± 0.18 cm^2 compared with 0.06 ± 0.16 cm^2 for those treated with a statin ($P = .03$). In multivariate analysis, statin usage was a significant independent predictor of a smaller decrease in valve area ($P = .01$) and a lesser increase in peak gradient ($P = .02$). In this study, the statin-treated patients, despite a higher risk profile for progression, had reduced aortic stenosis progression compared with those who were not treated with a statin.

The beneficial effect of statins seen in patients with aortic stenosis could be the result of their anti-inflammatory properties. Serum levels of C-reactive protein, a sensitive marker of systemic inflammation, are elevated in patients with established aortic stenosis.[82] Statins have recently been shown to lower the median level of CRP in a prospective, randomized, community-based, double-blind trial.[83]

ATHEROSCLEROSIS-RELATED EVENTS IN DIABETES MELLITUS

Patients with diabetes mellitus are at unusually high risk for CAD-related events, including MI and death.[84,85] In fact, the risk for subsequent myocardial infarction is equal or higher in patients with diabetes mellitus without CHD than in patients with a prior history of myocardial infarction. The risk for a recurrent event is nearly doubled in patients with CHD in the presence of diabetes. National Cholesterol Education Program (NCEP) guidelines thus consider diabetes mellitus a coronary risk equivalent and emphasize the concept of aggressive treatment with an LDL cholesterol goal of lower than 100 mg/dL. Patients with diabetes mellitus have been included in all the major clinical trials discussed earlier, and the benefit of statin treatment in the diabetic subpopulation has been well recognized. In the 4S study, use of simvastatin decreased the incidence of major CHD events (CHD death and nonfatal myocardial infarction) by 55%.[86] Simvastatin also reduced the risk for total mortality and CHD mortality in diabetic patients by 43% and 36%, respectively. Similar data regarding the impact of statins are seen in other trials. The Prospective Pravastatin Pooling Project used data from three major trials (WOSCOPS, CARE, and LIPID).[87] In a subpopulation of 1444 diabetic patients, pravastatin significantly reduced risk for CHD death or nonfatal myocardial infarction by 19% and risk for CHD death, nonfatal myocardial infarction, or revascularization by 26% in the diabetic patients. Most recently, the results of another landmark study, the Heart Protection Study, confirmed the benefit of aggressive lipid-lowering in diabetic patients.[8] In a subpopulation of 5963 diabetics in this study, a 26% reduction in major CHD events was noted. In the subgroup of diabetic patients who also had CHD, a 12% reduction in relative risk for major vascular events was seen among those receiving simvastatin. The incidence of new-onset diabetes was reduced by 30% in patients receiving statins in the WOSCOPS study. This may relate to some ancillary benefits of statins. However, in the HPS study, there was no difference in the development of diabetes.

ATHEROSCLEROSIS-RELATED EVENTS IN CHRONIC RENAL DISEASE

Cardiovascular mortality rates are 10 to 20 times higher in patients with end-stage renal disease (ESRD) than in people without renal disease.[88] This disparity is more marked in younger individuals with ESRD. The role of statins in the primary prevention of atherosclerosis-related events in patients with ESRD needs further emphasis.

Patients with even mild chronic kidney disease are at high risk for cardiovascular events. According to the National Kidney Foundation, all patients with chronic renal disease should be considered in the highest risk group for cardiovascular disease regardless of traditional risk factors.[89,90]

Data from the 1994 National Health and Nutrition Examination Survey (NHANES) showed that an estimated 3% of the U.S.

population had elevated serum creatinine levels,[91] and this rose to 10% to 25% for persons over the age of 69 years.[92] Although renal insufficiency frequently culminates in renal failure, it is more likely that patients with chronic kidney disease will develop CHD and die before they reach dialysis. In the Cardiovascular Health Study, the prevalence of either subclinical or clinical CHD was greater than 48% for patients whose creatinine clearance was lower than 40 mL/min/1.73 m^2.[92] Similarly, in the Women's Ischemia Syndrome Evaluation Study, women with a mildly elevated creatinine (1.2 to 1.9) were 3.2 times more likely to have significant angiographic CAD, after controlling for age, homocysteine, and other risk factors.[93] Patients with a moderately reduced glomerular filtration rate are more likely to develop a future myocardial infarction after controlling for traditional risk factors and angiographic disease.[94] Dyslipidemia is common in patients with chronic kidney disease. Statins are the most effective drugs to lower LDL cholesterol in chronic renal disease and are generally safe. They should be the agents of first choice in chronic renal diseases, but dosage reduction and additional monitoring may be needed. Large randomized clinical trials of statins have excluded patients with established significant renal disease. Hence, the suggestion of potential benefits of statins in this group comes from large epidemiologic data.

Elevated lipid levels are also associated with faster progression of proteinuric renal disease. Data from small trials and results of a meta-analysis suggest that treatment of the hyperlipidemia may slow progression of renal disease.[95] However, the main reason to treat hyperlipidemia remains a high incidence of CHD in chronic renal disease. The National Kidney Foundation has recommended that chronic renal disease be considered a CAD risk equivalent, setting an LDL cholesterol goal of lower than 100 mg/dL (as mentioned earlier for diabetes mellitus).[88] Although the current NCEP ATP III guidelines do not include chronic renal disease as a CAD risk equivalent, the available evidence suggests that treatment with statins in patients with chronic renal disease not only may prevent atherosclerosis-related cardiovascular events, but also may slow the progression of proteinuric kidney disease.

EFFECTS OF STATINS ON RENAL TRANSPLANTATION

Lipid disorders after renal transplantation play a major role in the pathogenesis of atherosclerosis, and chronic renal allograft rejection is circumstantial. The absolute rate of clinical vascular disease and cardiovascular complications in transplant patients, the high prevalence of an atherogenic lipid profile, and the evidence from the large statin regression trials in the general population suggest that lipid-lowering treatment is necessary in most patients undergoing renal transplantation. Furthermore, animal models and observational studies in patients have found correlations between plasma lipid levels and both acute and chronic rejection. Animal transplant models and clinical trials in heart transplant patients also suggest that statin treatment decreases the incidence of chronic rejection in a manner that may also be independent of lipid lowering. Although the mechanisms behind this protective effect remain unclear, statins may be the first agents to be effective in preventing chronic rejection and in reducing the rate of cardiovascular complications in renal transplant recipients.

Trimarchi and colleagues[96] performed a retrospective analysis to assess the immunosuppressive activity of statins in kidney transplantation and to determine their effects on serum cholesterol and triglyceride levels after transplantation, on the incidence of acute rejection episodes, and on renal function. They found that kidney function was significantly better in patients who received statins early after transplantation. The data suggested that statins exerted immunosuppressive effects and reduced the number of acute rejection episodes, and that these agents improved allograft survival and kidney function.

Current evidence suggests that, despite our lack of understanding about the mechanisms of the nephroprotective effect of statins in both native and allograft kidney transplants, the role of statins in this setting is interesting: even if there is no direct atherosclerotic event, possible mediation of the benefits through modulation of lipids is likely.

STATINS IN CONGESTIVE HEART FAILURE AND LEFT VENTRICULAR REMODELING

Congestive heart failure is frequently a result of an atherosclerosis-related event such as myocardial infarction. Recurrent MI, chronic ischemia, and ventricular remodeling add to the progression of heart failure. Hence, statin-induced prevention of atherosclerosis-related events such as MI and hibernating myocardium reduces the incidence of ischemic cardiomyopathy and CHF.

Increased left ventricular mass is common in patients with hypertension and is a powerful predictor of future cardiovascular events. It is interesting that the addition of pravastatin to anti-hypertensive treatment led to a greater reduction in left ventricular mass in patients with hypertension and hyerlipidemia in one study, suggesting an interaction of the renin-angiotensin system and hyperlipidemia.[97] This effect may be related to attenuation of an angiotensin II–mediated increase in left ventricular mass.

Recent studies have in fact shown the potential benefit of statins in ameliorating the angiotensin II–mediated organ damage. The known interaction of statins in attenuating angiotensin II–induced cellular signaling and the involvement of angiotensin II in left ventricular remodeling after myocardial infarction led to the study of the effect of cerivastatin in rats with heart failure after MI by Bauersachs and colleagues.[98] In this study, the authors were able to demonstrate the benefit of cerivastatin in improving left ventricular remodeling and function in rats with heart failure. This effect was associated with an attenuated left ventricular expression of fetal myosin heavy-chain isoenzymes and collagen I, suggesting that statin treatment may retard the progression of heart failure. Similarly, using angiotensin II–dependent models of rats transgenic for human rennin and angiotensinogen, Dechend and co-workers[99] demonstrated the amelioration of angiotensin II–induced cardiac injury by cerivastatin. In this study, the use of statins decreased the angiotensin II–induced hypertension, cardiac hypertrophy, fibrosis, and remodeling independent of cholesterol reduction. Although the clinical significance remains uncertain, the results suggest that statins interfere with angiotensin II–induced signaling and transcription factor activation, thereby reducing end-organ damage, and thus these agents may have a more direct effect on the prevention and progression of CHF in addition to the reduction of myocardial damage by MI. Subset analysis of the Evaluation of Losartan in the Elderly (ELITE II) trial of the Losartan Heart Failure Survival Study also demonstrated that the risk for death was reduced by nearly 40% in patients receiving statins in addition to an ACE inhibitor or angiotensin receptor blocker.[100] Independent clinical indications for the use of statins in CHF, however, have not been made.

INTERACTION OF DYSLIPIDEMIA AND HYPERTENSION

Hypercholesterolemia and hypertension are major risk factors for coronary heart disease, and both are often present in the same patient. It is thought that interactions between dyslipidemia and activation of neurohumoral systems, such as the renin-angiotensin system, may not only explain the frequent coexistence of hypertension and dyslipidemia but may also play an important role in the pathogenesis of atherosclerosis. Experimental data suggest that the effects of angiotensin II and lipoproteins on atherogenic risk are not independent. Accumulating data from recent experimental and clinical studies suggest that the pathways by which angiotensin II and dyslipidemia lead to vascular disease may frequently overlap. Interventions directed at lowering total and LDL cholesterol and triglycerides and raising HDL cholesterol result in a reduction in cardiovascular events. Control of blood pressure similarly results in a decrease in cardiovascular events. Acetylcholinesterase (ACE) inhibitors or angiotensin II type 1 (AT_1) receptor blockers modulate the renin-angiotensin system and are beneficial in reducing cardiovascular events in patients with vascular disease. There is a suggestion that the use of cholesterol-lowering drugs combined with agents that modulate the renin-angiotensin system may have additive benefits in the prevention and treatment of CAD, hypertension, and heart failure.

Using macrophages harvested from the peritoneum after injection of angiotensin II, Keidar and colleagues were able to demonstrate that angiotensin II dramatically increased macrophage cellular cholesterol biosynthesis with no significant effect on blood pressure or on plasma cholesterol levels.[101] The ACE inhibitor fosinopril and the AT_1 receptor blocker losartan decreased cholesterol biosynthesis in response to angiotensin II. Furthermore, in cells that lack the AT_1 receptor angiotensin II did not increase cellular cholesterol synthesis. These observations confirm the role of the AT_1 receptor in angiotensin II–mediated cholesterol synthesis by macrophages.

The angiotensin II–mediated increase in macrophage cholesterol influx has been demonstrated and attributed to the oxidant stress contributing to and facilitating LDL cholesterol oxidation by arterial wall components.[102] Angiotensin II can also bind to LDL and form modified lipoprotein, which is taken up at an enhanced rate by the scavenger receptors of macrophages, leading to cellular cholesterol accumulation.[103] Li and co-workers[104] have studied the kinetics of oxidized LDL cholesterol (ox-LDL) uptake in endothelial cells, and they observed that angiotensin II, in a concentration-dependent fashion, enhanced the uptake of ^{125}I-labeled ox-LDL in these cells. The AT_1 receptor blocker losartan, but not the AT_2 receptor blocker PD 123319, blocked the enhanced uptake of ox-LDL. Fluvastatin, a competitive inhibitor of HMG-CoA reductase, blocks the stimulatory effect of angiotensin II on macrophages.

Increased oxidative stress is now regarded as an important feature of hypercholesterolemic atherosclerosis. LDL cholesterol enhances AT_1 receptor expression in cultured smooth muscle cells,[105] and atherosclerotic lesions are associated with increased ACE expression,[106] which may serve as a source for local production of angiotensin II and ultimately increase stimulation of superoxide anion production.

Experimental studies have shown that dyslipidemia enhances renin-angiotensin system activity. All components of increased renin-angiotensin system activation have been identified in hyperlipidemic atherosclerotic lesions. These include, in particular, increased expression of ACE and the AT_1 receptor.[107,108] A number of recent studies in human atherosclerotic tissues have confirmed the up-regulation of ACE and the AT_1 receptors, particularly in the regions that are prone to plaque rupture.[109] Importantly, these same areas show extensive inflammatory cell deposits, macrophage accumulation, and apoptosis.

In vitro studies have shown that incubation of vascular smooth muscle cells with LDL increases expression of the AT_1 receptors.[110] Li and colleagues examined the expression of angiotensin II receptors in human coronary artery endothelial cells, and they observed that ox-LDL increases the mRNA and protein for AT_1, but not AT_2, receptors, implying that ox-LDL increases AT_1 expression at the transcriptional level.[111] In this process, activation of the redox-sensitive transcription factor nuclear factor kappa B (NF-κB) plays a critical role. In recent studies, investigators showed that ox-LDL also enhances ACE expression in human coronary artery endothelial cells.[112] To define the relationship of the renin-angiotensin system and lipids in humans, Nickenig and co-workers administered angiotensin II to normocholesterolemic and hyper-cholesterolemic men.[113] They found that blood pressure was exaggerated in the hypercholesterolemic group and that this response could be blunted by LDL cholesterol–lowering agents. Furthermore, these investigators found that there was a linear relationship between AT_1 receptor density on platelets and LDL cholesterol concentration in plasma. In addition, treatment with statins decreased AT_1 receptor density. Statin-mediated down-regulation of AT_1 receptor expression has also been noted in vascular smooth muscle cells.[114] One study has indeed shown that statins directly decrease AT_1 receptor expression in endothelial cells.[115]

Activation of the renin-angiotensin system with the formation of angiotensin II and activation of angiotensin II receptors, particularly AT_1 receptors, have been implicated in the pathobiology of atherosclerosis, plaque rupture, and subsequent myocardial ischemic dysfunction and congestive heart failure.[116] Several studies have shown that ACE inhibitors decrease the progression of atherosclerosis in a variety of animal species.[117,118] Because a number of different ACE inhibitors exert similar antiatherosclerotic effects, it can be assumed that this represents a class effect. In concurrence with a slowing of the progression of atherosclerosis, ACE inhibitors decrease markers of inflammation and LDL cholesterol oxidation in the atherosclerotic regions.

Atherosclerosis is inhibited by fosinopril and losartan in animal studies, suggesting that the antiatherosclerotic effects of the renin-angiotensin system inhibitors may be due, at least in part, to direct inhibition of LDL cholesterol oxidation and other actions of angiotensin II in the vessel wall.

The role of angiotensin II in promoting atherosclerotic lesions and aortic aneurysms in apolipoprotein E–deficient mice has been recently examined by Daugherty and colleagues.[119] These investi-gators showed that a 1-month infusion of angiotensin II enhanced the severity of aortic atherosclerotic lesions compared with placebo. Interestingly, there was extensive formation of abdominal aortic aneurysms in apoE-deficient mice infused with angiotensin II. Furthermore, the presence of hyperlipidemia was necessary for the development of aneurysms. These observations suggest that increased plasma concentrations of angiotensin II have profound effects on vascular pathology when combined with hyperlipidemia, and inhibitors of the renin-angiotensin system may have a therapeutic benefit, especially in the hyperlipidemic state.

Endothelial dysfunction in hypercholesterolemic animals has been shown to be improved by ACE inhibitors.[120] Mancini and co-workers showed that treatment of CAD patients with the ACE inhibitor quinapril improved coronary vasomotion.[121] Quinapril had greater efficacy in improving endothelial function in patients with an LDL cholesterol level of higher than 130 mg/dL than in patients with an LDL cholesterol level of lower than 130 mg/dL.

We have recently identified high-affinity lectin-like receptors for ox-LDL (LOX-1) in cultured human coronary artery endothelial cells by the reverse transcriptase–polymerase chain reaction (RT-PCR), Western blot, and radioligand binding.[122] Native LDL does not bind to this receptor. Vascular endothelial cells in vitro[123] and in vivo[124] internalize and degrade ox-LDL through this putative receptor-mediated pathway, which does not seem to involve the classic macrophage scavenger receptor. Recent studies show that the cytokine tumor necrosis factor α (TNF-α)[125] and fluid shear stress[126] markedly up-regulate LOX-1 gene expression. LOX-1 activation is involved in apoptosis (programmed cell death) in response to ox-LDL,[127,128] mitogen-activated protein kinase 1 (MAPK-1) activation, and expression of adhesion molecules and attachment of monocytes to activated endothelial cells.[129] There is a critical role of NF-κB in the effects of ox-LDL on endothelial cells.[130] The proapoptotic effect of angiotensin II in human coronary artery endothelial cells and the role of AT$_1$ receptor and protein kinase C (PKC) activation have also been shown by our group.[131]

Li and colleagues from our laboratory have demonstrated that angiotensin II up-regulates LOX-1 expression as well as the uptake of ox-LDL in human coronary artery endothelial cells via activation of the AT$_1$ receptor.[132] The effects of angiotensin II were blocked by the AT$_1$ receptor blockers losartan and candesartan, but not by the AT$_2$ receptor blocker PD 213319. Angiotensin II and ox-LDL exerted a cumulative cell injurious effect, measured as LDH release and cell viability. Again, AT$_1$ receptor blockers reduced the cumulative injurious effect of angiotensin II and ox-LDL. Importantly, the chain-breaking antioxidant α-tocopherol also attenuated the injurious effects of ox-LDL and angiotensin II, emphasizing the importance of redox-sensitive pathways in the crosstalk between the renin-angiotensin system and dyslipidemia.[133] The crosstalk between ox-LDL and angiotensin II is further evident from the work of Chen and co-workers, who showed intense immunostaining and up-regulation of the gene for LOX-1 in the atherosclerotic tissue of rabbits fed a high-cholesterol diet.[134] Losartan therapy not only reduced atherosclerosis but also blocked the up-regulation of LOX-1. Recent studies from our laboratory show a marked up-regulation of LOX-1 in concert with apoptosis in human atherosclerotic plaques, particularly in the regions that are prone to rupture.

ROLE OF STATINS IN BLOOD PRESSURE CONTROL

The association of hypertension with hyperlipidemia has been noted in several population studies. The prevalence of hypertension is greater in populations with high cholesterol.[135] Dyslipidemia may be another metabolic factor that influences blood pressure. Sung and colleagues examined the blood pressure response to a standard mental arithmetic test in 37 healthy normotensive subjects with hypercholesterolemia and 33 normotensive subjects with normal cholesterol levels.[136] The blood pressure response during the arithmetic test was significantly higher in the hypercholesterolemic group than in the normocholesterolemic group. In a double-blind, crossover-design study, treatment with statins was associated with lower mean systolic blood pressure prior to and during the arithmetic test. These observations suggest that individuals with hypercholesterolemia have exaggerated systolic blood pressure responses to mental stress and the lipid lowering improves systolic blood pressure response to stress. Nazzaro and co-workers made an interesting observation of combined and distinct effects of ACE inhibitors and statins on blood pressure.[137] They examined the effects of lipid lowering on blood pressure in a study of 30 subjects with coexisting hypertension and hypercholesterolemia. The combination of statins and ACE inhibitor achieved greater blood pressure reduction than either alone. These observations suggest a close interplay of the renin-angiotensin system and lipid metabolism, perhaps a crosstalk between dyslipidemia and the renin-angiotensin system relative to vascular dynamics.

Several other small studies have shown that lipid-lowering treatment with statins may have a blood pressure–lowering effect. Some of these important studies are summarized in Table 4-6.

EVIDENCE FOR CLINICAL BENEFIT OF RENIN-ANGIOTENSIN SYSTEM MODULATION AND DYSLIPIDEMIA

As discussed earlier, epidemiologic studies have shown that elevated levels of LDL cholesterol are associated with the onset of hypertension and atherosclerosis.[145] Furthermore, ACE inhibitors have been shown to promote regression and even prevent atherosclerosis, suggesting a link between atherosclerosis and the renin-angiotensin system.[146]

Studies demonstrating benefits from simultaneous modulation of the renin-angiotensin system and dyslipidemia in the clinical setting are summarized in Table 4-7. Indirect evidence for an interaction between dyslipidemia and the renin-angiotensin system comes from some clinical studies such as ELITE[100] and the Lipoprotein and Coronary Atherosclerosis Study (LCAS).[150] Other studies suggest that the renin-angiotensin system may affect

Table 4-6

Evidence for Blood-Pressure-Lowering Effect of Lipid-Lowering Treatment

Author (Reference No.)	Study Outline	Drug Used	Final Outcome
O'Callaghan et al[138]	25 patients with hypertension and hyperlipidemia	Pravastatin vs. placebo for 12 wk	Pravastatin did not lower blood pressure.
Abetel et al[139]	23 patients with hypertension and hyperlipidemia	Fluvastatin 40 mg for 3 mo	Fluvastatin lowered blood pressure by 8-16 mm Hg.
Glorioso et al[140]	25 patients with hypertension and hyperlipidemia	Pravastatin 20-40 mg vs. placebo for 32 wk	Pravastatin decreased systolic blood pressure by 8 mm Hg.
Sposito et al[141]	Patients with hypertension and hyperlipidemia	ACE inhibitor (enalapril or lisinopril) alone or with statin (lovastatin or pravastatin)	Additive blood-pressure-lowering effect of the combination compared to ACE inhibitor alone
Borghi et al[142]	Patients with hypertension and hyperlipidemia	Statins (pravastatin or simvastatin) in addition to antihypertensive treatment	Additive benefit of statins in blood pressure lowering shown
Tonolo et al[143]	26 microalbuminuric hypertensive type 2 diabetic patients	Simvastatin in addition to antihypertensive treatment	Simvastatin exerted additional blood pressure–lowering effect and also reduced 24-hr urinary albumin excretion;
Jonkers et al[144]	17 patients with hypertriglyceridemia and hypertension	Bezafibrate	bezafibrate reduced systolic blood pressure by 5 mm Hg.

ACE, angiotensin-converting enzyme.

Table 4-7

Summary of the Results of Clinical Trials Suggesting Interaction between RAS and Dyslipidemia

Clinical Trials (Reference No.)	Study Objective	Results
TREND[147]	Effects of ACE inhibitor (quinapril) in acetylcholine-induced endothelial response of coronary artery according to LDL cholesterol level	Quinapril 40 mg/day had a greater efficacy in improving endothelial function in the group with LDL cholesterol > 130 mg/dL than in the group with LDL cholesterol < 130 mg/dL.
QUIET[148,149]	Effect of ACE inhibitor (quinapril) on ischemic events and angiographic progression of coronary disease assessed in patients who underwent percutaneous intervention	Overall effect on the primary ischemic and angiographic endpoints was neutral. However, patients with LDL cholesterol > 130 mg/dL had significantly less progression of disease compared to patients with LDL cholesterol < 130 mg/dL.
LCAS[150]	Effect of statin (fluvastatin) on minimal luminal diameter assessed by quantitative coronary angiography according to ACE genotype. LDL reduction according to ACE genotype was analyzed.	There was a significant difference in the reduction of LDL cholesterol according to ACE genotype. Subjects with DD, ID, or II genotype achieved reductions of 31%, 25%, and 21%, respectively.
ELITE II[100]	Effect of captopril and losartan on cardiac events in older adult patients with CHF	Both captopril and losartan decreased crude mortality similarly. However, patients who were on statins had an additional ~50% reduction in mortality.

ACE, angiotensin-converting enzyme; ELITE, Evaluation of Losartan in the Elderly; LCAS, Lipid and Coronary Atherosclerosis Study; QUIET, Quinapril Ischemic Event Trial; RAS, renin-angiotensin system; TREND, Trial on Reversing Endothelial Dysfunction.

4

responses to lipid-lowering agents. Observations from unpublished data and from studies such as the ELITE trial do support the hypothesis that combination treatment with ACE inhibitors and statins may have incremental benefits in reducing mortality.

Data from preclinical studies suggest that the renin-angiotensin system may be up-regulated by abnormal lipids, most likely via production of ox-LDL. On the other hand, activation of the renin-angiotensin system leads to the release of reactive oxygen species and transcriptional up-regulation of LDL cholesterol and ox-LDL uptake in macrophages, smooth muscle cells, and endothelial cells. These findings extend our understanding of the interplay among risk factors to synergistically increase cardiovascular risk and of the antiatherosclerotic effects of local ACE inhibition to reduce cardiovascular risk. Trials aimed at modifying the renin-angiotensin system, along with drugs that lower total and LDL cholesterol and inhibitors of oxidative modification of LDL cholesterol, will address the clinical relevance of this biologic interaction.

COST-EFFECTIVENESS AND SAFETY

The cost-effectiveness of pravastatin therapy, based on the WOSCOPS trial, was analyzed for various countries. Over a broad range of inputs, cost-effectiveness ratios were below $25,000 per life-years gained, regardless of the country; cost-effectiveness was better in groups with higher baseline risk.[151]

In the AFCAPS/TexCAPS trial, the cost of lovastatin treatment was $4654 per patient.[152] However, over the duration of the study, lovastatin decreased the frequency of cardiovascular hospitalization by 28% and cardiovascular diagnostic and therapeutic procedures (angioplasty and bypass surgery) by 23% and 32%, respectively. The net effect was that cardiovascular health care costs were reduced by 27% with lovastatin compared with placebo, offsetting the cost of the drug by $524 per patient. A cost-effectiveness study for primary prevention of CHD found that treatment with lovastatin at a dose of 20 mg/day was cost-effective for middle-aged men and women, with baseline total cholesterol levels of 258 mg/dL (6.67 mmol/L) or higher.[153] Higher doses (above 20 mg/day with lovastatin) appeared to be progressively less cost-effective unless the serum cholesterol was above 300 mg/dL (7.8 mmol/L), probably because of a progressively smaller increase in effect.

IMPACT OF NCEP GUIDELINES (ATP III) IN THE USE OF LIPID-LOWERING AGENTS

The Third Report of the Expert Panel on Detection, Evaluation and Treatment of High Blood Cholesterol in Adults (ATP III) has summarized the current recommendations for the management of high serum cholesterol.[154] These guidelines are based on epidemiologic observations that showed a graded relationship between the total cholesterol concentration and coronary risk and the evidence for benefit in treating hyperlipidemia. These updated clinical guidelines for cholesterol testing and management are based on clinical trial data and other evidence that have become available since the previous guidelines were published in 1993. They are influenced by the absence (primary prevention) or presence (secondary prevention) of preexisting CHD.[4] A meta-analysis of 38 primary and secondary prevention trials found that for every 10% reduction in serum cholesterol, CHD mortality was reduced by 15% and total mortality risk by 11%.[31] No increase in non-CHD mortality was seen.

Emphasis on Multiple Risk Factors

ATP III has focused on multiple risk factors in primary prevention. Whereas the category of highest risk in ATP II was limited to patients with known CHD or other manifestations of atherosclerotic disease, the new guidelines recognize CHD risk equivalents that raise the risk for a CHD event in patients without known CHD to that of patients who have established CHD. Diabetes mellitus is a CHD risk equivalent, and patients with diabetes mellitus, most of whom have multiple risk factors, should be treated as aggressively as patients with known CHD. This change is based on the fundamental concept that the intensity of therapy should be matched to the risk for CHD. Because epidemiologic studies have shown that adults with diabetes have the same risk for CHD as patients who have already had a CHD event, it is logical that diabetics be treated just as intensively as patients with CHD.

Among patients with multiple (two or more) risk factors, the intensity of treatment should be directed by the Framingham estimate of absolute risk for a CHD event in the next 10 years. The presence of multiple risk factors conferring a 10-year CHD risk of greater than 20% is a CHD risk equivalent, and these patients should be treated as aggressively as patients with known CHD. Patients whose 10-year CHD risk is 10% to 20% are identified for intensive treatment, with drug therapy considered for patients with an LDL cholesterol level higher than 130 mg/dL, whereas the drug initiation cut-point remains over 160 mg/dL in patients with a 10-year risk of lower than 10%. ATP III recognizes as a secondary target of therapy the *metabolic syndrome*, a constellation of risk factors that include abdominal obesity, atherogenic dyslipidemia (elevated triglyceride level, small LDL cholesterol particles, low HDL cholesterol, elevated blood pressure, insulin resistance (with or without glucose intolerance), and a prothrombotic and proinflammatory state. Intensified therapeutic lifestyle changes should be initiated, including weight reduction and increased physical activity, with the combined objective of reducing underlying causes of the metabolic syndrome and treating lipid and nonlipid risk factors associated with the metabolic syndrome.

LIMITATIONS OF APPLYING CONTROLLED TRIALS TO CLINICAL PRACTICE

Although lipid-lowering therapy is effective for primary prevention, it is uncertain if the results of these trials can be applied to a general population. Several types of patients were not included, such as those with desirable total cholesterol but low HDL cholesterol levels, average total cholesterol and average or high HDL cholesterol levels, and those with hypertriglyceridemia as the major dyslipidemia. In a report from the Framingham Heart Study, as many as 40% of men and 80% of women had lipid profiles that have not been studied in these large trials; importantly, 25% of men and 66% of women who developed CHD during follow-up would not have been eligible for these trials, primarily because of isolated hypertriglyceridemia.[155]

An important question that must be addressed is the applicability of these observations to the primary care setting. On the basis of the data from most clinical trials, it is becoming clear that there is a 25% to 35% relative risk reduction in major coronary events in both primary and secondary prevention trials. Thus, patients at highest risk for coronary events are likely to derive more benefit in absolute terms. The benefit seen in WOSCOPS and the AFCAPS/TexCAPS study translated to an absolute reduction of only 2% to 3%. Currently, we have no way of predicting who these two to three patients out of 100 are who will derive the benefit. The other 97 to 98 out of 100 will not derive major benefits. Not knowing which patients are likely to benefit, our current recommendation is to treat everyone at risk. Identification of those patients likely to have future events may change the way we treat patients in the future. Several new developments, including genomic studies, may eventually be helpful.

Despite recognition of atherosclerosis as a disease that starts early, we have no scientific data to suggest how soon in life treatment should be started. Should young patients (younger than 20 years of age) be tested routinely and those at high risk be treated early? Will the benefit of treatment outweigh potential risks of treatment for a prolonged period of time? Most of our current primary prevention strategies are directed at individuals who already bear the burden of subclinical atherosclerotic disease, and our aim is to reduce the adverse events. In principle, it would be prudent to prevent the atherosclerotic disease in the early stage rather than to reduce secondary events alone.

As outlined earlier, many clinical studies have not included patients who are at high risk for coronary events. For example, management of patients with low HDL cholesterol but normal total and LDL cholesterol remain enigmatic. Should we further reduce LDL cholesterol anyway, particularly when we do not have an effective way of treating low HDL cholesterol? Development of drugs that target an increasing HDL cholesterol may help address some of these issues.

Racial and ethnic differences in treatment benefits may exist. The goals and intensity of treatment may vary for people of different ethnic and racial origins. For now we have generalized data available from clinical studies, which have mostly included white populations. Similarly, the risk for adverse events may also differ by race.

Cost-effectiveness of treatment remains a primary concern, particularly when we identify nearly 35 million Americans needing pharmacologic intervention. Because the overall event rate is relatively low in low-risk patients, the absolute benefit will be very limited despite an impressive relative risk reduction of about 35%. In a low-risk patient population, the cost of reducing one event may exceed $125,000, whereas the cost may be around $25,000 in a high-risk patient population. The cost of saving one life may indeed exceed $1,000,000 in a very-low-risk patient population. Such cost containment issues will need to be addressed by society. Thus, further risk stratification may help avoid treating some patients unnecessarily. Technologies such as high-sensitivity C-reactive protein, electron beam computed tomography (to find the coronary calcium score), and genomic studies may evolve in the future to redefine our treatment strategy.

Above all, emphasis on therapeutic lifestyle changes (e.g., in dietary habits) will need to be emphasized to the most vulnerable, the adolescents, and the patients of tomorrow. Evidence from prospective cross-cultural, cohort, and interventional studies in the prevention of CHD by diet and lifestyle changes have been reviewed in the literature.

CONCLUSIONS

Significant advances have been made in the recognition and treatment of atherosclerotic risk factors. Therapeutic lifestyle changes should continue to play a central role in the prevention and treatment of this disorder. Availability of statins has led to a significant improvement in the treatment of hyperlipidemia. Many controlled clinical trials have helped to establish guidelines for evidence-based medicine. Several limitations remain, particularly in identifying those patients who will specifically benefit with statin treatment. Until more is known, we will continue to treat all patients who are at risk for adverse coronary events.

References

1. Stamler J, Wentworth D, Neaton JD: Is the relationship between serum cholesterol and risk of premature death from coronary heart disease continuous and graded? Findings in 356,222 primary screenees of the Multiple Risk Factor Intervention Trial (MRFIT). JAMA 256:2823-2828, 1986.
2. The Expert Panel: Second Report of the Expert Panel on Detection,

Evaluation, and Treatment of High Blood Cholesterol in Adults. JAMA 269(23):3015-3023, 1993.

3. Muldoon MF, Manuck SB, Mendelsohn AB, et al: Cholesterol reduction and non-illness mortality: Meta-analysis of randomized clinical trials. BMJ 322:11-15, 2001.

4. Shepherd J, Cobbe SM, Ford I, et al: Prevention of coronary heart disease with pravastatin in men with hypercholesterolemia. N Engl J Med 333:1301-1307, 1995.

5. West of Scotland Coronary Prevention Study Group: Baseline risk factors and their association with outcome in the West of Scotland Coronary Prevention Study. Am J Cardiol 79:756-762, 1997.

6. Downs JR, Clearfield M, Weis S, et al, for the AFCAPS/TexCAPS Research Group: Primary prevention of acute coronary events with lovastatin in men and women with average cholesterol levels: Results of AFCAPS/TexCAPS. JAMA 279:1615-1622, 1998.

7. Randomised trial of cholesterol lowering in 4444 patients with coronary heart disease: The Scandinavian Simvastatin Survival Study (4S). Lancet 344:1383-1389, 1994.

8. Heart Protection Study Collaborative Group: MRC/BHF Heart Protection Study of cholesterol lowering with simvastatin in 20536 high-risk individuals: A randomized controlled trial. Lancet 360:1623-1630, 2002.

9. ASCOT-LLA: Prevention of coronary and stroke events with atorvastatin in hypertensive patients who have average or lower-than-average cholesterol concentrations, in the Anglo-Scandinavian Cardiac Outcome Trial—Lipid Lowering Arm (ASCOT-LLA): A multicentre randomized controlled trial. Lancet 361:1149-1158, 2003.

10. The ALLHAT Officers and Coordinators for the ALLHAT Collaborative Research Group: Major outcomes in moderately hypercholesterolemic, hypertensive patients randomized to pravastatin vs usual care. JAMA 288:2998-3007, 2002.

11. The Cholesterol and Recurrent Events Trial Investigators: The effect of pravastatin on coronary events after myocardial infarction in patients with average cholesterols. N Engl J Med 335:1001-1009, 1996.

12. The Long-term Intervention with Pravastatin in Ischaemic Disease (LIPID) Study Group: Prevention of cardiovascular events and death with pravastatin in patients with coronary heart disease and a broad range of initial cholesterol levels. N Engl J Med 339:1349-1357, 1998.

13. Athyros VG, Papageorgiou AA, Mercouris BR, et al: Treatment with atorvastatin to the National Cholesterol Education Program goal versus 'usual' care in secondary coronary heart disease prevention. The GREek Atorvastatin and Coronary-heart-disease Evaluation (GREACE) study. Curr Med Res Opin 18:220-228, 2002.

14. PROSPER Study Group: Pravastatin in elderly individuals at risk of vascular disease (PROSPER): A randomized controlled trial. Lancet 360:1623-1630, 2002.

15. LaRosa JC, He J, Vupputuri S: Effect of statins on risk of coronary disease: A meta-analysis of randomized controlled trials. JAMA 282:2340-2346, 1999.

16. Lemaitre RN, Psary BM, Heckbert SR, et al: Therapy with hydroxymethylglutaryl coenzyme A reductase inhibitors (statins) and associated risk of incident cardiovascular event in older adults: Evidence from the Cardiovascular Health Study. Arch Intern Med 162:1395-1400, 2002.

4

17. Hachinski V, Graffagnino C, Beaudry M, et al: Lipids and stroke: A paradox resolved. Arch Neurol 53:303-308, 1996.
18. Koren-Morag N, Tanne D, et al: Low- and high-density lipoprotein cholesterol and ischemic cerebrovascular disease: The bezafibrate infarction prevention registry. Arch Intern Med 162:993-999, 2002.
19. Horenstein RB, Smith DE, Mosca L: Cholesterol predicts stroke mortality in the Women's Pooling Project. Stroke 33:1863-1868, 2002.
20. Prospective Studies Collaboration: Cholesterol, diastolic blood pressure, and stroke: 13000 strokes in 450000 people in 45 prospective cohorts. Lancet 346:1647-1652, 1995.
21. Marmot MJ, Poulter NR: Primary prevention of stroke. Lancet 344:344-347, 1992.
22. Goode GK, Miller JP, Heagery AM: Hyperlipidemia, hypertension, and coronary heart disease. Lancet 345:362-364, 1995.
23. Krumholz HM, Seeman TE, Merrill SS, et al: Lack of association between cholesterol and coronary heart disease mortality and morbidity and all-cause mortality in persons older than 70 years. JAMA 272:1335-1340, 1994.
24. Anderson KM, Castelli WP, Levy D: Cholesterol and mortality: 30 years of follow-up from the Framingham Study. JAMA 257:2176-2180, 1987.
25. Eastern Stroke and Coronary Heart Disease Collaborative Research Group: Blood pressure, cholesterol and stroke in Eastern Asia. Lancet 352:1801-1807, 1998.
26. Law MR, Thomson SG, Wald NJ: Assessing possible hazards of reducing serum cholesterol. BMJ 308:373-379, 1994.
27. Iso H, Jacobs DR, Wentworth D, et al: Serum cholesterol levels and six-year mortality from stroke in 350977 men screened for the multiple risk factor intervention trial. N Engl J Med 320:904-910, 1989.
28. Ridker PM, Cushman M, Stampfer MJ, et al: Inflammation, aspirin, and the risk of cardiovascular disease in apparently healthy men. N Engl J Med 336:973-979, 1997.
29. Rerkasem K, Shearman CP, Williams JA, et al: C-reactive protein is elevated in symptomatic compared with asymptomatic patients with carotid artery disease. Eur J Vasc Endovasc Surg 23:505-509, 2002.
30. MIRACL, Waters DD, Schwartz GG, et al: Effects of atorvastatin on stroke in patients with unstable angina or non-Q-wave myocardial infarction: A Myocardial Ischemia Reduction with Aggressive Cholesterol Lowering (MIRACL) substudy. Circulation 106:1690-1695, 2002.
31. Gotto AM Jr, Farmer JA: Reducing the risk for stroke in patients with myocardial infarction: A Myocardial Ischemia Reduction with Aggressive Cholesterol Lowering (MIRACL) substudy. Circulation 106:1595-1598, 2002.
32. Pfeffer MA, Keech A, Sacks FM, et al: Safety and tolerability of pravastatin in long-term clinical trials: Prospective Pravastatin Pooling (PPP) Project. Circulation 105:2341-2346, 2002.
33. Plehn JF, Davis BR, Sacks FM, et al: Reduction of stroke incidence after myocardial infarction with pravastatin: The cholesterol and Recurrent Events (CARE) study. The Care Investigators. Circulation 99:216-223, 1999.
34. Hebert PR, Gaziano JM, Chan KS, Hennekens CH: Cholesterol lowering with statin drugs, risk of stroke, and total mortality: An overview of randomized trials. JAMA 278:313-321, 1997.

4

35. Crouse JR 3rd, Byington RP, Hoen HM, Furberg CD: Reductase inhibitor monotherapy and stroke prevention. Arch Intern Med 157:1305-1310, 1997.
36. Bucher HC, Griffith LE, Guyatt GH: Effect of HMGcoA reductase inhibitors on stroke. A meta-analysis of randomized trials. Ann Intern Med 128:89-95, 1998.
37. Warshafsky S, Packard D, Marks SJ, et al: Efficacy of 3-hydroxy-3-methylglutaryl coenzyme A reductase inhibitors for prevention of stroke. J Gen Intern Med 14:763-774, 1999.
38. Di Mascio R, Marchioli R, Tognoni G: Cholesterol reduction and stroke occurrence: An overview of randomized clinical trials. Cerebrovasc Dis 10:85-92, 2000.
39. Byington RP, Davis BR, Plehn JF, et al: Reduction of stroke events with pravastatin: The Prospective Pravastatin Pooling (PPP) Project. Circulation 103:387-392, 2001.
40. Sirol M, Bouzamondo A, Sanchez P, et al: Does statin therapy reduce the risk of stroke? A meta-analysis. Ann Med Interne (Paris) 152:188-193, 2001.
41. Corvol JC, Bouzamondo A, Sirol M, et al: Differential effects of lipid-lowering therapies on stroke prevention: A meta-analysis of randomized trials. Arch Intern Med 163:669-676, 2003.
42. Callahan A: Cerebrovascular disease and statins: A potential addition to the therapeutic armamentarium for stroke prevention. Am J Cardiol 88:33J-37J, 2001.
43. Cholesterol Treatment Trialists (CTT) Collaboration: Protocol for a prospective collaborative overview of all current and planned randomized trials of cholesterol treatment regimens. Am J Cardiol 75:1130-1134, 1995.
44. Brayne C, Gill C, Huppert FA, et al: Incidence of clinically diagnosed subtypes of dementia in an elderly population: Cambridge Project for Later Life. Br J Psychiatr 167:255-262, 1995.
45. Snowdon DA, Grenier LH, Mortimer JA, et al: Brain infarction and the clinical expression of Alzheimer disease: The Nun Study. JAMA 277:813-817, 1997.
46. Jick H, Zornberg GL, Jick SS, et al: Statins and the risk of dementia. Lancet 356:1627-1631, 2000.
47. Sawada N, Itoh H, Nakao K: Novel actions of HMG-CoA reductase inhibitors (statins): Vascular and cerebral protection through inhibition of small GTPase Rho. Nippon Rinsho 59:2470-2475, 2001.
48. Wolozin B, Kellman W, Ruosseau P, et al: Decreased prevalence of Alzheimer disease associated with 3-hydroxy-3-methylglutaryl coenzyme A reductase inhibitors. Arch Neurol 57:1439-1443, 2000.
49. Pederson TR, Kjekshus J, Pyorala K, et al: Effect of simvastatin on ischemic signs and symptoms in the Scandinavian Simvastatin Survival Study (4S). Am J Cardiol 81:333-335, 1998.
50. Mayer O, Hromadka M: Statins in the treatment of patients with arterial occlusive disease of the lower extremities. Vnitr Lek 47:664-669, 2001.
51. McDermott MM, Guralnik JM, Greeland P, et al: Statin use and leg functioning in patients with and without lower-extremity peripheral arterial disease. Circulation 107:757-761, 2003.
52. Takemoto M, Liao JK: Pleiotropic effects of 3-hydroxy-3-methylglutaryl coenzyme A reductase inhibitors. Arterioscler Thromb Vasc Biol 11:1712-1719, 2001.

53. Van Haelst PL, vanDoormaal JJ, May JF, et al: Secondary prevention with fluvastatin decreases levels of adhesion molecules, neopterin and C-reactive protein. Eur J Intern Med 12:503-509, 2001.
54. Rikitake Y, Kawashima S, Takeshita S, et al: Anti-oxidative properties of fluvastatin, an HMG-CoA reductase inhibitor, contribute to prevention of atherosclerosis in cholesterol-fed rabbits. Atherosclerosis 154:87-96, 2001.
55. Hernandez-Perera O, Perez-Sala D, Navarro-Antolin J, et al: Effects of the 3-hydroxy-3-methylglutaryl-CoA reductase inhibitors, atorvastatin and simvastatin, on the expression of endothelin-1 and endothelial nitric oxide synthase in vascular endothelial cells. J Clin Invest 101:2711-2719, 1998.
56. Huhle G, Abletshauser C, Mayer N, et al: Reduction of platelet activity markers in type II hypercholesterolemic patients by a HMG-CoA reductase inhibitor. Thromb Res 95:229-234, 1999.
57. Pekkanen J, Linn S, Heiss G, et al: Ten-year mortality from cardiovascular disease in relation to cholesterol level among men with and without preexisting cardiovascular disease. N Engl J Med 322:1700-1707, 1990.
58. Kurowska EM: Nitric oxide therapies in vascular diseases. Curr Pharm Des 8:155-166, 2002.
59. Stamler JS, Loh E, Reddy MA, et al: Nitric oxide regulates basal systemic and pulmonary vascular resistance in healthy humans. Circulation 91:1314-1319, 1994.
60. Roberts WC: The senile cardiac calcification syndrome. Am J Cardiol 58:572-574, 1986.
61. Edwards JE: On the etiology of calcific aortic stenosis. Circulation 26:17-18, 1962.
62. Sarig S, Weiss TA, Katz, et al: Detection of cholesterol associated with calcium mineral using confocal fluorescence microscopy. Lab Invest 71:782-787, 1994.
63. Watson KE, Bostrom K, Ravindranath R, et al: TGF-b-1 and 25-hydroxycholesterol stimulate osteoblast-like vascular cells to calcify. J Clin Invest 93:2106-2113, 1994.
64. Mohler ER, Chawla MK, Chang AW, et al: Identification and characterization of calcifying valve cells from human and canine aortic valves. J Heart Valve Dis 8:254-260, 1999.
65. Mohler ER, Gannon FH, Reynolds C, et al: Bone formation and osteoblast remodeling in calcified cardiac valves: A clinical and pathologic analysis [abstract]. J Am Coll Cardiol 31:503A, 1998.
66. Mohler ER III: Are atherosclerotic processes involved in aortic-valve calcification? Lancet 356:524-525, 2000.
67. Mohler ER, Sheridan MJ, Nichols R, et al: Development and progression of aortic valve stenosis: Atherosclerosis risk factors: A causal relationship? A clinical morphologic study. Clin Cardiol 14:995-999, 1991.
68. Peter M, Hoffman A, Parker C, et al: Progression of aortic stenosis: Role of age and concomitant coronary artery disease. Chest 103:1715-1719, 1993.
69. Bahler RC, Desser DR, Finkelhor RS, et al: Factors leading to progression of valvular aortic stenosis. Am J Cardiol 84:1044-1048, 1999.
70. Rosenhek R, Binder T, Porenta G, et al: Predictors of outcome in severe, asymptomatic aortic stenosis. N Engl J Med 343:611-617, 2000.

71. Hoagland PM, Cook EF, Flatley M, et al: Case-control analysis of risk factors for presence of aortic stenosis in adults. Am J Cardiol 55:744-747, 1985.
72. Aronow WS, Ahn C, Kronzon I, et al: Association of coronary risk factors and use of statins with progression of mild valvular aortic stenosis in older persons. Am J Cardiol 88:693-695, 2001.
73. Stewart BF, Siscovick D, Lind BK, et al: Clinical factors associated with calcific aortic valve disease. J Am Coll Cardiol 29:630-634, 1997.
74. Wilmhurst PT, Stevenson RN, Griffiths H, et al: A case-control investigation of the relation between hyperlipidemia and calcific aortic valve stenosis. Heart 78:475-479, 1997.
75. Boon A, Cheriex E, Lodder J, Kessells F: Cardiac valve calcification: Characteristics of patients with calcification of the mitral annuls or aortic valve. Heart 78:472-474, 1997.
76. Palta S, Pai AM, Gill KS: New insights into the progression of aortic stenosis: implications for secondary prevention. Circulation 101:2497-2502, 2000.
77. Nassimiha D, Aronow WS, Ahn C, et al: Association of risk factors with progression of valvular aortic stenosis in older persons. Am J Cardiol 87:1313-1314, 2001.
78. Otto CM, Lind BK, Kitzman DW, et al: Association of aortic-valve sclerosis with cardiovascular mortality and morbidity in the elderly. N Engl J Med 341:142-147, 1999.
79. Pohle K, Maffert R, Ropers D, et al: Progression of aortic valve calcification: Association with coronary atherosclerosis and cardiovascular risk factors. Circulation 104:1927-1932, 2001.
80. Shavelle DM, Takasu J, Budoff M, et al: HMG CoA reductase inhibitor (statin) and aortic valve calcium. Lancet 359:1125-1126, 2002.
81. Novaro GM, Tiong IY, Pearce GL, et al: Effect of hydroxymethylglutaryl coenzyme A reductase inhibitors on the progression of calcific aortic stenosis. Circulation 104:2205-2209, 2001.
82. Galante A, Pietroiusti A, Vellini M, et al: C-reactive protein is increased in patients with degenerative aortic valvular stenosis. J Am Coll Cardiol 38:1078-1082, 2001.
83. Albert MA, Danielson E, Rifai N, et al, for the PRINCE investigators: Effect of statin therapy on C-reactive protein levels. JAMA 286:64-70, 2001.
84. Krolewski AS, Warran JH, Valsani P, et al: Evolving natural history of coronary artery disease in diabetes mellitus. Am J Med 90:56-61S, 1991.
85. Stamler J, Vaccaro O, Neaton JD, et al: Diabetes, other risk factors, and 12-yr cardiovascular mortality for men screened in the multiple risk factor intervention trial. Diabetes Care 16:434-444, 1993.
86. Pyorala K, Pederson TR, Kjekshus J, et al: Cholesterol lowering with simvastatin improves prognosis of diabetic patients with coronary heart disease: A subgroup analysis of the Scandinavian Simvastatin Survival Study (4S). Diabetes Care 20:614-620, 1997.
87. Sacks FM, Tonkin AM, Shepherd J, et al: Effect of pravastatin on coronary disease events in subgroups defined by coronary risk factors: The Prospective Pravastatin Pooling Project. Circulation 102:1893-1900, 2000.
88. Levey AS, Beto JA, Coronado BE, et al: Controlling the epidemic of cardiovascular disease in chronic renal disease: What do we know? What do we need to learn? Where do we go from here? Am J Kidney Dis 32:853-906, 1998.

4

89. Sarnak MJ, Levey AS: Cardiovascular disease and chronic renal disease: A new paradigm. Am J Kidney Dis 35:S117-S131, 2000.
90. Kasiske BL: Hyperlipidemia in patients with chronic renal disease. Am J kidney Dis 32:S142-S156, 1998.
91. Coresh J, Wei L, McQuillan G, et al: Prevalence of high blood pressure and elevated serum creatinine level in the United States: Findings from the Third National Health and Nutrition Examination Survey (1988-1994). Arch Intern Med 161:1207-1216, 2001.
92. Culleton BF, Larson MG, Evans JC, et al: Prevalence and correlates of elevated serum creatinine levels: The Framingham Heart Study. Arch Intern Med 159:1785-1790, 1999.
93. Reis SE, Olson MB, Fried L, et al: Mild renal insufficiency is associated with angiographic coronary artery disease in women. Circulation 105:2826-2829, 2002.
94. Beddhu S, Allen-Brady K, Cheung AK, et al: Impact of renal failure on the risk of myocardial infarction and death. Kidney Int 62:1776-1783, 2002.
95. Fried LF, Orchard TJ, Kasiske BL: The effect of lipid reduction on renal disease progression: A meta-analysis. Kidney Int 59:260-269, 2001.
96. Trimarchi HM, Brennan S, Gonzalez JM, et al: Effects of statins in kidney transplantation. Medicina (B Aires). 60:457-465, 2000.
97. Su SF, Hsiao CL, Chu CW, et al: Effects of pravastatin on left ventricular mass in patients with hyperlipidemia and essential hypertension. Am J Cardiol 86:514-518, 2000.
98. Bauersachs J, Galuppo P, Fraccarollo D, Christ M: Improvement of left ventricular remodeling and function by hydroxymethylglutaryl coenzyme a reductase inhibition with cerivastatin in rats with heart failure after myocardial infarction. Circulation 104:982-985, 2001.
99. Dechend R, Fiebeler A, Park JK, et al: Amelioration of angiotensin II-induced cardiac injury by a 3-hydroxy-3-methylglutaryl coenzyme A reductase inhibitor. Circulation 104:576-581, 2001.
100. Pitt B, Poole-Wilson PA, Segal R, et al: Effect of losartan compared with captopril on mortality in patients with symptomatic heart failure: Randomized trial—the Losartan Heart Failure Survival Study ELITE II. Lancet 355:1582-1587, 2000.
101. Keidar S, Attias J, Heinrich R, et al: Angiotensin II atherogenicity in apolipoprotein E deficient mice is associated with increased cellular biosynthesis. Atherosclerosis 146:249-257, 1999.
102. Keidar S: Angiotensin, LDL peroxidation and atherosclerosis. Life Sci 63:1-11, 1998.
103. Keidar S, Kaplan M, Aviram M: Angiotensin II-modified LDL is taken up by macrophages via the scavenger receptor, leading to cellular cholesterol accumulation. Arterioscler Thromb Vasc Biol 16:97-105, 1996.
104. Li DY, Zhang YC, Philips MI, et al: Upregulation of endothelial receptor for oxidized low-density lipoprotein (LOX-1) in cultured human coronary artery endothelial cells by angiotensin II type 1 receptor activation. Circ Res 84:1043-1049, 1999.
105. Nickenig G, Sachinidis A, Michaelsen F, et al: Upregulation of vascular angiotensin II receptor gene expression by low-density lipoprotein in vascular smooth muscle cells. Circulation 95:473-478, 1997.
106. Diet F, Prat RE, Berry GH, et al: Increased accumulation of tissue ACE in human atherosclerotic coronary artery disease. Circulation 94:2756-2767, 1996.

4

107. Mitanchi H, Bandoh T, Kumura M, et al: Increased activity of vascular ACE related to atherosclerosis lesions in hyperlipidemic rabbits. Am J Physiol 271:H1065-H1071, 1996.
108. Yang BC, Phillips MI, Mohuczy D, et al: Increased angiotensin II type 1 receptor expression in hypercholesterolemic atherosclerosis in rabbits. Arterioscler Thromb Vasc Biol 18:1433-1439, 1998.
109. Schieffer B, Schieffer E, Hilfiker-Kleiner D, et al: Expression of angiotensin II and interleukin 6 in human coronary atherosclerotic plaques: Potential implications for inflammation and plaque instability. Circulation 101:1372-1378, 2000.
110. Nickenig G, Sachinidis A, Seewald S, et al: Influence of oxidized low-density lipoprotein on vascular angiotensin II receptor expression. J Hypertens 15:S27-S30, 1997.
111. Li D, Saldeen T, Romeo F, Mehta JL: Oxidized LDL upregulates angiotensin II type 1 receptor expression in cultured human coronary artery endothelial cells: The potential role of transcription factor NF-kappa B. Circulation 102:1970-1976, 2000.
112. Li D, Singh RM, Liu, et al: Oxidized-LDL through LOX-1 increases the expression of angiotensin converting enzyme in human coronary artery endothelial cells. Cardiovasc Res 57:238-243, 2003.
113. Nickenig G, Baumer AT, Temur Y, et al: Distinct and combined vascular effects of ACE blockade HMG-CoA reductase inhibition in hypertensive subjects. Hypertension 33:719-725, 1999.
114. Wassman S, Nickenig G, Bohm M: HMG-CoA reductase inhibitor atorvastatin downregulates AT1 receptor gene expression and cell proliferation in vascular smooth muscle cells. Kidney Blood Press Res 21:392-393, 1999.
115. Nickenig G, Baumer AT, Temur Y, et al: Statin-sensitive dysregulated AT_1 receptor function and density in hypercholesterolemic men. Circulation 100:2131-2134, 1999.
116. Griendling KK, Murphy TJ, Alexander RW: Molecular biology of the renin-angiotensin system. Circulation 87:1816-1828, 1993.
117. Hayek T, Attias J, Coleman R, et al: The angiotensin-converting enzyme inhibitor, fosinopril, and the angiotensin II receptor antagonist, losartan, inhibit LDL oxidation and attenuate atherosclerosis independent of lowering blood pressure in apolipoprotein E deficient mice. Cardiovasc Res 44:579-587, 1999.
118. Leif SJ, Karin P, Gunnar A, et al: Antiatherosclerotic effects of the angiotensin-converting enzyme inhibitors captopril and fosinopril in hypercholesterolemic minipigs. J Cardiovasc Pharmacol 24:670-677, 1994.
119. Daugherty A, Manning MW, Cassis LA: Angiotensin II promotes atherosclerotic lesions and aneurysms in apolipoprotein E-deficient mice. J Clin Invest 105:1605-1612, 2000.
120. Becker RH, Wiemer G, Linz W: Preservation of endothelial function by ramipril in rabbits on a long-term atherogenic diet. J Cardiovasc Pharmacol 18:S110-S115, 1991.
121. Mancini GB, Henry GC, Macaya C, et al: Angiotensin-converting enzyme inhibition with quinapril improves endothelial vasomotor dysfunction in patients with coronary artery disease: The TREND (Trial on Reversing Endothelial Dysfunction). Circulation 94:258-265, 1996.
122. Mehta JL, Li D: Identification, regulation and function of a novel lectin like oxidized low-density lipoprotein receptor. J Am Coll Cardiol 39:1429-1435, 2002.

4

123. Kume N, Arai H, Kawai C, Kita T: Receptors for modified low density lipoproteins on human endothelial cells: Different recognition for acetylated low-density lipoprotein and oxidized low-density lipoprotein. Biochem Biophys Acta 1091:63-67, 1991.

124. Kume N, Sawamura T, Moriwaki H, et al: Inducible expression of LOX-1, a novel lectin-like receptor for oxidized low density lipoprotein, in vascular endothelial cells. Circ Res 83:322-327, 1998.

125. Moriwakitt H, Kume N, Kataoka H, et al: Expression of lectin-like oxidized low density lipoprotein receptor-1 in human and murine macrophages: Upregulated expression by TNF-alpha. FEBS Lett 440:29-32, 1998.

126. Murase T, Kume N, Korenaga R, et al: Fluid shear stress transcriptionally induces lectin-like oxidized LDL receptor-1 in vascular endothelial cells. Circ Res 83:329-333, 1998.

127. Li DY, Yang BC, Mehta JL: Ox-LDL induces apoptosis in cultured human coronary artery endothelial cells: Role of PKC, PTK, bcl-2, and Fas. Am J Physiol 275:H568-H576, 1998.

128. Li D, Mehta JL: Upregulation of endothelial receptor for oxidized LDL (LOX-1) by oxidized LDL and implications in apoptosis of human coronary artery endothelial cells: Evidence from use of antisense LOX-1 mRNA and chemical inhibitors. Arterioscler Thromb Vasc Biol 20:1116-1122, 2000.

129. Li D, Mehta JL: Antisense to LOX-1 inhibits oxidized -mediated upregulation of monocyte chemoattractant protein-1 and monocyte adhesion to human coronary artery endothelial cells. Circulation 101:2889-2895, 2000.

130. Li D, Saldeen T, Romeo F, Mehta JL: Oxidized LDL upregulates angiotensin II type 1 receptor expression in cultured human coronary artery endothelial cells: The potential role of transcription factor NF-kappa B. Circulation 102:1970-1976, 2000.

131. Li D, Yang B, Philips MI, Mehta JL: Pro-apoptotic effects of Ang II in human coronary artery endothelial cells: role of AT_1 receptor and PKC activation. Am J Physiol 276:H786-792, 1999.

132. Li DY, Zhang YC, Philips MI, et al: Upregulation of endothelial receptor for oxidized low-density lipoprotein (LOX-1) in cultured human coronary artery endothelial cells by angiotensin II type 1 receptor activation. Circ Res 84:1043-1049, 1999.

133. Mehta JL, Li D: Facilitative interaction between angiotensin II and oxidized LDL in cultured human coronary artery endothelial cells. J Ren Ang Ald Syst 2:D70-S76, 2001.

134. Chen H, Li D, Sawamura T, et al: Upregulation of LOX-1 expression in aorta of hypercholesterolemic rabbits: Modulation by losartan. Biochem Biophys Res Commun 276:1100-1104, 2000.

135. Lloyd-Jones DM, Evans JC, Larson MG, et al: Cross-classification of JNC VI blood pressure stages and risk groups in the Framingham Heart Study. Arch Intern Med 159:2206-2212, 1999.

136. Sung BH, Izzo JI, Wilson MF: Effects of cholesterol reduction on BP response to mental stress in patients with high cholesterol. Am J Hypertens 10:592-599, 1997.

137. Nazzaro P, Manzari M, Merlo M, et al: Distinct and combined vascular effects of ACE blockade and HMG-CoA reductase inhibition in hypertensive subjects. Hypertension 33:719-725, 1999.

138. O'Callaghan CJ, Krum H, Conway EL, et al: Short-term effects of

pravastatin on blood pressure in hypercholesterolaemic hypertensive patients. Blood Press 3:404-406, 1994.

139. Abetel G, Poget PN, Bonnabry JP: Hypotensive effect of an inhibitor of cholesterol synthesis (fluvastatin): A pilot study. Schweiz Med Wochenschr 128:272-277, 1998.

140. Glorioso N, Troffa C, Filigheddu F, et al: Effect of the HMG-CoA reductase inhibitors on blood pressure in patients with essential hypertension and primary hypercholesterolemia. Hypertension 34:1281-1286, 1999.

141. Sposito AC, Mansur AP, Coelho OR, et al: Additional reduction in blood pressure after cholesterol-lowering treatment by statins (lovastatin or pravastatin) in hypercholesterolemic patients using angiotensin-converting enzyme inhibitors (enalapril or lisinopril). Am J Cardiol 83:1497-1499, A8, 1999.

142. Borghi C, Prandin MG, Costa FV, et al: Use of statins and blood pressure control in treated hypertensive patients with hypercholesterolemia. J Cardiovasc Pharmacol 35:549-555, 2000.

143. Tonolo G, Melis MG, Formato M, et al: Additive effects of simvastatin beyond its effects on LDL cholesterol in hypertensive type 2 diabetic patients. Eur J Clin Invest 30:980-987, 2000.

144. Jonkers IJ, de Man FH, van der Laarse A, et al: Bezafibrate reduces heart rate and blood pressure in patients with hypertriglyceridemia. J Hypertens 19:749-755, 2001.

145. Steinberg D: Lipoproteins and atherogenesis. JAMA 264:3047-3052, 1990.

146. Becker RH, Wiemer G, Linz W: Preservation of endothelial function by ramipril in rabbits on a long-term atherogenic diet. J Cardiovasc Pharmacol 18:S110-S115, 1991.

147. Pitt B, Pepine C, O'Neill B, et al, for the TREND investigators: Modulation of ACE inhibitor efficacy on coronary endothelial dysfunction by low-density lipoprotein cholesterol [abstract]. J Am Coll Cardiol 29:70A, 714-715, 1997.

148. Cashin-Hemphill L, Dinsmore RE, Chan RC, et al, for the QUIET Investigators: LDL cholesterol and angiographic progression in the QUIET trial [abstract]. J Am Coll Cardiol 29:85A, 725-721, 1997.

149. Pitt B, O'Neill B, Feldman R, et al: The Quinapril Ischemic Event Trial (QUIET): Evaluation of chronic ACE inhibitor therapy in patients with ischemic heart disease and preserved left ventricular function. Am J Cardiol 87:1058-1063, 2001.

150. Marian AJ, Safavi F, Ferlic L, et al: Interactions between angiotensin-I converting enzyme insertion/deletion polymorphism and response of plasma lipids and coronary atherosclerosis to treatment with fluvastatin: The lipoprotein and coronary atherosclerosis study. J Am Coll Cardiol 35(1):89-95, 2000.

151. Caro J, Klittich W, McGuire A, et al, for the WOSCOPS Economic Analysis Committee: International economic analysis of primary prevention of cardiovascular disease with pravastatin in WOSCOPS. Eur Heart J 20:263-268, 1999.

152. Gotto AM, Boccuzzi SJ, Cook JR, et al: Effect of lovastatin on cardiovascular resource utilization and costs in the Air Force/Texas Coronary Atherosclerosis Prevention Study (AFCAPS/TexCAPS). AFCAPS/TexCAPS Research Group. Am J Cardiol 86:1176-1181, 2000.

153. Perreault S, Hamilton VH, Lavoie F, et al: Treating hyperlipidemia for the primary prevention of coronary disease: Are higher doses of lovastatin cost effective? Arch Intern Med 157:375-381, 1998.

4

154. Expert Panel on Detection, Evaluation, and Treatment of High Blood
     Cholesterol in Adults: Executive Summary of the Third Report of the
     National Cholesterol Education Program (NCEP) (Adult Treatment
     Panel III). JAMA 285:2486-2497, 2001.
155. Lloyd-Jones DM, O'Donnell CJ, D'Agostino RB, et al: Applicability of
     cholesterol lowering primary prevention trials to a general
     population: The Framingham Heart Study. Arch Intern Med 161:949-
     954, 2001.

4

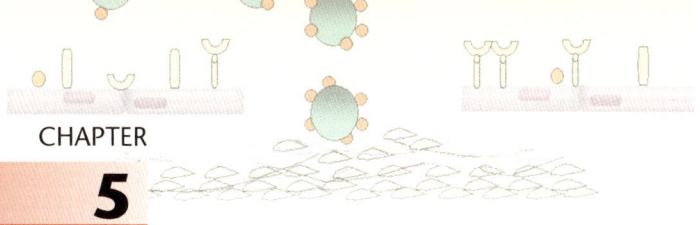

CHAPTER

5

Secondary Prevention of Atherosclerosis and Related Events by Statins

John Kjekshus

The important relationship between elevated cholesterol and cardiovascular disease was recognized as early in 1938.[1] But not until the development of effective lipid-reducing drugs was it possible to demonstrate beyond doubt that the reduction of low-density-lipoprotein (LDL) cholesterol was able to cut all-cause mortality exclusively by reducing cardiovascular deaths.[2] Initial studies with quantitative angiography as well as ultrasound measurements of intima media thickness demonstrated small but significant slowing of the progression, and even regression, of atheromatous plaques in the coronary and carotid arteries.[3-5] The alleged mechanism of benefit is not as much debulking of the atheromatous plaque as it is a reduction of the inflammation in the vascular wall and improvement of endothelial function. The result is reduced vascular remodeling and stabilization of the vulnerable plaques. As yet, we do not know if this is a specific statin effect or a consequence of the changes in the lipoprotein profile. Furthermore, the statin effect is not limited to the arterial vasculature. The post–coronary artery bypass graft (post-CABG) trial demonstrated protective effects on saphenous venous bypass grafts by comparing a more aggressive with a moderate lipid reduction.[6] Reduction of LDL cholesterol with treatment to between 2.4 and 2.5 mmol/L (93 and 97 mg/dL) compared to only 3.37 to 3.49 mmol/L (130 to 135 mg/dL) resulted in less progression of graft stenosis, 27% compared to 39%.

Several prospective, randomized, placebo-controlled trials have established the fundamental role of statin treatment of athero-sclerotic disease, including coronary heart disease, stroke, and peripheral vascular disease, in so-called primary and secondary prevention studies.[2,7-13] Statin treatment has therefore become the cornerstone in the management of atherosclerotic disease in clinical practice. The improved survival occurs over a large range of baseline total and LDL cholesterol concentrations.[14,15] The relative reduction of cardiovascular events (fatal and nonfatal) with statins is independent of risk and has generally ranged around 30% in most studies. This number may be misleading because it does not consider absolute risk. The absolute risk for an event is highest in secondary high-risk and lowest in primary preventive (low-risk) trials. Several studies have developed risk criteria; most are based on the Framingham criteria (age, fasting LDL cholesterol, high-density-lipoprotein [HDL] cholesterol, blood pressure, diabetes, and smoking status).[16,17] Although the risk criteria differ somewhat between studies and cannot be readily transferred from one population to another, the basic idea has important clinical implications.

The number of events accumulates almost linearly over time. Most guidelines accept a threshold for aggressive lipid-lowering treatment—when the future risk exceeds a 10% chance of a major cardiovascular event (sudden death, fatal or nonfatal myocardial infarction [MI], stroke, and need for revascularization) over the next 5 years.[18,19] The higher the absolute risk in terms of an index or a congregate of risk markers, the more an individual has to gain from treatment.

When estimated risk is taken into account, the benefit of statin treatment in terms of absolute risk reduction is described by a curvilinear relationship. Definition of risk has therefore strong bearings on indications for and cost-effectiveness of statin treatment.[20,21] The cost per life saved with statin treatment is 2 to 6 times higher in low-risk than in high-risk patients.

Although several risk factors contribute to the risk of cardiovascular events, a history of myocardial infarction has been the most decisive risk factor. Even in the low-risk West of Scotland Coronary Prevention Study (WOSCOPS), which included only patients without known coronary risk factors, the findings of nonspecific minor electrocardiographic abnormalities identified a subset with markedly elevated risk.[22] The relationship between the absolute cardiovascular risk and absolute risk reduction is linear. Therefore, dichotomization into primary and secondary preventive treatments is obsolete, and it has now been recognized that a much broader stratification panel, based on global risk factor definition, is necessary. That is, any evidence of cardiovascular disease, a history of myocardial infarction or a peripheral vascular event, angina pectoris, silent ischemia, or peripheral vascular disease puts a patient at high risk for a cardiovascular event. In these patients, the benefits of statin therapies are relatively consistent regardless of the risk factors present, and other risk factors are irrelevant in determining indications for statin treatment.[23] In patients without a history of cardiovascular disease, the presence of other established risk factors have to be taken into considerations (age, sex, smoking, blood pressure, heart rate, glucose intolerance, inheritance, lipid profile, Lp(a) lipoprotein, and homocysteine). These risk factors work independently, and the relative risk reduction with statin treatment is unchanged or increased for all of them. Thus, the absolute risk and benefit in terms of lives saved are markedly increased.

PROSPECTIVE CLINICAL TRIALS IN HIGH-RISK PATIENTS

Since 1994, a total of six prospective, double-blind, placebo-controlled, randomized trials with statin treatment in high-risk patients have been published (Table 5-1). They are the Scandinavian Simvastatin Survival Study (4S),[2] the Cholesterol and Recurrent Events (CARE) trial,[7] Long-term Intervention with Pravastatin in Ischemic Disease (LIPID),[9] the Heart Protection Study (HPS),[11] the Prospective Study of Pravastatin in the Elderly at Risk (PROSPER),[10] and the Anglo-Scandinavian Cardiac Outcomes Trial—Lipid-Lowering Arm (ASCOT-LLA).[12] All of these trials were analyzed according to the intention-to-treat principle. Results are shown in Tables 5-2 and 5-3.

In addition, two other relevant studies in high-risk patients have been published. Both were open, one comparing pravastatin and the other atorvastatin treatment to usual care in high-risk patients. They are the Antihypertensive and Lipid-Lowering Treatment to Prevent Heart Attack trial (ALLHAT)[24] and the Greek Atorvastatin and Coronary Heart Disease Evaluation (GREACE) study.[25]

The 4S Trial

The 4S was the first successful trial to study the effect of a marked reduction of cholesterol on overall mortality.[2] The trial included patients with a history of stable angina or a previous MI. A total of 4444 men and women with a cholesterol level between 5 mmol/L (192 mg/dL) and 8 mmol/L (308 mg/dL) were randomized to take simvastatin, 20 mg, or placebo, with titration to 40 mg if the goal of cholesterol lower than 5 mmol/L (192 mg/dL) was not reached. The investigators were blinded to the results of the titration, and the placebo arm was equally up-titrated. Follow-up was 5.4 years.

Total and LDL cholesterol levels were reduced by 25% and 35%, respectively. After 37% of the patients had their daily dose raised from 20 to 40 mg, 72% reached the treatment goal of cholesterol, 5.2 mmol/L (200 mg/dL). Triglycerides decreased by 10%, and HDL increased by 8%. All-cause mortality was reduced by 30%, almost exclusively by a reduction in coronary heart disease mortality of 42%. The curves started to dissociate after 6 months and continued to diverge during the follow-up period. The benefit was consistent, and subgroup analysis demonstrated similar benefit regardless of sex, age, smoking habits, and diabetes. The treatment was particularly effective in reducing sudden cardiac death (death within 1 hour and presumed to be arrhythmic) by 41%.

Table 5-1

Baseline Characteristics of 4S, CARE, LIPID, HPS, PROSPER, and ASCOT-LLA

	4S	CARE	LIPID	HPS	PROSPER	ASCOT-LLA
Number	4444	4159	9014	20,536	5804	10,305
Study drug (mg)	Simvastatin (20–40)	Pravastatin (40)	Pravastatin (40)	Simvastatin (40)	Pravastatin (40)	Atorvastatin (10)
Follow-up, yr	5.4	5.0	6.1	5.0	3.2	3.3
Age, mean (±SD)	58 (7)	59 (9)	31–75	40–80	75 (3.3)	63 (8.5)
Women, %	19	14	17	25	52	19
BMI, kg/m^2 (±SD)	NA	28 (4)	—	NA	27 (4.2)	29 (4.6)
Coronary disease, %	100	100	100	65	27	0
History of MI, %	79	100	64	41	13	0
Diabetes, %	4	14	9	19	11	25
Hypertension, %	26	42	42	41	62	100
Smoking, %	27	21	10	15	27	33
Current Treatment						
Beta-blocker, %	57	40	47	26	NA	39
Aspirin, %	37	83	83	63	NA	17
ACE inibitor, %	NA	15	83	19	NA	32
Dropouts, %	12	10	23	32	14	13

4S, Scandinavian Simvastatin Survival Study; CARE, Cholesterol and Recurrent Events trial; LIPID, Long-term Intervention with Pravastatin in Ischemic Disease; HPS, Heart Protection Study; PROSPER, Prospective Study of Pravastatin in the Elderly at Risk; ASCOT-LLA, Anglo Scandinavian Cardiac Outcomes Trial—Lipid-Lowering Arm; ACE, angiotensin-converting enzyme; BMI, body mass index; MI, myocardial infarction; NA, not available.

The effects on the survival curves were independent of the LDL at baseline but dependent on the reduction of LDL. Retrospective analysis revealed unexpectedly a significant reduction in fatal and nonfatal cerebral vascular events, with a relative risk reduction of 30%.

In a subgroup analysis, patients were defined according to quartiles of HDL cholesterol and triglycerides.[26] Patients in the quartile with the lowest HDL cholesterol and highest triglycerides, "the lipid triad," were compared to a matched group with isolated high LDL cholesterol, but high HDL cholesterol and low triglycerides, with the objective of examining the role of the two lipid fractions with regard to efficacy. LDL cholesterol was comparable between the groups. The quartile with the lipid triad had a much higher event rate in the placebo group and the greatest event reduction by simvastatin treatment.

Substudies confirmed that elevated levels of Lp(a), or homocysteine each carried an independent risk. Although simvastatin did not change the levels of Lp(a)[27] and homocysteine,[28] there was a clear benefit of treatment in all patients exposed to these risk factors.

Recently, data from the 4S trial were reexamined after a follow-up period of 7.4 years. It was found that the survival benefit was maintained, bringing forward the 30% reduction of all-cause mortality.[29] The follow-up did not reveal any safety concerns. There was a trend in the direction of less cancer in the simvastatin group.

The CARE Trial

The CARE trial included 4159 men and women, all with myocardial infarction but a total cholesterol level below 2.6 mmol/L (240 mg/dL).[8] The patients were randomized to pravastatin, 40 mg, or matching placebo and were followed for an average of 5 years. Total cholesterol was reduced by 20%, LDL cholesterol by 28%, and triglycerides by 14%. HDL cholesterol increased by 5%.

The primary endpoint, the combination of nonfatal MI, coronary heart disease, or death, was reduced by 24%. Myocardial revascularization was reduced by 27%, and fatal and nonfatal vascular events were reduced by 31%. The effect of pravastatin on all-cause mortality amounted to an insignificant 9% reduction. As in the 4S trial, the benefit extended to diabetic patients, women, and older adults. The number of strokes was reduced by 31%.

However, in a substudy, the overall benefit was shown to be restricted to patients with a reduction in LDL concentration to 3.2 mmol/L (125 mg/dL). Concentrations below that were not associated with further benefit, and the investigators questioned the benefit of more aggressive treatment.

The LIPID Trial

The LIPID trial included patients with a history of MI or hospitalization for a previously unstable angina and with a total cholesterol

Table 5-2

Lipoproteins, Baseline, and Percentage Change on Treatment

Lipoproteins	4S		CARE		LIPID		HPS		PROSPER		ASCOT-LLA	
	BASELINE	CHANGE (%)	BASELINE	CHANGE (%)	BASELINE	CHANGE (%)	BASELINE	CHANGE (%)	BASELINE	CHANGE (%)	BASELINE	CHANGE (%)
Total cholesterol												
mmol/L	6.75	−25	5.4	−20	5.7	−18	5.9	−20	5.7	NA	5.5	−19
mg/dL	261		209		218		228		220		212	
LDL cholesterol												
mmol/L	4.9	−35	3.6	−28	3.9	−25	3.4	−29	3.8	−27	3.4	−29
mg/dL	188		139		150		131		(147)		131	
HDL cholesterol												
mmol/L	1.19	+8	1.0	+5	0.90	+5	1.06	3	1.3	+5	1.3	0
mg/dL	46		39		36		41		50		50	
Triglyceride												
mmol/L	1.51	−10	1.75	−14	1.58	−11	2.1	−14	1.5	−12	1.7	−14
mg/dL	132		155		140		186		133		150	

4S, Scandinavian Simvastatin Survival Study; CARE, Cholesterol and Recurrent Events trial; LIPID, Long-term Intervention with Pravastatin in Ischemic Disease; HPS, Heart Protection Study; PROSPER, Prospective Study of Pravastatin in the Elderly at Risk; ASCOT-LLA, Anglo-Scandinavian Cardiac Outcomes Trial—Lipid-Lowering Arm; LDL, low-density lipoprotein; HDL, high-density lipoprotein.

5

between 4 and 7 mmol/L (155 and 271 mg/dL).[9] A total of 9014 men and women were randomized to treatment. The study compared pravastatin, 40 mg, with placebo and was followed for 6.1 years. Total and LDL cholesterol were reduced by 18% and 25%, respectively. Triglycerides were reduced by 11% and HDL cholesterol increased by 5%. The reduction in total LDL cholesterol was less than optimal because of the large crossover in treatments during the study. The primary endpoint was coronary mortality, which was reduced by 24%. Total mortality was reduced by 22%. There was also a significant (19%) reduction in the incidence of stroke, confirming the outcomes in the 4S and the CARE trials.

The HPS Trial

The HPS was a megatrial including 20,536 high-risk patients between the ages of 40 and 80 years.[11] The patients were eligible to join the study if they were at high risk as defined by coronary artery disease, peripheral vascular disease, diabetes, or hypertension. The patients were randomized to simvastatin, 40 mg, or placebo. Cholesterol at entry had to be 3.5 mmol/L (135 mg/dL) or higher; there was no upper limit. Of the patients, 25% were women, 35% had no known coronary disease, and 29% were diabetics. A relatively large number of patients, averaging 18%, in the placebo group received statins during follow-up. Accordingly, the difference in LDL cholesterol between the two treatment groups was less than planned, and was reduced from 1.2 to 0.75 mmol/L (46 to 29 mg/dL) over the follow-up period. After a follow-up of 5 years, there was a significant 12% reduction in all-cause mortality, resulting mainly from a 17% reduction in cardiovascular deaths. The combined endpoint of coronary heart disease death and nonfatal MI was reduced by 27%. There was also a consistent reduction in stroke rates (25%) and in coronary revascularization rates (30%).

The benefit was seen regardless of sex, age, prior cardiovascular disease, hypertension, or diabetes. The benefit was also independent of baseline LDL cholesterol. Thus, the same relative risk reduction was observed in patients with baseline LDL cholesterol levels below and above 3.0 mmol/L (116 mg/dL). That the HPS patients were at high risk was reflected in the observed event rate in the placebo group: 14.7% died over 5 years, compared to 11.5% in the 4S. Vascular deaths occurred in 9.1% compared to 9.3% in the 4S. The number of fatal and nonfatal coronary events was lower in HPS—11.8% compared to 27.6% in the 4S. This reflects the importance of an expanded risk evaluation without regard to LDL cholesterol. In contrast to the CARE experience, the HPS expanded the target for lipid lowering to all high-risk patients and confirmed that in these patients, any cholesterol level is probably too high, and that these patients will benefit from reduction of the lipid level.

Table 5–3

Incidence of Endpoints, Absolute and Relative Risk Reduction, and Number Needed to Treat to Avoid One Event

	4S	CARE	LIPID	HPS	PROSPER	ASCOT-LLA
Mortality						
Placebo, N (%)	256 (11.5)	196 (9.4)	633 (14.1)	1507 (14.7)	306 (10.5)	212 (4.1)
Annual, N (%)	47 (2.1)	39 (1.9)	103 (2.3)	301 (2.9)	95 (3.2)	64 (1.2)
ARR (%)	3.3	0.8	3.1	1.8	0.2	0.5
RRR (95% CI)	0.70 (0.58-0.85)	0.91 (0.88-1.26)	0.78 (0.69-0.87)	0.87 (0.81-0.94)	0.97 (0.83-1.14)	0.87 (0.71-1·06)
NNT, 5 yr	32	130	40	57	231	126
Fatal CHD + Nonfatal MI						
Placebo, N (%)	622 (28)	274 (13.2)	715 (15.9)	1212 (11.8)	356 (12.2)	154 (3.0)
Annual, N (%)	115 (5.2)	55 (2.6)	117 (2.6)	242 (2.4)	111 (3.8)	46 (0.9)
ARR (%)	9	3.0	3.2	3.1	2.1	1.1
RRR (95% CI)	0.66 (0.59-0.75)	0.76 (0.64-0.91)	0.76 (0.68-0.85)	0.73 (0.67-0.79)	0.81 (0.69-0.94)	0.64 (0.50-0.83)
NNT, 5 yr	13	33	35	33	28	63
Stroke, Fatal + Nonfatal						
Placebo, N (%)	98 (4.4)	78 (3.8)	204 (4.5)	585 (5.7)	131 (4.5)	121 (2.4)
Annual, N (%)	18 (0.8)	16 (0.8)	33 (0.7)	117 (1.1)	41 (1.4)	36 (0.7)
ARR (%)	1.3	1.2	0.8	1.4	-0.2	0.7
RRR (95% CI)	0.70 (0.52-0.96)	0.69 (0.48-0.97)	0.81 (0.66-1.0)	0.75 (0.66-0.85)	1.03 (0.81-1.31)	0.73 (0.56-0.96)
NNT, 5 yr	86	87	161	73	—	108
NNH, 5 yr, NNT	—	—	—	—	463	—

Table 5–3—cont'd
Incidence of Endpoints, Absolute and Relative Risk Reduction, and Number Needed to Treat to Avoid One Event

	4S	CARE	LIPID	HPS	PROSPER	ASCOT-LLA
Revascularization						
Placebo, N (%)	383 (17.2)	391 (18.8)	708 (15.7)	725 (7.1)	48 (1.6)	NA
Annual, N (%)	71 (3.2)	78 (3.8)	116 (2.6)	145 (1.4)	15 (0.5)	NA
ARR (%)	5.9	4.7	2.7	2.1	0.3	NA
RRR (95%, CI)	0.63 (0.54-0.74)	0.73 (0.63-0.85)	0.80 (0.72-0.90)	0.70 (0.62-0.77)	0.82 (0.54-1.26)	NA
NNT, 5 yr	18	21	45	48	206	NA
Any Major Vascular Event (Fatal Cardiovascular Death, Nonfatal MI, Fatal and Nonfatal Stroke, Revascularization)						
Placebo, N (%)	1220 (54.9)	743 (35.7)	1627 (36.0)	2585 (25.2)	523 (18.0)	486 (9.5)
Annual, N (%)	225 (10.2)	149 (7.1)	267 (5.9)	517 (5.0)	163 (5.6)	147 (2.9)
ARR (%)	18.7	8.8	7.0	5.4	2.3	2.0
RRR (95% CI)	0.67	0.75	0.81	0.76 (0.72-0.81)	0.85 (0.75-0.97)	0.79 (0.69-0.90)
NNT, 5 yr	6	11	17	19	27	35

4S, Scandinavian Simvastatin Survival Study; CARE, Cholesterol and Recurrent Events trial; LIPID, Long-term Intervention with Pravastatin in Ischemic Disease; HPS, Heart Protection Study; PROSPER, Prospective Study of Pravastatin in the Elderly at Risk; ASCOT-LLA, Anglo-Scandinavian Cardiac Outcomes Trial—Lipid-Lowering Arm; ARR, absolute risk reduction; NA, not available; NNH, number needed to hurt; NNT, number needed to treat; RRR, relative risk reduction; MI, myocardial infarction; CHD, cardiac heart disease.

The ASCOT-LLA Trial

The ASCOT-LLA trial was part of an antihypertensive study in high-risk patients who were not conventionally dyslipidemic.[12] Patients were hypertensive, with a systolic blood pressure of 160 mm Hg or higher, a diastolic blood pressure of 100 mm Hg or higher, or both, or with previously treated hypertension with a systolic blood pressure of at least 140 mm Hg.

In addition, the patients had at least three of the following cardiovascular risk factors: left ventricular hypertrophy, electro-cardiographic abnormality, type 2 diabetes, peripheral arterial disease, previous stroke, transient ischemic attack, male sex, age 55 years or older, smoking, a ratio of total to HDL cholesterol of 6 or higher (plasma), or a family history of premature coronary disease. A total of 1305 patients with nonfasting total cholesterol concentrations of 6.5 mmol/L or lower were randomized to atorvastatin, 10 mg, or placebo.

Atorvastatin reduced total and LDL cholesterol by 24% and 35%, respectively. Because of a 13% rate of dropout in the active group and 9% crossover in the placebo group, the relative decreases at the end of the study were 19% and 29%, respectively. Compared with placebo, atorvastatin reduced triglycerides by about 14% at study completion, whereas HDL cholesterol was actually unchanged at the end of the follow-up.

The study was planned for 5 years but was stopped after 3.3 years, when the primary combined endpoint of nonfatal MI and fatal coronary heart disease was significantly reduced in the treatment arm. In the atorvastatin group, 100 primary events occurred, compared with 154 events in the placebo group, a risk reduction of 36%. Fatal and nonfatal strokes were reduced by 27%. All-cause mortality was not significantly reduced (13%). There was, however, no effect on fatal and nonfatal heart failure, new onset of diabetes mellitus, or renal impairment. However, the numbers were small and subject to chance findings.

The high-risk profile of the included patients is reflected in the fact that the combined total cardiovascular and procedural event rates amounted to 9.5% over 3.3 years. Assuming a linear relationship, the cumulative events are converted to an annual rate of 2.9%, well above the guideline threshold.[19]

A subgroup analysis of hypertensive patients in the 4S demonstrated an effect slightly in excess of the overall result in the 4S with respect to relative risk reduction. However, because the overall cardiovascular event rate is higher in hypertensive patients, the absolute benefit is larger.

The ASCOT study plus the subgroup analyses in previous trials have clearly demonstrated that the effects of statins are additional to the effects obtained by blood pressure control. This underscores the importance of global reassessment of risk in these patients. Importantly, no negative interaction was observed between statin treatment and the overall use of blood pressure–lowering regimens.

The PROSPER Trial

The PROSPER trial was undertaken to the test the efficacy of statins in older adults at high risk for vascular disease.[10] The study included 5804 older adults between 70 and 82 years of age with a history of or risk factors for vascular disease. Cholesterol concentrations at baseline ranged from 4.0 to 9.0 mmol/L (154 to 347 mg/dL). The patients were randomized to pravastatin, 40 mg, or placebo and followed for 3.2 years. The primary endpoint was a composite of coronary death, nonmyocardial infarction, and fatal and nonfatal strokes. The average age was 75 years. The mean total cholesterol at baseline was 5.7 mmol/L (220 mg/dL), LDL cholesterol 3.8 mmol/L (147 mg/dL), HDL cholesterol 1.3 mmol/L (50 mg/dL), and triglycerides 1.5 mmol/L (133 mg/dL). LDL cholesterol was reduced by 27% in the entire cohort. The primary endpoint was reduced by 15%. Fatal coronary heart disease and nonfatal MI were reduced by 19%. Stroke and transient ischemic attack were not significantly reduced, but the trend was in favor of pravastatin treatment.

Overall, there was 25% more cancer in the pravastatin treatment group than in the placebo group. However, the numbers were small and subject to chance. The result is at variance with a meta-analysis of all trials.[30] No evidence of any effect on dementia or cognitive impairment was observed in this cohort. However, the observation period was probably too short to be able to identify any effect on cognitive impairment. The efficacy was not related to LDL concentrations, and there was a strong treatment effect among patients with low HDL cholesterol levels, which concurs with the data observed in the 4S.

OTHER STUDIES
The ALLHAT-LLA Trial

The ALLHAT was an open study examining the effect of statin treatment specifically among 10,355 hypertensive patients.[24] Pravastatin (40 mg) was compared to usual care. The demographics of the patients included in the ALLHAT trial differed markedly from those of patients in the ASCOT trial in that there were more blacks, fewer with diabetes, and a lower mean systolic blood pressure. Relatively few patients had a history of previous coronary disease. No significant benefit in terms of all-cause mortality, coronary, or stroke events was obtained. Because the trial was open, the study was flawed by a substantial increase in the use of statins in the usual care group, leading to differences in total and LDL cholesterol of only 9% and 17%, respectively. The lipid reduction was therefore too low to anticipate a significant reduction in overall or cardiovascular events. However, the point estimate of the trial was on the regression line for all trials comparing efficacy to lowering of LDL cholesterol.[24]

5

The GREACE Trial

Sixteen hundred patients with coronary heart disease were randomized either (1) to aggressive lipid lowering with atorvastatin (10 to 80 mg/day) with the specific goal of lowering LDL cholesterol to lower than 2.6 mmol/L (100 mg/dL) or (2) to usual care with lifestyle intervention as well as treatment considered necessary by the physician, including lipid-lowering drugs.[25] The mean dose of atorvastatin was 24 mg/day. LDL cholesterol was reduced by 46%, triglycerides were reduced by 31%, and HDL cholesterol was increased by 7%. The lipid goal was reached by 95% of the aggressively treated patients, in contrast to only 3% in the usual care group. Only 14% of the patients in the usual care group received cholesterol-lowering drugs. After 2 years, 24.5% of the patients on usual care experienced an event (death, nonfatal myocardial infarction, unstable angina, congestive heart failure, revascularization, or stroke) compared to 12% on atorvastatin. An impressive relative risk reduction of 51% was observed in the aggressively treated group. The results were consistent for all subgroups in the composite endpoint.

Although the study was open, and for some reason two independent groups classified the endpoints, one for each treatment group, which invites bias, three important points can be made. First, the study demonstrates that it is possible to attain the National Cholesterol Education Program (NCEP) lipid goal of an LDL cholesterol level lower than 2.6 mmol/L (100 mg/dL) in almost all patients by dose titration in a dedicated clinical setting. Second, this trial resulted in a 50% reduction in coronary events, which represented the largest decrease in risk in any trial to date and virtually without side effects. Finally, the use of lipid-lowering drugs in usual care is disappointingly low.

ACUTE CORONARY SYNDROMES

In all published trials that include patients in stable condition, the statin effect on coronary events appeared after more than a year of treatment. Although prospective survival studies on patients with acute coronary syndrome have not been performed to show this, functional improvement from statins related to inflammatory markers and endothelial dysfunction appears to be early, usually after days or a few weeks.[31,32]

Formerly, the recommendation for patients with acute coronary syndrome was to try dietary counseling for 6 months before considering statin treatment. However, these patients are at particular risk for a recurrent event and are therefore a special target population for early treatment. Implementation of statin treatment during the hospital stay has been very effective in establishing treatment in patients at risk; postponing statin use by 6 months results is a gross underutilization of treatment.

5

Several observational studies have suggested that statin therapy in patients admitted to the coronary care unit benefit by receiving a statin before discharge. In a retrospective analysis of the GUSTO 2B trial (Global Use of Streptokinase or Tissue Plasminogen Activator for Occluded Coronary Arteries) and the PURSUIT trial (Platelet Glycoprotein 2B/3A in Unstable Angina: Receptor Suppression Using Integrilin Therapy), 17,156 patients without discharge statin therapy were compared to 3653 patients on statin therapy at discharge. At the 6-month follow-up, the relative reduction of mortality was 33% after adjusting for confounding factors.[33]

Identical findings were obtained in a Swedish prospective cohort study.[34] Patients with a first registry-recorded acute MI and discharged alive from 58 Swedish hospitals were reexamined after 1 year to identify the relative risk of 1-year mortality according to statin treatment. Early statin treatment before discharge was associated with a relative risk reduction of 25% when adjusted for confounding factors at baseline. The reduction in mortality started early after discharge and was consistent in all subgroups, based on age, sex, baseline characteristics, previous disease manifestations, and medications.

Early mortality benefit was also observed in a retrospective analysis from the OPTIMAAL trial (Optimal Trial in Myocardial Infarction with the Angiotensin II Antagonist Losartan).[35] The 5477 patients included were within 14 days of an acute MI and had signs and symptoms of heart failure. Lipid-lowering treatment by simvastatin reduced coronary heart disease events by 51%, which was still significant after adjustment for risk variables during hospitalization (14%). This benefit was additional to and independent of the benefit obtained by beta-blocker treatment at discharge.

In contrast, a retrospective analysis of SYMPHONY and SYMPHONY II (Sibrafiban versus Aspirin to Yield Maximum Protection from Ischemic Heart Events Post-acute Coronary Syndromes) did not confirm the previous findings.[36] After adjustments for variables at baseline, the result did not show any difference between statin treatment ($N = 3952$) and no-statin treatment ($N = 8413$) at discharge.

In the PRISM trial (Platelet Receptor Inhibition of Ischemic Syndrome Management), patients with unstable coronary syndrome were analyzed retrospectively for potential benefit of statin treatment.[37] When statin treatment was initiated before discharge, incident death and nonfatal MIs were significantly reduced compared to these outcomes in patients who did not receive statin at or during the 30 days after discharge. Relative risk was 0.49 (confidence interval [CI], 0.21 to 0.86; $P < .004$). There was also less need for revascularization among the statin-treated patients. However, if the treatment was stopped during the hospital stay, the immediate postdischarge event rate increased markedly compared to that in patients on statin treatment (hazard ratio, 2.93 [CI, 1.51-5.92]).

The MIRACL trial (Myocardial Ischemia Reduction with Acute Cholesterol Lowering) tested in a prospective manner the use of statin immediately after an acute coronary event.[38] Within 96 hours after hospital admission, 3806 patients with unstable angina were randomly assigned to atorvastatin, 80 mg/day, or placebo. In the placebo group, LDL cholesterol during treatment was 3.49 mmol/L (135 mg/dL) compared to 1.87 mmol/L (72 mg/dL) in patients on atorvastatin. The main endpoint was a composite of death, nonfatal MI, resuscitated cardiac arrest, or worsening angina requiring hospitalization. The composite endpoint was significantly reduced (from 17.4% to 14.8%), and the relative risk reduction was 16% ($P < .048$). Although marginally positive, the difference was small and the result was exclusively driven by worsening angina. This small study points to the necessity to carry out larger prospective controlled clinical trials to avoid confounding bias.

USE OF STATINS IN ELECTIVE ANGIOPLASTY

Two small studies have addressed the effect of statin treatment on patients scheduled for elective angioplasty. In the AVERT trial (Atorvastatin versus Revascularization Treatment) atorvastatin, 80 mg/day, was compared to usual care with balloon angioplasty (percutaneous coronary intervention [PCI]) and lipid-reducing treatment at the investigator's discretion.[39] Atorvastatin reduced LDL cholesterol by 46% compared to 18% in the PCI group, and the cardiovascular events were reduced by 36% during the follow-up of 18 months.

The LIPS (Lescol Intervention Prevention Study) included patients undergoing PCI.[40] The patients were randomized to early statin therapy or placebo. At hospital discharge, 844 patients received fluvastatin, 8 mg/day, and 833 patients received placebo. The patients were followed for 3.9 years. Fluvastatin reduced LDL cholesterol levels by 27%, and the corresponding reduction in major cardiac events was 22%. The effect in this trial was independent of LDL cholesterol at baseline but in accordance with the risk assessment at baseline.

USE OF STATINS IN HEART FAILURE

The progression of coronary arteriosclerosis and thrombosis is the main cause of heart failure, and statin treatment has been shown to reduce the development of heart failure.[41] However, patients with heart failure have always been excluded from clinical trials with lipid-lowering drugs. As of today, we do not have the information from prospective trials to recommend statins for patients with established heart failure. Heart failure is characterized by polypharmacy and adding another drug may cause unwanted interactions. Statins reduce coenzyme Q10, and this may have a detrimental effect on the maintenance of myocardial function. Patients with heart failure also differ from those without it by having increased levels of endotoxins, shown to depress myocardial function and to accelerate atherosclerosis.[42,43] Lipoproteins have been shown to neutralize endotoxins, which may explain the finding that low cholesterol levels portend a poor prognosis in heart failure patients.[44] Studies are underway to clarify this issue.

CURRENT GUIDELINES

The ubiquity of the statin effect is reflected in the finding that relative risk reduction among low-risk patients is similar to that in high-risk patients, yet the absolute risk is small (Fig. 5-1).[7,13] Several guidelines have therefore focused on risk assessment and on establishing treatment goals on the basis of large prospective clinical trials.[18,19] According to the National Cholesterol Education

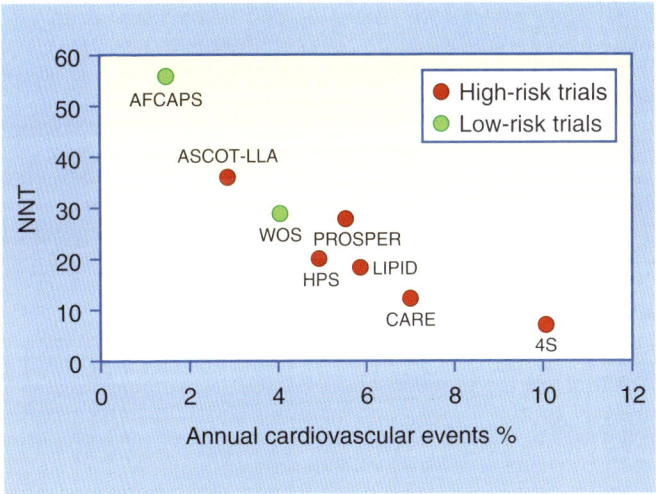

Figure 5-1 **Relationship between percentage of annual major cardiovascular events in the placebo arm of large statin trials (primary and secondary prevention) and numbers needed to treat (NNT).** Major cardiovascular events included cardiovascular death, nonfatal myocardial infarction, fatal and nonfatal strokes, and coronary revascularization. 4S, Scandinavian Simvastatin Survival Study; AFCAPS, Air Force Coronary Atherosclerosis Prevention Study; ASCOT-LLA, Anglo-Scandinavian Cardiac Outcomes Trial—Lipid-Lowering Arm; CARE, Cholesterol and Recurrent Events trial; HPS, Heart Protection Study; LIPID, Long-term Intervention with Pravastatin in Ischemic Disease; PROSPER, Prospective Study of Pravastatin in the Elderly at Risk; WOS, West of Scotland Coronary Prevention Study.

Program (NCEP) Adult Treatment Panel (ATP III) guidelines,[18] high-risk patients are those with coronary heart disease or risk equivalents. The optimal goal of statin treatment is an LDL cholesterol level of lower than 2.6 mmol/L (100 mg/dL). The revised European guidelines recommend a cutoff level of 2.5 mmol/L (116 mg/dL).[50] The treatment recommendation also includes patients without coronary heart disease (CHD). The guidelines define CHD equivalents as diabetes, other forms of atherosclerotic disease, peripheral arterial disease, abdominal aortic aneurysm, symptomatic carotid stenosis, and risk factors such as cigarette smoking, family history of premature coronary heart disease, age older than 45 years, hypertension, and low HDL cholesterol (<1.0 mmol/L [40 mg/dL]). In the European guidelines, the focus is on an expected 10-year risk for a cardiovascular event, estimated at 20%. If the LDL cholesterol is higher than 3.4 mmol/L (130 mg/dL), the effect on mortality and morbidity can be identified very early after discharge. It is therefore recommended that an immediate assessment of lipid status be made in all patients hospitalized for a coronary syndrome so that treatment can be initiated before they are discharged. Overall compliance to treatment is also better maintained when initiated before discharge. If LDL cholesterol is low, the benefit depends more on other risk factors present, and clinical judgment, based on a global risk factor evaluation, applies. However, the HPS study has demonstrated a clear benefit, even when LDL cholesterol is below 2.6 mmol/L (100 mg/dL). Several studies have also confirmed the extra risk associated with low HDL cholesterol, especially in combination with elevated triglycerides.[26] These patients receive extra benefit from statin treatment. The results of these trials will probably change the guidelines in the future.

CONCLUSIONS

The vast experience with and rapidly accumulating knowledge of the use of statins in the treatment of cardiovascular disease are reflected in the rapid succession of guidelines for treating cardiovascular disease. Data from several trials have confirmed that the benefits of statin treatment are not limited to middle-aged patients with coronary heart disease but can also be seen in stroke reduction,[45] older adults,[10,11,46] patients with diabetes[11,47,48] and hypertension,[2,12,24] and those at risk because of high Lp(a)[27] and homocysteine.[28] Treatment with statins also slows the progression of peripheral arterial disease.[49]

In practical terms, this means that all CHD and CHD-equivalent individuals should be considered as candidates for early statin treatment regardless of their baseline LDL cholesterol levels. The most recent trials have confirmed earlier assumptions that the goal of treatment should an LDL cholesterol level that is as low as possible; the recommended level of lower than 2.6 mmol/L (100 mg/dL) is attainable by careful titration of patients at risk.

The role of statins in severe heart failure still awaits final clarification. The effects of statins on inflammation, vascular function, and hemostasis may be of importance, but as yet it is not clearly defined how much of the benefit of statins is related to their specific properties and how much to the overall consequences of the lipid lowering.

References

1. Müller C: Angina pectoris in hereditary xanthomatosis. Arch Intern Med 64:675-700, 1939.
2. Scandinavian Simvastatin Survival Study Group: Randomised trial of cholesterol lowering in 4444 patients with coronary heart disease: The Scandinavian Simvastatin Survival Study Group (4S). Lancet 344:1383-1389, 1994.
3. MAAS Investigators: Effect of simvastatin on coronary atheroma: The Multicentre Anti-Atheroma Study (MAAS). Lancet 344:633-638, 1994.
4. Jukema JW, Bruschke AVG, van Boven AJ, et al: Effects of lipid lowering by pravastatin on progression and regression of coronary artery disease in symptomatic men with normal to moderately elevated serum cholesterol levels. Circulation 91: 2528-2540, 1995.
5. Smilde TJ, van Wissen S, Wollersheim H, et al: Effects of aggressive lipid lowering on atherosclerosis progression in familial hypercholesterolaemia (ASAP): A prospective, randomised, double-blind trial. Lancet 357:577-581, 2001.
6. Post-Coronary Artery Bypass Graft Trial Investigators: The effects of aggressive lowering of low-density lipoprotein cholesterol levels and low-dose anticoagulation on obstructive changes in saphenous-vein coronary-artery bypass grafts. N Engl J Med 336;153-162, 1997.
7. Shepherd J, Cobbe SM, Ford I, et al: Prevention of coronary heart disease with pravastatin in men with hypercholesterolemia: West of Scotland Coronary Prevention Study Group. N Engl J Med 333:1301-1307, 1995.
8. Sacks FM, Pfeffer MA, Moye LA, et al: The effect of pravastatin on coronary events after myocardial infarction in patients with average cholesterol levels: Cholesterol and Recurrent Events Trial Investigation. N Engl J Med 335:1001-1009, 1996.
9. The Long-term Intervention with Pravastatin in Ischaemic Disease (LIPID) Study Group: Prevention of cardiovascular events and death with pravastatin in patients with coronary heart disease and a broad range of initial cholesterol levels. N Engl J Med 339:1349-1357, 1998.
10. Shepherd J, Blauw GJ, Murphy MB, et al: Pravastatin in elderly individuals at risk of vascular disease (PROSPER): A randomised controlled trial. Lancet 360;1623-1630, 2002.
11. Heart Protection Collaborative Group: MRC/BHF Heart Protection Study of cholesterol lowering with simvastatin in 20536 high risk individuals: A randomised placebo-controlled trial. Lancet 360:7-22, 2002.
12. Sever PS, Dahløf B, Poulter NR, et al: Prevention of coronary and stroke events with atorvastatin in hypertensive patients who have average or lower-than-average cholesterol concentrations, in the Anglo-Scandinavian Cardiac Outcomes Trial-Lipid Lowering Arm (ASCOT-LLA): A multicentre randomised controlled trial. Lancet 361:1149-1158, 2003.

5

13. Downs JR, Clearfield M, Weis S, et al: Primary prevention of acute coronary events with lovastatin in men and women with average cholesterol levels. Results of AFCAPS/TexCAPS. Air Force/Texas Coronary Atherosclerosis Prevention Study. JAMA 279:1615-1622, 1998.

14. Scandinavian Simvastatin Survival Study Group: Baseline serum cholesterol and treatment effect in the Scandinavian Simvastatin Survival Study (4S) Lancet 345:1274-1275, 1995.

15. West of Scotland Coronary Prevention Study Group: Influence of pravastatin on plasma lipids on clinical events in the West of Scotland Coronary Prevention Study (WOSCOPS). Circulation 97:1440-1445, 1998.

16. Lloyd-Jones DM, Larson MG, Beiser A, Levy D: Lifetime risk of developing coronary heart disease. Lancet 353:89-92, 1999.

17. Wilson PW, D'Agostino RB, Levy D, et al: Prediction of coronary heart disease using risk factor categories. Circulation 97:1837-184, 1998.

18. Expert Panel on Detection, Evaluation, and Treatment of High Blood Cholesterol in Adults: Executive Summary of the Third Report of the National Cholesterol Education Program (NCEP) Expert Panel on Detection, Evaluation, and Treatment of High Blood Cholesterol in Adults (Adult Treatment Panel III). JAMA 285:2486-2497, 2001.

19. Task Force Report: Prevention of coronary heart disease in clinical practice. Eur Heart J 19:1434-1503, 1998.

20. Johannesson M, Jønsson B, Kjekshus J, et al: Cost effectiveness of simvastatin treatment of lower cholesterol levels in patients with coronary heart disease. New Engl J Med 336:332-336, 1997.

21. Caro J, Klittich W, McGuire A, et al: The West of Scotland coronary prevention study: Economic benefit analysis of primary prevention with pravastatin. BMJ 315:1577-1582, 1997.

22. West of Scotland Coronary Prevention Study Group: West of Scotland Coronary Prevention Study: Identification of high-risk groups and comparison with other cardiovascular intervention trials. Lancet 348:1339-1342, 1996.

23. Grover SA, Paquet S, Levington C, et al: Estimating the benefits of modifying risk factors of cardiovascular disease. A comparison of primary vs secondary prevention. Arch Intern Med 158:655-662, 1998.

24. The ALLHAT Collaborative Research Group: Major outcomes in moderately hypercholesterolemic, hypertensive patients randomised to pravastatin vs usual care: The antihypertensive and lipid-lowering treatment to prevent heart attack trial (ALLHAT-LLT). JAMA 288:2998, 2002.

25. Athyros VG, Papageorgiou AA, Mercouris BR, et al: Treatment with atorvastatin to the national cholesterol educational program goal versus 'usual' care in secondary coronary heart disease prevention. Curr Med Res Opin 18:220-228, 2002.

26. Ballantyne CM, Olsson AG, Cook TJ, et al: Influence of low/high-density lipoprotein cholesterol and elevated triglyceride on coronary heart disease events and response to simvastatin therapy in 4S. Circulation 104:3046-3051, 2001.

27. Berg K, Chrisophersen B, Cook T, et al: Lp(a) lipoprotein level predicts survival and major coronary events in the Scandinavian Simvastatin Survival Study. Clin Genet 52:254-261, 1997.

28. Nygard O, Refsum H, Kjekshus J, et al: Total homocysteine levels

predict major coronary events and mortality in simvastatin treated patients of 4S. Circulation 104:S550, 2001.

29. Pedersen TR, Wilhelmsen L, Færgeman O, et al. on behalf of the Scandinavian Simvastatin Survival Study (4S) Group: Follow-up study of patients randomized in the Scandinavian Simvastatin Survival Study (4S) of cholesterol lowering. Am J Cardiol 86:257-262, 2000.

30. Bjerre LM, Lelorier J: Do statins cause cancer? A meta-analysis of large randomized clinical trials. Am J Med 110:716-723, 2001.

31. O'Driscoll G, Green D, Taylor RR: Simvastatin, an HMG-coenzyme A reductase inhibitor, improves endothelial function within 1 month. Circulation 95:1126-1131, 1997.

32. Plenge JK, Hernandez TL, Weil KM, et al: Simvastatin lowers C-reactive protein within 14 days. Circulation 106:1447-1457, 2002.

33. Aronow HD, Topol EJ, Roe MT, et al: Effect of lipid lowering therapy on early mortality after acute coronary syndromes: An observational study. Lancet 357:1063-1068, 2001.

34. Stenestrand U, Wallentin L: Early statin treatment following acute myocardial infarction and 1-year survival. JAMA 285:430-436, 2001.

35. Hognestad A, Myhre E, Snapinn S, Kjekshus J: Early lipid lowering and beta-blockade during acute myocardial infarction reduce death and nonfatal myocardial infarction in heart failure patients. Circulation 104(Suppl II):762, 2002.

36. Newby LK, Kristinsson A, Bhapkar MV, et al: Early statin initiation and outcomes in patients with acute coronary syndromes. JAMA 287:3087-309, 2002.

37. Heeschen C, Hamm CW, Laufs U, et al: Withdrawal of statins increases event rates in patients with acute coronary syndromes. Circulation 105:1446-1452, 2002.

38. Schwartz GG, Olsson AG, Ezekowitz MD, et al: Effects of atorvastatin on early recurrent ischemic events in acute coronary syndromes: The MIRACL study: A randomized controlled trial. JAMA 285:1711-1718, 2001.

39. Pitt B, Waters D, Brown WV, et al: Aggressive lipid-lowering therapy compared with angioplasty in stable coronary artery disease: Atorvastatin versus revascularisation treatment investigators N Engl J Med 341:70-76, 1999.

40. Serruys PW, de Feyter P, Macaya C, et al: Fluvastatin for prevention of cardiac events following successful first percutaneous coronary intervention: A randomized controlled trial. JAMA 287:3215-3222, 2002.

41. Kjekshus JK, Pedersen TR, Olsson AG, et al: The effects of simvastatin on the incidence of heart failure in patients with coronary heart disease. J Card Fail 3:249-254, 1997.

42. Niebauer J, Volk HD, Kemp M, et al: Endotoxin and immune activation in chronic heart failure: A prospective cohort study Lancet 353:1938-1842, 1999.

43. Rauchhaus M, Coats AJ, Anker SD: The endotoxin-lipoprotein hypothesis. Lancet 356:930-933, 2000.

44. Rauchhaus M, Doehner W, Davos CH, et al: Serum total cholesterol high density lipoprotein and prognosis in patients with chronic heart failure. J Am Coll Cardiol (Suppl):156A, 2001.

45. DiNapoli P, Taccardi AA, Oliver M, DeCaterina R: Statins and stroke: Evidence for cholesterol-independent effects. Eur Heart J 23:1908-1921, 2002.

46. Mietinen TA, Pyorala K, Olsson AG, et al: Cholesterol lowering therapy in women and elderly patients with myocardial infarction or angina pectoris: Findings from the Scandinavian Simvastatin Survival Study (4S). Circulation 96:4211-4218, 1997.
47. Pyorala K, Pedersen TR, Kjekshus J, et al: Cholesterol lowering with simvastatin improves prognosis of diabetic patients with coronary heart disease. Diabetes Care 4:614-620, 1997.
48. Freeman DJ, Norrie J, Sattar N, et al: Pravastatin and development of diabetes mellitus: Evidence for a protective treatment effect in the West of Scotland Coronary Prevention Study. Circulation 103:357-362, 2001.
49. Pedersen TP, Kjekshus J, Pyorala K, et al: Effect of simvastatin on ischemic signs and symptoms in the Scandinavian Simvastatin Survival Study (4S). Am J Cardiol 81:333-335, 1998.
50. De Backer G, Ambrosioni E, Borch-Johnson K, et al: European guidelines on cardiovascular disease prevention in clinical practice: Third Joint Task Force of European and Other Societies on Cardiovascular Disease Prevention in Clinical Practice. Eur J Cardiovasc Prev Rehabil 10:S1-S10, 2003.

5

Statins and Reduction of Stroke: Cholesterol-Lowering versus Pleiotropic Effects

Raffaele De Caterina, Francesco Palma, and Pericle Di Napoli

Many drugs, even when they modulate only a single target or metabolic step, have multiple effects because of the different functions that the target pathway or function plays in different organs or tissues. Therefore, pleiotropy (from the Greek *pleio* for "multiple" and *tropos* for "direction, or turn") is common in pharmacology. Far from being ideal (e.g., Paul Ehrlich's "magic bullets"), drugs usually exert multiple effects on an organism. These may be related or unrelated to the primary mode of action of the drug. Pleiotropic effects may emerge during preclinical and clinical studies in drug development but, more often, are discovered a posteriori, long after the therapeutic agent is marketed. They may be undesirable and recognized as adverse side effects, they may be neutral, or they may be beneficial, enhancing the desirable effect of the drug.

In recent years, major clinical trials and ancillary mechanistic studies have provided growing evidence that part of the impressive effects of statins, the most widely prescribed lipid-lowering agents, on the occurrence or recurrence of vascular events could be ascribed to their pleiotropism. As discussed in this chapter, the effects of statins on stroke are likely to be the manifestations of statins' pleiotropy, and pleiotropy, in contrast with cholesterol lowering, may play different roles in different cardiovascular diseases. The reduction of stroke by statins is most likely a manifestation of a cholesterol-independent effect, contrary to the better known effect of statins on events attributable to coronary heart disease (CHD).

6

BACKGROUND: STROKE AS AN IMPORTANT TARGET FOR PREVENTION IN THE AGING POPULATION

Stroke is the third leading cause of death in the United States after heart disease and cancer. An estimated 500,000 to 600,000 first strokes occur in the United States each year, and approximately 160,000 of these are fatal, with considerable long-term disability among survivors.[1] Stroke is also a major cause of death across Europe. Recently mortality rates from stroke appear to have decreased in the most affluent western European countries, but they are increasing in central and eastern European countries.[2,3] Although it is not clear whether these changes in mortality reflect variation in death certification, medical management, or true variations in incidence,[4] life expectancy is increasing and the population of the Western world is aging: the proportion of people older than 60 years is expected to rise in Europe from 20% in 2000 to 37% in 2050. Because of the aging of the population, the proportion of individuals at risk for stroke will increase. Stroke is a major cause of disability and is responsible for the most disability-adjusted life-years lost among people 60 years and older.[5] Approximately 20% of patients having their first stroke will die within the first month,[4] and a third of those surviving up to 6 months will be dependent on others for their daily activities. Consequently, stroke places a large burden on healthcare and social service resources, and methods of preventing strokes or improving outcomes are required to reduce this burden.

Many of the risk factors for the development of CHD are also risk factors for stroke. It may be that controlling these risk factors will also reduce the incidence of stroke. One main exception in this pattern is hypercholesterolemia. Although the role of hypercholesterolemia in the pathogenesis of CHD has been clearly established, its contribution to the incidence of stroke and the benefits of lipid-lowering therapy are less well defined. Recently, the potential benefit of one class of cholesterol-lowering compounds, statins, in preventing stroke has been strongly supported by data in the literature. This effect is likely to be the result of ancillary properties of statins, other than those leading to cholesterol reduction, and it may lead to the use of statins (possibly as neuroprotective agents) for stroke.

HISTORY OF STATINS

First introduced into clinical practice in the late 1980s, several years after the discovery of their lipid-lowering effects,[6] the 3-hydroxy-3-methylglutaryl coenzyme A (HMG-CoA) reductase inhibitors (statins) reduce cholesterol synthesis through a competitive inhibition of HMG-CoA reductase, an enzyme that catalyzes the rate-limiting conversion step of HMG-CoA to mevalonate.[7] This leads to increased expression of low-density-lipoprotein (LDL) receptors,[8] ultimately leading to the reduction of LDL plasma concentration.

Ample epidemiologic data have suggested that hypercholesterolemia is a powerful risk factor for CHD.[9,10] In addition, different cholesterol-lowering drugs or nonpharmacologic treatments can significantly reduce morbidity from CHD,[11-19] thus proving a causal role for cholesterol in coronary events. Cholesterol seems, however, to play little or no role in the pathogenesis of cerebrovascular accidents, including stroke.[20,21] Recent clinical trials and surrogate endpoint data, however, strongly suggest that statins protect against stroke.[14,19,22-27] We will analyze this apparent paradox here and review the evidence for pleiotropic effects of statins playing a substantial role in preventing stroke and cerebrovascular accidents.

STATINS EXERT MOST OF THEIR EFFECTS ON CHD BY REDUCING CHOLESTEROL

The Framingham Heart study,[9] the Multiple Risk Factor Intervention Trial (MRFIT),[28] and the Prospective Cardiovascular Münster (PROCAM) study all established a positive relationship between elevated serum cholesterol concentrations and CHD. Data from the MRFIT and Pooling Project[29] have clearly established that there is an exponential increase in the risk for CHD with an increase of plasma cholesterol. Subsequently, large-scale lipid-lowering intervention trials, predominantly in patients with established CHD, demonstrated that lowering plasma cholesterol, and specifically, LDL cholesterol, can halt the progression and even induce some regression of preexisting coronary atherosclerosis[30-32] and significantly decrease the risk for clinical coronary events.[33-39] The effectiveness of lipid-lowering therapy in reducing CHD morbidity was first established in a series of intervention trials using either dietary interventions or first-generation hypolipidemic drugs (now less used), such as fibrates, niacin, or colestipol.[11,40,41]

The strongest and most compelling evidence about the impact of lipid-lowering therapy on progression (and even regression) of preexisting coronary atherosclerosis and decreased risk for clinical coronary events has come, however, from intervention trials with statins.[30,31,42] Here, for the first time, intervention trials with a lipid-lowering treatment have shown a significant reduction in coronary and all-cause mortality. This important conclusion is most likely possible because of the large size of recent statin trials and the magnitude of the cholesterol reduction achieved. A comparative meta-analysis of six statin and nine nonstatin trials, in both primary and secondary prevention, indeed showed that the degree of cholesterol lowering is an excellent predictor of cardiovascular event reduction, independent of the intervention (statin or nonstatin).[43] This conclusion is unchanged with the inclusion of the more recent Air Force/Texas Coronary Atherosclerosis Prevention Study (AFCAPS/TexCAPS),[42] the MIRACL trial,[26] the Antihypertensive and Lipid-Lowering Treatment to Prevent Heart Attack Trial—Lipid-Lowering Treatment Arm (ALLHAT-LLT),[44] and the Anglo-Scandinavian Cardiac Outcomes Trial Lipid-Lowering Arm (ASCOT-LLA).[45]

A subanalysis of AFCAPS/TexCAPS based on the levels of C-reactive protein (CRP) at entry has recently shown the efficacy of lovastatin in patients with below-median LDL cholesterol at entry but above-median CRP levels.[46] Although it may be that inflammation, reflected by high levels of CRP, may mark an increased cardiovascular risk, which can be reduced by lovastatin through cholesterol-independent mechanisms, such conclusions still would pertain to patients with a low HDL/LDL ratio, which may mark a statin-sensitive subset of patients even in the presence of "normal" LDL cholesterol levels.[47]

Figure 6-1 shows that the beneficial effect of statins (percentage reduction of CHD events as a function of percentage reduction of cholesterol) is on a similar regression line as that of other, nonstatin, cholesterol-lowering interventions and therefore fully explained by cholesterol lowering.[48,49] Data obtained from recent meta-analyses[50,51] suggests that the relationship between total cholesterol concentration and coronary events is curvilinear or log-linear with no further decrease in events expected below 150 mg/dL (corresponding to an LDL cholesterol concentration of 110 mg/dL), a result that is very similar to that found in the Cholesterol and Recurrent Events (CARE) trial. When LDL cholesterol levels are in this range, further lowering with statin therapy elicits diminishing returns in terms of CHD event rates.

The results obtained from more recent trials involving mixed (primary and secondary) prevention confirm the relevance of the reduction in total and LDL cholesterol in preventing cardiovascular events. The Heart Protection Study (HPS) included 20,536 patients with previous CHD or with a high risk for cardiovascular events with normal cholesterol levels or mild to moderate hypercholesterolemia.[27] It confirmed that simvastatin, 40 mg/day, reduces all-cause death (12.9% versus 14.7% in the placebo group, $P = .0003$) and cardiovascular death (5.7% versus 6.9% in the placebo group, $P = .0005$) during the 5-year follow-up, with a 20% reduction in total cholesterol also in patients with normal cholesterol at baseline (lower than 5 mmol/L [193 mg/dL]).

Another recent trial, the Prospective Study of Pravastatin in the Elderly at Risk (PROSPER), included 5804 patients with a history of, or risk factors for, vascular disease, and a mean total cholesterol of 6.1 mmol/L (221 mg/dL) during the 3.2 years of follow-up.[52] This trial reported that pravastatin treatment (40 mg/day) reduced primary endpoints (coronary death, nonfatal myocardial infarction, and stroke) to 408 events compared with

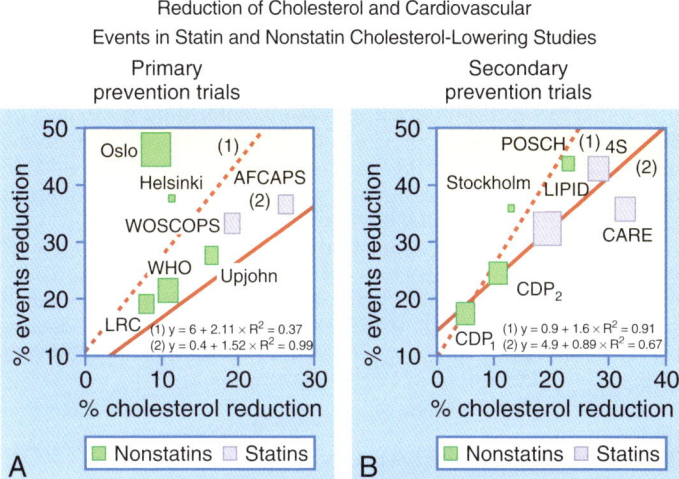

Reduction of Cholesterol and Cardiovascular
Events in Statin and Nonstatin Cholesterol-Lowering Studies

Figure 6-1 **Linear regression analysis between percentage reduction of cholesterol and cardiovascular events in statin and nonstatin cholesterol-lowering studies, subdivided into primary prevention (*A*) and secondary prevention (*B*) trials.** The area of each *square* is proportional to the sample size in the corresponding study. Note that the slope of the regression line is similar in statin and nonstatin studies. (Data collected from Lipid Research Clinics [LRC], Upjohn Trial, World Health Organization Clofibrate Trial [WHO], Oslo study, Helsinki Heart study, West of Scotland Coronary Prevention Study [WOSCOPS] Trial, and Air Force/ Texas Coronary Atherosclerosis Prevention Study [AFCAPS/TexCAPS] [primary prevention trials]; Coronary Drug Project with niacin [CDP$_1$] or clofibrate [CDP$_2$], Stockholm Ischaemic Heart Disease Trial, Program on the Surgical Control of the Hypercholesterolemia [POSCH] study, Scandinavian Simvastatin Survival Study [4S], Cholesterol and Recurrent Events [CARE] Trial, Long-term Intervention with Pravastatin in Ischemic Disease [LIPID] study [secondary prevention trials]. Cardiovascular events include coronary CHD deaths and nonfatal myocardial infarction [all trials], unstable angina, sudden cardiac death as first event [AFCAP/TexCAPS], resuscitated cardiac arrest [4S]. Data from the recent MIRACL study were not included because of the considerably shorter follow-up [16 weeks] and the difference in the definition of cardiovascular events, here also including objectively documented recurrent symptomatic myocardial ischemia requiring emergency rehospitalization.) Dotted lines (1) are the regression lines based on nonstatin cholesterol-lowering studies. Solid lines (2) are the regression lines based on statin studies.

473 in patients on placebo (hazard ratio 0.85, confidence interval [CI] 0.74-0.97, *P* = .014). Pravastatin lowered LDL cholesterol concentrations by 34% and total cholesterol by 23.4%.

Similar results, though in apparent contradiction, were seen in the recently published ALLHAT-LLT. In this trial, pravastatin treatment (40 mg/day) in 10,355 adults, with a mean age of 66 years and hypertension and moderate hypercholesterolemia (mean total cholesterol, 224 mg/100 dL, LDL cholesterol, 146 mg/100 dL) was unable to significantly reduce all-cause or CHD mortality when compared with usual care in patients with well-controlled hypertension and moderate hypercholesterolemia. However, the observed reduction of cholesterol was limited (17% in the pravastatin group and 9% in the usual-care group), and in dyslipidemic patients (28% of patients) the usual care also included other statins, fibrates, and a lipid-lowering diet.[44]

Overall, data are consistent in pointing to cholesterol reduction as a key explanation for the benefit of all cholesterol-lowering agents in coronary heart disease, with statins producing more significant benefits than other pharmacologic or dietary interventions because of their greater potency in achieving cholesterol reduction.

THE UNCERTAIN RELATIONSHIP OF CHOLESTEROL AND STROKE

In contrast to their established roles in the pathogenesis of CHD, raised plasma cholesterol and LDL cholesterol levels are less well established as important risk factors for cerebrovascular disease.[21,51,53,54] The reasons are likely to be many. Although nearly all CHD events are linked to coronary atheroma, less than half of strokes are due to large-vessel atheroma. Nonatheromatous causes of strokes, such as cardiac arrhythmias leading to cerebral emboli, cardiomyopathies, or intracranial vessel diseases, are responsible for most of the rest. Still, the majority of ischemic strokes are caused by thromboemboli arising from atheromatous disease (outside the brain, either from the carotid arteries or the aortic arch), in which hypercholesterolemia is commonly present. The contention that cholesterol lowering is effective in reducing carotid atheroma is supported by ultrasound measurements of carotid artery intima media thickness, independently shown to be a predictor of the occurrence of stroke.[55] Such measurements indeed show that reductions of plasma LDL cholesterol by 25% or more prevented any detectable progress in carotid intima media thickness and reduced the development of new lesions both in asymptomatic people and in patients younger than 75 years—as for coronary atheroma. Thus, the reduction of CHD with cholesterol-lowering therapy would still be expected to be accompanied by some reduction in the incidence of stroke.

Yet several studies suggest that raised total cholesterol levels do not predict stroke-related death. In some studies, cholesterol levels are actually inversely related to stroke death.[57] In the Framingham Heart study, total cholesterol level was related positively to stroke mortality only in women younger than 55 years.[9] In that study, there was actually an inverse relationship between cholesterol and short-term mortality from stroke for women older than 70 years. In a study from Israel, patients with stroke had lower cholesterol levels.[58]

This apparent contradiction may be a result of the composite etiology of stroke and the fact that, in earlier studies, thrombotic and hemorrhagic strokes were not differentiated. Indeed, epidemiologic data from the MRFIT[28] and the Helsinki Heart Study[59] suggest that hypercholesterolemia is a risk factor for nonhemorrhagic stroke. Observational data from the Honolulu Heart Program[60] and the MRFIT[61] suggested that there is a J-shaped relationship between serum cholesterol and total stroke, with increased risk only at very low and very high cholesterol. One explanation for this relationship may be that high cholesterol levels predispose an individual to atherothrombotic cerebral infarct, whereas low cholesterol levels may independently increase the risk for the less common variety of hemorrhagic stroke. However, the relationship between low cholesterol levels and hemorrhagic stroke needs further support,[36] and it has also been somewhat related to the presence of elevated blood pressure. When stroke etiologies are not classified but are simply pooled, there is clearly no relationship between cholesterol levels and stroke. An analysis of 45 prospective observational cohorts, reporting 13,397 strokes (independent of etiology) in 450,000 people, showed no independent association of baseline total cholesterol level and the cumulative risk for stroke.[62] In aggregate, even the relationship between raised total cholesterol and isolated thrombotic stroke is far less strong than between raised total cholesterol and CHD.[21]

CHOLESTEROL LOWERING AND STROKES—THE STATIN PARADOX

Two meta-analyses have reviewed the results of trials reported before 1995 and have suggested that lowering serum cholesterol through dietary modification or nonstatin drugs does not reduce stroke mortality or morbidity. Clofibrate, which has a more potent triglyceride-lowering and HDL-elevating effect than other cholesterol-lowering drugs, actually appeared to increase the risk for fatal stroke (odds ratio 2.64, 95% CI 1.42-4.92, $P = .002$) in spite of an 8% reduction of total serum cholesterol.[63] In the Program on the Surgical Control of the Hypercholesterolemia (POSCH) study, an intervention with partial ileal bypass surgery in patients with hypercholesterolemia and a previous myocardial infarction significantly reduced total and LDL cholesterol levels (by 23.3% and 37.7%, respectively) and the combined double endpoint (death due to CHD and confirmed nonfatal myocardial infarction) by 35% ($P < .001$). However, it failed to show any trend toward reduced cerebrovascular accidents ($P = .69$).[12]

In contrast, data from all the major statin trials indicate convincingly that these drugs reduce the incidence of stroke. In the Scandinavian Simvastatin Survival Study (4S, a secondary prevention trial), there was a significant reduction in the total number of fatal and nonfatal strokes (70 versus 98) in the simvastatin compared to the placebo group, although the numbers of deaths due to cerebrovascular accident were similar. Ischemic nonembolic strokes and transient ischemic attacks were reduced by 51% and 35%, respectively.[64] In the CARE trial, the pravastatin group had a 31% lower incidence of all strokes (P = .03), although again the incidence of fatal strokes was about the same. Of note, there was no increase in the rate of hemorrhagic stroke.[24] In the Long-term Intervention with Pravastatin in Ischemic Disease study (LIPID), a secondary prevention trial, pravastatin significantly reduced the incidence of stroke (19%, P = .022).[19,25] Only in the West of Scotland Coronary Prevention Study (WOSCOPS), a primary prevention trial, was the number of strokes similar in the pravastatin and in the placebo groups (46 versus 51, respectively; P = .67).[16] The reduction of strokes by statins was also confirmed in some short-term clinical studies.[22,23] Levels of total cholesterol lower than 160 mg/dL (4.16 mmol/L), which in MRFIT were associated with a higher risk for hemorrhagic stroke, did not lead to any increase in hemorrhagic stroke in the statin trials.

More recent trials have provided further strong evidence that statin therapy reduces stroke (Table 6-1). The MIRACL study has shown that atorvastatin, initiated 24 to 96 hours after an acute coronary event, reduces recurrent ischemic events in the first 16 weeks. In this trial, involving 3086 patients, there were no significant differences in the risk of death, nonfatal myocardial infarction, and cardiac arrest between the atorvastatin group (N = 1538) and the placebo group (N = 1548), although the atorvastatin group had a lower risk for symptomatic ischemia requiring emergency rehospitalization (6.2% versus 8.4%; relative risk 0.74, 95% CI, 0.57-0.95, P = .02). More interesting, and significantly, there were 50% fewer strokes in the atorvastatin than in the placebo group (12 versus 24, respectively; P = .045).[26,65]

The Heart Protection Study (HPS) also confirmed the reduction of stroke by simvastatin, 40 mg/day, and it suggested the absence of a relationship between cholesterol levels at entry and the reduction of stroke. In 20,536 patients with a high risk for vascular events, simvastatin treatment significantly reduced the risk for all-cause stroke (relative risk reduction 25%, CI 0.66-0.85, P < .00001). This also occurred in patients with relatively low levels of LDL cholesterol (<116 mg/dL [3.0 mmol/L]) and of total cholesterol (<193 mg/dL [5.0 mmol/L]).[27]

The PROSPER study recently reported that pravastatin treatment reduced the risk for coronary events but not for stroke.[52] However, it was noted that the stroke rate in PROSPER was half that predicted, and therefore the study was probably underpowered for a detection of a beneficial effect of statin treatment.[52] A small reduction in transient ischemic attacks (TIAs), of borderline statistical significance (P = .051), was observed in PROSPER, indicating that pravastatin may have had an effect on the cerebral

Table 6–1

Characteristics of the Newer Statin Trials

Study	Year	Prevention Type	Follow-Up (yr)	Total Cholesterol Reduction (%)	Sample Size (T/C)	All Stroke (T/C)	TIA (T/C)	Stroke Reduction (%)	95% CI
MIRACL[65]	2001	Secondary	0.3	34	1.538/1.548	12/24	—	50	0.49 (0.2-0.98), P < .0001
HPS[27]	2002	Mixed	5	20	10.269/10.267	444/585	—	25	0.75 (0.66-0.85), P < .0001
ALL-HAT[44]	2002	Mixed	8	9.6	5.170/5.185	209/231	—	10	0.91 (0.75-1.09), P = .31
PROSPER[52]	2002	Mixed	3.2	23	2.891/2.913	135/131	77/102 RRR –25%, P = .051	—	—
ASCOT-LLA[45]	2003	Mixed	3.3	24	5.168/5.137	89/121	—	27	0.73 (0.56-0.96), P = .024

C, control; CI, confidence interval; RRR, relative risk reduction; T, treatment; TIA, transient ischemic attack.

6

circulation. The ability of statins to prevent TIAs is also suggested in a small case report study.[66] The effectiveness of statins in preventing stroke in patients with a prior cerebrovascular event has yet to be demonstrated in prospective randomized trials. An ongoing trial, the Stroke Prevention by Aggressive Reduction of Cholesterol Levels (SPARCL), is now examining the effect of statin treatment on cerebrovascular events in patients with prior stroke or TIA.

The recently published data from the ALLHAT-LLT study are somewhat in conflict with this general pattern. Here, pravastatin treatment (40 mg/day) given to 10,355 adults (mean age, 66 years) with hypertension and moderate hypercholesterolemia (total cholesterol 224 mg/100 dL, LDL cholesterol 146 mg/100 dL) was unable to significantly reduce all-cause mortality, coronary heart disease, or stroke when compared with usual care in patients with well-controlled hypertension and moderate hypercholesterole-mia.[44] However, the lack of benefit observed in the ALLHAT-LLT study may reflect reduced patient adherence to therapy, high crossover rates, and the lower risk status of the participants.[67]

Recent meta-analyses have accumulated the numbers of strokes in all trials using statins to prevent CHD (Table 6-2). In aggregate, statin treatment appears to reduce the risk for stroke significantly. Secondary prevention trials demonstrated a significant reduction in cerebrovascular events, whereas primary prevention trials showed only trends toward reductions in the stroke rate, probably because of the lower risk for stroke in this setting.[71] In one meta-analysis comprising 21,303 patients, statin treatment significantly reduced all-cause death (−24%) and nonfatal strokes (−32%), although the numbers of fatal strokes were similar in the treatment group and in the placebo group.[69]

These benefits of statin therapy appear largely unrelated in magnitude to cholesterol reduction,[72] as shown—for both statin and nonstatin trials—in Figure 6-2. From a comparison with Figure 6-1, one can appreciate the difference between the slopes of regression lines in CHD and those in stroke, which argues against a role of cholesterol in explaining any of the effects of interventions in stroke. Yet the question of the causal relationship between cholesterol reduction and the occurrence of stroke remains open and incompletely resolved. Quite controversial are the recent data obtained from the meta-analysis of Corvol and colleagues, where the effect of cholesterol reduction on stroke is evident.[70] Here the reduction of relative risk (29%) with cholesterol lowering is evident, but this appears to be stronger when the total cholesterol level is decreased to lower than 232 mg/100 dL (6.0 mmol/L). This magnitude of reduction is easily obtained using only statins as lipid-lowering agents. Occasionally, some reduction of stroke is shown with nonstatin drugs, such as fibrates, but in this case it is not clearly related to cholesterol reduction. The Veterans Affairs High-Density Lipoprotein Cholesterol Intervention Trial (VA-HIT)

Table 6–2

Statin Therapy and Stroke: Results from Main Meta-Analyses

Reference	Sample Size		Strokes (Fatal and Nonfatal)		Relative Reduction in Rates (%)	95% CI
	Statin	Placebo	Statin	Placebo		
Crouse et al.[71]						
PPT	3,908	3,900	48	56	15	0.27-0.42 (P = .48)
SPT	5,862	5,848	134	192	31	0.13-0.45 (P = .001)
PSPT	9,770	9,748	182	248	27	0.11-0.40 (P = .001)
Hebert et al.	16,826	11,875	193	261	29	0.59-0.88 (P = .001)
Ross et al.[69]	10,387	10,199	74	97	23	0.57-1.04 (fatal stroke)
			106	159	33	0.54-0.88 (nonfatal stroke)
Blauw et al.[68]	10,314	10,124	181	261	31	0.57-0.83 (P < .001)
Corvol et al.[70]	39,943	43,218	672	939	29	0.66-0.87 (P < .001)

CI, confidence interval; PPT, primary prevention trials; SPT, secondary prevention trials; PSPT, primary and secondary prevention trials.

Reduction of Cholesterol and All-Cause Strokes
in Statin and Nonstatin Cholesterol-Lowering Studies

Nonstatin trials

Statin trials

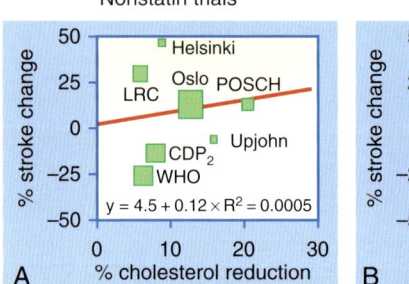

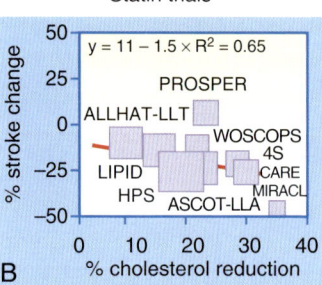

Figure 6-2 **Linear regression analysis between percentage reduction of cholesterol and all-cause strokes in nonstatin (A) and statin (B) cholesterol-lowering studies.** The area of each *square* is proportional to the sample size of the corresponding study. Note the absence of any relationship between cholesterol reduction and all-cause strokes, in both nonstatin and statin trials. Thus, despite the reduction of stroke in statin trials (see text), it appears unlikely that these favorable effects are mediated by cholesterol reduction. (Data collected from Lipid Research Clinics [LRC], Upjohn Trial, World Health Organization Clofibrate Trial [WHO], Oslo Study, Helsinki Heart Study, West of Scotland Coronary Prevention Study [WOSCOPS] Trial, Program on the Surgical Control of the Hypercholesterolemia [POSCH] Study, Air Force/Texas Coronary Atherosclerosis Prevention Study [AFCAPS/TexCAPS], Coronary Drug Project [CDP], Stockholm Ischaemic Heart Disease Trial, Scandinavian Simvastatin Survival Study [4S], Cholesterol and Recurrent Events [CARE] Trial, Long-term Intervention with Pravastatin in Ischemic Disease [LIPID] study, Myocardial Ischemia Reduction with Aggressive Cholesterol Lowering [MIRACL] study, Antihypertensive and Lipid-lowering Treatment to Prevent Heart Attack Trial [ALLHAT-LLT], Prospective Study of Pravastatin in the Elderly at Risk [PROSPER] study, Heart Protection study [HPS], and Anglo-Scandinavian Cardiac Outcomes Trial—Lipid-Lowering Arm [ASCOT-LLA].)

6

recently demonstrated that, despite a reduction of total cholesterol of only 4.4% in 1267 patients with coronary artery disease and low levels of high-density-lipoprotein (HDL) cholesterol, gemfibrozil treatment reduced all-cause strokes by 37%.[73] These findings, apparently in contradiction with previous data on fibrates, await further confirmation. Overall, it appears wise to consider other ways by which statins might protect against strokes.

CHOLESTEROL-INDEPENDENT NEUROPROTECTIVE PROPERTIES OF STATINS

Statins competitively inhibit HMG-CoA reductase, an early step of cholesterol biosynthesis, thus decreasing the production of

Schematic Representation of the Mevalonate Pathway and the Origin of Isoprenoids

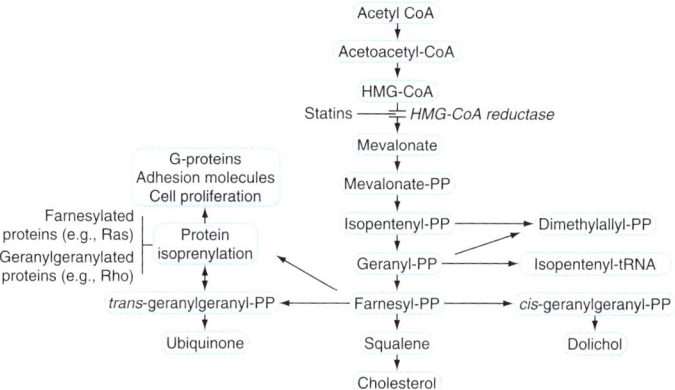

Figure 6-3 **Schematic representation of the mevalonate pathway and the origin of isoprenoids.** Isoprenoids are derivatives of intermediates in cholesterol biosynthesis and have a number of actions, including effects on G proteins, adhesion molecules, and cell proliferation. Isopentenyl pyrophosphate is involved in transfer RNA synthesis; dolichol in plasma membrane fluidity; ubiquinone in mitochondrial respiration; and geranyl and farnesyl pyrophosphate in the posttranslational modification of a number of intracellular regulatory proteins. HMG-CoA, hydroxymethylglutaryl coenzyme A; PP, pyrophosphate.

mevalonate and other subsequent intermediates in the mevalonate pathway (Fig. 6-3). These include isopentenyl pyrophosphate, involved in transfer-RNA synthesis; dolichol, which is involved in plasma membrane fluidity; ubiquinone, involved in mitochondrial respiration; and geranyl and farnesyl pyrophosphate, which are involved in the posttranslational modification of a number of intracellular regulatory proteins.[8,74] Therefore, the inhibition of HMG-CoA reductase will probably have multiple effects (see Fig. 6-3). Some of these are likely candidates to explain statin effects in stroke prevention and in reduction of brain damage (Table 6-3).[75-77]

Statin effects that help explain protection from stroke are those causing stabilization or regression of atherosclerosis in both the coronary and carotid arteries ("cholesterol-dependent" effects), and effects on endothelial function and the inflammatory response elicited by ischemic and peroxidative damage ("cholesterol-independent" effects)[75-78] (Fig. 6-4).

These can be grouped into (1) effects explained by the influence of statins on nitric oxide bioavailability, (2) anti-inflammatory effects, (3) anti-thrombotic effects, and (4) antioxidant effects.

Table 6–3

Main Neuroprotective Properties of Statins in Cerebral Ischemia and Stroke

Cholesterol-Lowering–Dependent Effects
Stabilization/regression of atherosclerosis outside the brain
Favorable hemorrheologic and antithrombotic properties
Cholesterol-Lowering–Independent Effects
Endothelium
Modulation of eNOS, nNOS, and iNOS
   Inhibition of leukocyte and platelet adhesion
   Vasodilation
   Maintenance of a thromboresistant interface between the
     bloodstream and the vessel wall
   Favorable hemorrheologic and antithrombotic properties
Inflammatory Processes
Reduction of monocyte adhesion molecules (CD 11b/CD 18-Mac-1)
   Reduced isoprenylation of leukocyte G proteins
   Reduced isoprenoid-dependent anchoring
   Reduced dimerization of adhesion molecules such as CD11b/CD18
     on monocytes
Reduction of other cellular adhesion molecules (CAM) (P-selectin,
   VCAM-1, and ICAM-1)
Modulation of central nervous system cytokine production by
   decreasing isoprenylation of proteins involved in intracellular
   signaling and inflammation
   Modulation of adhesion molecule expression on cerebral
     endothelium and inflammatory cells
   Inhibition of inflammatory cell migration
   Reduction of thrombogenesis through inhibition of tissue factor
     expression
   Reduction of interleukin (IL)-1β, tumor necrosis factor
     (TNF)-α–induced neuronal apoptosis
Antioxidant Effects
Reduction of lipoprotein oxidation and amelioration of free radical
   injury
   Increase of α-tocopherol-to-total cholesterol ratio
   Preservation of superoxide dismutase (SOD) activity
   Preservation of the paraoxonase system

Nitric Oxide–Dependent Neuroprotective Effects of Statins

Among the various cholesterol-independent statin effects, those on nitric oxide (NO) are likely to be highly clinically relevant. In the cerebral endothelium and parenchyma, statins may regulate all the different isoforms of nitric oxide synthase (NOS).[75,77,79] NO produced by the constitutive endothelial NOS (eNOS, NOS III) has a protective role in ischemic conditions, regulating leukocyte and platelet adhesion and activation, inducing vasodilation and reducing postischemic hyperpermeability,[76] and maintaining the antithrombotic properties of the vessel wall (Fig. 6-5). The

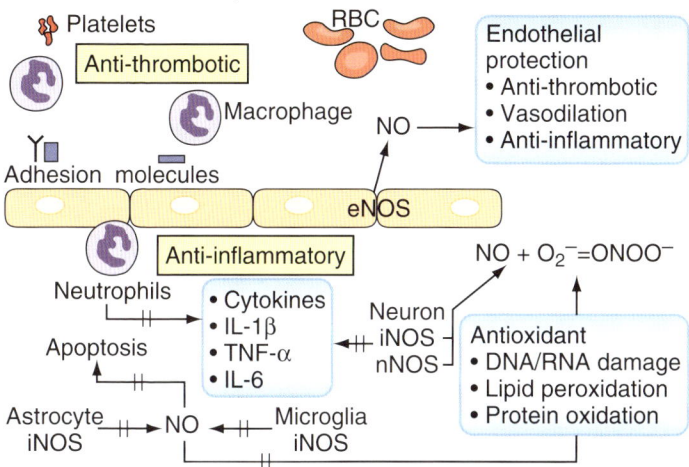

Figure 6-4 **Neuroprotective action of statins.** Statins preserve endothelial function and exert antioxidant, anti-inflammatory, antiapoptotic, and antithrombotic effects that are neuroprotective during cerebral hypoxia, ischemia, and reperfusion. eNOS, endothelial nitric oxide synthase; IL, interleukin; iNOS, inducible nitric oxide synthase; nNOS, neuronal nitric oxide synthase; NO, nitric oxide; O_2^-, superoxide anion; $ONOO^-$, peroxynitrite; RBC, red blood cells; TNF, tumor necrosis factor.

importance of eNOS activity in the cerebral circulation is shown by the fact that eNOS knockout mice (lacking the gene for this enzyme) have larger cerebral infarcts after middle cerebral artery occlusion, and the administration of nitro-L-arginine induces a reduction of infarct size. In spontaneously hypertensive rats, enhanced NO availability, either by the administration of NO donor (3-morpholinosydnonimine)[80] or the eNOS substrate L-arginine,[83] also confers protection from stroke. The inducible form of NOS (iNOS, NOS II), produced by astrocytes, neutrophils, and the microglia after stimulation with a series of proinflammatory mediators, also contributes to the inflammatory response in conjunction with cytokines such as tumor necrosis factor-α (TNF-α), interleukin (IL)-1β, and IL-6.[79,84,85] Iadecola and co-workers have reported that mice lacking the iNOS gene have a significant reduction in the volume of cerebral infarcts.[86] Excessive NO production after inflammatory stimulation leads to an enhanced reaction of NO with superoxide anion,[76] with increased production of peroxynitrite, and may in turn be responsible for increased peroxidative damage in the brain parenchyma and the vascular wall. This occurs through enhanced neuronal and endothelial cell apoptosis and the promotion of oxidative damage of cellular DNA and RNA, proteins, and membrane lipids.[76,79,87] The neuronal NOS

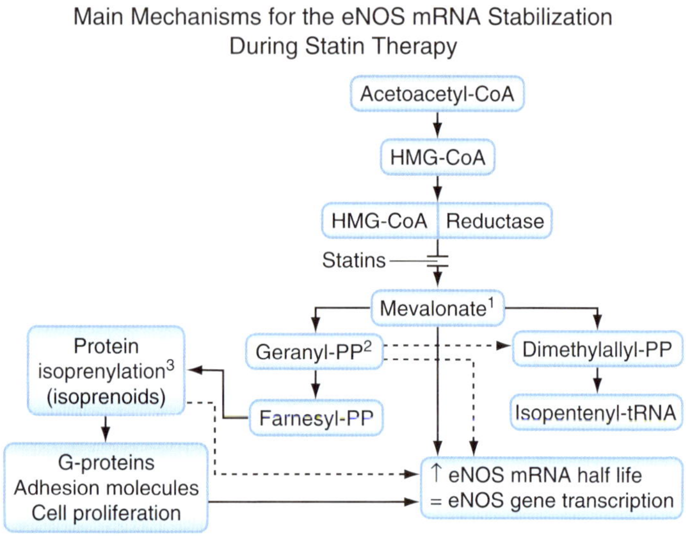

Main Mechanisms for the eNOS mRNA Stabilization
During Statin Therapy

Figure 6-5 Schematic representation of the main mechanisms for eNOS mRNA stabilization during statin therapy. Three main mechanisms contribute to eNOS mRNA instabilization through the mevalonate pathway: (1) L-mevalonate stimulates proteins that bind to a sequence motif (AUUUA) in the 3'-untranslated region of eNOS mRNA, (2) geranyl-geranylation is necessary for the proper function of Rho GTPases, favoring eNOS mRNA degradation, and (3) isoprenoids contribute to cell proliferation, which favors eNOS mRNA degradation (eNOS mRNA stability is cell cycle dependent). By inhibiting these mechanisms, statins stabilize eNOS mRNA, leaving eNOS mRNA synthesis unaltered. The net result is an increase in eNOS mRNA steady-state concentration and protein. eNOS, endothelial nitric oxide synthase; HMG-CoA, 3-hydroxy-3-methylglutaryl coenzyme A; PP, pyrophosphate.

(nNOS, NOS I) is also actively involved in ischemia and reperfusion injury of brain parenchyma, being able to promote oxidative damage and glutamate-mediated cytotoxicity.[88] Morikawa and colleagues have reported that nNOS contributes to the development of ischemic brain necrosis.[83]

Statin therapy favorably modifies the balance of NO production. Statins augment cerebral blood flow, reducing cerebral infarct size and improving neurologic outcome in normocholesterolemic mice; this is concomitant with increased eNOS activity, without any changes in nNOS expression. The blood flow and neuroprotective effects of statins, evident also in stroke-prone strains of normocholesterolemic rodents, are completely absent in eNOS-deficient mice, indicating that enhanced eNOS activity by HMG-CoA reductase inhibitors is the predominant mechanism by which these agents protect against cerebral injury.

Experimental studies also suggest that statin therapy reduces the cytokine-mediated up-regulation of iNOS.[89] This inhibition may suppress the inflammatory response accompanying acute ischemia, which contributes to the ischemic damage of brain parenchyma. These observations are consistent with those in several experimental models of ischemia or hypoxia. In human endothelial cells exposed to hypoxia, statins increase NO production by modulating eNOS mRNA stability.[90,91] In normocholesterolemic rat hearts, statins decrease polymorphonucleate adhesion after ischemia and reperfusion.[92] Statins also reduce myocardial damage in isolated perfused working hearts from normocholesterolemic rats by increasing eNOS and reducing iNOS expression.[93] These effects on NOS and cerebral microvasculature may also contribute to the explanations for the recent observed reduction of the risk for dementia in patients treated with statins.[1,94]

These effects of statins on NOS are likely to result from a modulation of isoprenoid synthesis. Isoprenylation is important for the vesicular targeting of membrane proteins, including eNOS.[95] In particular, farnesylation is necessary for the anchoring of G proteins, such as p21^{ras}, to cell membrane. This modulates receptor-mediated eNOS activity through effects on membrane fluidity and cell growth.[96] Farnesylation of the γ subunit of certain G proteins may also be involved in the modulation of Ca^{2+} entry, an important step in reperfusion injury.[97] Among G proteins, small GTPases are an important target for pleiotropic effects of statins.[98] These GTPases, among which are Rho, Rac, and Cdc42, act as molecular switches, capable of regulating cell function, polarity, protrusion and adhesion (cytoskeletal response), synthesis and migration of DNA, phospholipase D activation, sensitivity of cell responses to Ca^{2+}, and myocyte hypertrophy. Rho proteins, in particular, have a role in accelerating eNOS mRNA degradation.[99] An inhibition of rho occurs by reduced prenylation, as a consequence of HMG-CoA reductase inhibition by statins, and therefore leads to a reduced eNOS mRNA degradation and higher levels of eNOS protein and activity.[100,101] The eNOS mRNA stabilization by statins may also be caused by L-mevalonate stimulation of proteins that bind to a sequence motif (AUUUA) in the 3′–untranslated region of eNOS mRNA, which is known to mediate mRNA destabilization via protein-mRNA interactions.[102] In addition, because eNOS mRNA stability is cell cycle dependent, statins may stabilize eNOS mRNA indirectly by regulating the cell cycle of vascular endothelial cells.[90]

Anti-Inflammatory and Antiatherothrombotic Effects of Statins

The relationship between inflammation and atherosclerosis and its complications have received increasing attention. Inflammatory cell infiltration is commonly observed in atherosclerotic plaques. A variety of circulating markers of inflammation, including CRP, serum amyloid A protein (SAA), heat shock protein 65, IL-6, and a number of leukocyte adhesion molecules,[103-106] have been shown to predict either the extent of atherosclerosis or the risk of vascular events. Atherosclerosis is prevented when genes of some mediators of the inflammatory response (such as monocyte chemoattractant protein-1 [MCP-1], IL-8, or macrophage–colony-stimulating factor [M-CSF]) are eliminated by gene knockout in atherosclerosis-prone dyslipidemic mice.[107,108]

A pivotal role in the origin, progression, and destabilization of atheroma is played by several protein families involved in the adhesion and activation of inflammatory cells in vessel walls, such as selectins, intercellular adhesion molecule-1 (ICAM-1), and vascular cell adhesion molecule-1 (VCAM-1).[108] Inflammatory cells play a key role in promoting plaque destabilization: they stimulate matrix degradation and inhibit smooth muscle cell (SMC) function or survival, and they may lead to thrombosis by increasing tissue factor expression. Inflammatory cells can erode the fibrous cap of atheroma by releasing various matrix metalloproteinases and inhibiting matrix synthesis by SMCs. In particular, it has been shown that interferon-γ, an inflammatory cytokine produced by activated T cells, can down-regulate collagen synthesis by human SMCs in vitro.[109] Inflammatory cells are also cytotoxic to SMC and can induce apoptotic cell death.[108] There are also suggestions for a role of viral[110] or bacterial (e.g., *Helicobacter pylori*[111] or *Chlamydia pneumoniae*[112]) infections in promoting inflammation and plaque destabilization, but these need confirmation.[113,114]

HMG-CoA reductase inhibitors have been shown to inhibit several pathways in inflammatory processes that occur in plaque destabilization, cerebral hypoxia, ischemia, and reperfusion (see Table 6-3). Statins reduce leukocyte-endothelium interactions occurring either in hypercholesterolemic[115] or in normocholesterolemic conditions,[78,79] and they inhibit monocyte adhesion to the endothelium by reducing the endothelial expression of P-selectin, ICAM-1, and VCAM-1 as well as the number of monocytes expressing Mac-1, one of the ICAM-1 ligands.[103,116] In hypercholesterolemic humans, simvastatin and lovastatin reduce monocyte expression of CD11b/CD18, another ICAM-1 ligand.[116] These effects, mediated through reduced isoprenylation of leukocyte G proteins or reduced isoprenoid-dependent anchoring or dimerization of adhesion molecules such as CD11b/CD18 on monocytes, are involved in reducing ischemic cell damage after cerebral artery occlusion. These antiadhesion molecule effects appear to be dependent on enhanced NO production, because statins failed to ameliorate the high leukocyte rolling and adherence in eNOS-deficient mice. Anti-inflammatory effects of statins have been confirmed by recent data.[104] An analysis of the CARE study shows a reduction of cerebral and coronary ischemic events during pravastatin treatment, related to reduced CRP levels.[104] Similarly, CRP analysis of baseline and year 1 frozen sera from the AFCAPS/TexCAPS study has shown that CRP levels are significantly reduced by lovastatin treatment, 20 to 40 mg/day, in patients free of acute major coronary events ($P < .001$ between treatment group difference).[117] Data from the Pravastatin Inflammation/CRP Evaluation (PRINCE) indicate that statin treatment can significantly reduce serum CRP. Following 24 weeks of therapy with pravastatin, CRP levels were reduced by 13% in primary and secondary prevention populations, whereas placebo treatment of subjects in the primary prevention arm of the study had no effect ($P < .001$).[118] Although not always clearly demonstrated in normocholesterolemic conditions, these effects are likely to occur—at least in part—independently of cholesterol lowering[46] and the percentage change in CRP is not related to the percentage change in LDL cholesterol.[119]

Statins also modulate central nervous system production of cytokines such as TNF-α, IL-1β, and IL-6. The demonstration that these effects are reversible with the co-administration of mevalonate or farnesyl pyrophosphate also suggests the involvement of decreased isoprenylation by statins of proteins implicated in intracellular signaling and inflammation.[74] Recently, anti-inflammatory effects of statins have also been shown in human immune cells exposed to *Chlamydia pneumoniae*,[120] an agent linked to increased cardiovascular risk.

Antithrombotic Effects of Statins

Statins also exert beneficial antithrombotic effects. Acute ischemic stroke has been shown to be associated with elevation of prothrombotic markers such as fibrinogen, plasminogen activator inhibitor-1 (PAI-1), and thrombin–antithrombin III complexes.[76,121] Statins reduce enhanced platelet reactivity accompanying hyper-cholesterolemia, although it is not clear if such an effect occurs independently of cholesterol reduction,[122] and the thrombogenic potential of atheroma,[123] which is also independent of cholesterol levels.[124] Statins also directly influence the local fibrinolytic balance (inhibiting PAI-1 expression and increasing tissue type plasminogen activator, tPA, within the vessel wall), promoting fibrinolysis and thus reducing the thrombotic risk after plaque rupture.[125,126] By reducing the local expression of PAI-1 by SMCs within vascular lesions while increasing tPA expression by luminal endothelial cells, statins may tip the local fibrinolytic balance toward increased fibrinolysis, which would limit the extent of thrombus formation that follows plaque rupture. On the other hand, increased local fibrinolysis may also promote extracellular matrix degradation (activation of matrix metalloproteinases), which in turn may destabilize advanced atherosclerotic plaques.[126] However, most experimental results show that statins actually inhibit matrix metalloproteinase activity, thus probably leading also to a reduced risk for plaque rupture.[127]

Antioxidant Effects of Statins

Statins may also exert neuroprotection through antioxidant effects. These may contribute to reduced early atherogenesis, where LDL oxidation plays a key role in contributing to cholesterol accumulation in macrophages, foam cell formation, cytotoxicity, thrombosis, and inflammation.[128-130] Moreover, in the presence of oxidized LDL, the G-protein–dependent stimulation of NO release is interrupted, and the physiologic action of NO is directly blocked by lipid peroxidation products.[129] Oxidative injury is also directly involved in the development and progression of neuronal cell death in acute and chronic diseases of the central nervous system. Oxidative stress to the central nervous system predominantly causes enhanced lipid peroxidation because of the high content of lipids and, particularly, of polyunsaturated fatty acids, which are highly susceptible to oxidation. The central nervous system is particularly rich in the highly unsaturated docosahexaenoic acid, with six double bonds and therefore very liable to peroxidation.[131]

One important action of statins is their ability to scavenge oxygen-derived free radicals in a concentration-dependent manner. A variety of statins, including simvastatin, fluvastatin, atorvastatin, pravastatin, and cerivastatin, share this property.[78] Fluvastatin has also been claimed to scavenge hydroxyl radicals.[130] Some of the superoxide-scavenging actions of statins may be a result of their reduction in the biosynthesis of isoprenoids. Some superoxide-generating systems (e.g., the NAD(P)H oxidase system) are indeed isoprenylated proteins, and the inhibition of isoprenylation by statins would reduce the catalytic efficiency of these free radical generators.[75] Through still unclear mechanisms, statins have also been shown to reduce leukocyte-induced LDL oxidation,[132] increase the α-tocopherol-to-total cholesterol ratio,[133] and preserve the HDL-paraoxonase enzymatic system, which is consumed during HDL cholesterol oxidation.[133] Metabolites of atorvastatin have been shown to protect HDL cholesterol against oxidation and have a paraoxonase-sparing effect, protecting HDL cholesterol–associated paraoxonase activity against oxidative degradation.[134] Finally, statins may exert broader antioxidant effects through preservation of superoxide dismutase activity[135] and the inhibition of cytokine-mediated up-regulation of iNOS,[89] which would otherwise promote the inflammatory response and oxidative damage through the increased production of peroxynitrite that accompanies acute ischemia. These antioxidant effects have been considered as a possible explanation for the reported reduction of chronic cerebral degenerative diseases, such as Alzheimer's disease, by statins.[1,94,136]

CONCLUSIONS

There is persuasive evidence that statins protect from ischemic stroke. This effect is probably multifactorial and caused not only by atheroma stabilization in extracranial arteries and a reduction of CHD (reducing sources for thromboembolism), but also by direct neuroprotection. The latter appears to be largely independent of LDL cholesterol reduction and probably linked to reduction of isoprenoid intermediates in the mevalonate pathway.

Clinical and experimental data confirm the existence of endo-thelium-protective, anti-inflammatory, antithrombotic, and anti-oxidant properties of statins that could extend the usefulness of this class of drugs in the management of cerebrovascular disease in patients with or without hypercholesterolemia. The effects of statins on stroke are presently the best available evidence for the existence of clinically relevant cholesterol-independent "pleiotropic" effects of these drugs.

References

1. Vaughan C: Prevention of stroke and dementia with statins: Effects beyond lipid lowering. Am J Cardiol 91:23B-29B, 2003.
2. Sans S, Kesteloot H, Kromhout D: The burden of cardiovascular disease mortality in Europe. Eur Heart J 18:1231-1248, 1997.
3. Sarti C, Rastenyte D, Cepaitis Z, Tuomilehto J: International trends in mortality from stroke, 1968 to 1994. Stroke 31:1588-1601, 2000.
4. Warlow C: Epidemiology of stroke. Lancet 325:14-16, 1998.
5. Kalache A, Aboderin I: Stroke: The global burden. Health Policy Plan 10:1-21, 1995.
6. Endo A, Kuroda M, Tsujita Y: ML-236A, ML-236B, ML-236C: New inhibitors of cholesterogenesis produced by Penicillium citrinum. J Antibiot 29:1346-1348, 1976.
7. Grundy SM: HMG-CoA reductase inhibitors for treatment of hypercholesterolemia. N Engl J Med 319:24-33, 1988.
8. Goldstein JL, Brown MS: Regulation of mevalonate pathway. Nature 343:425-430, 1990.
9. Anderson KM, Castelli WP, Levy D: Cholesterol and mortality: 30 years of follow-up from the Framingham Study. JAMA 257:2176-2180, 1987.
10. Martin MJ, Hulley SB, Browner WS, et al: Serum cholesterol, blood pressure and mortality: Implications from a cohort of 361,662 men. Lancet 246:933-936, 1986.
11. Manninen V, Elo MO, Frick MH, et al: Lipid alteration and decline in the incidence of coronary artery disease in the Helsinki Heart Study. JAMA 260:641-651, 1988.
12. Buchwald H, Varco RL, Mattz JP, et al: Effect of partial ileal bypass surgery on mortality and morbidity from coronary heart disease in patients with hypercholesterolemia. N Engl J Med 323:946-955, 1990.
13. Ornish D, Brown S, Scherwitz L, et al: Can lifestyle changes reverse coronary heart disease? The Lifestyle Heart Trial. Lancet 336:624-626, 1990.
14. Scandinavian SSSG: Randomized trial of cholesterol lowering in 4444 patients with coronary artery disease. The Scandinavian Simvastatin Survival Study (4S). Lancet 344:1383-1389, 1994.
15. Byington RP, Jukema JW, Salonen JT, et al: Reduction in cardiovascular events during pravastatin therapy: Pooled analysis of

clinical events of the pravastatin atherosclerosis intervention program. 92:2419-2425, 1995.

16. West of Scotland Coronary Prevention Study Group: West of Scotland Coronary Prevention Study: Identification of high-risk groups and comparison with other cardiovascular intervention trials. Lancet 348:1339-1342 ,1996.

17. Sacks FM, Pfeffer MA, Moye LA, et al: The effect of pravastatin on coronary events after myocardial infarction in patients with average cholesterol levels: Cholesterol and Recurrent Events Trial Investigators. N Engl J Med 335:1001-1009, 1996.

18. de Faire U, Ericsson C, Grip L, et al: Secondary preventive potential of lipid-lowering drugs. The Bezafibrate Coronary Atherosclerosis Intervention Trial (BECAIT). Eur Heart J 17:37-42, 1996.

19. The Long-term Intervention with Pravastatin in Ischemic Disease (LIPID) Study Group: Prevention of cardiovascular events and death with pravastatin in patients with coronary artery heart disease and a broad range of initial cholesterol levels. N Engl J Med 339:1349-1357, 1998.

20. Tell G, Crouse J, Furberg C: Relation between blood lipids, lipoproteins and cerebrovascular atherosclerosis: A review. Stroke 19:423-430, 1988.

21. Oliver MF: Cholesterol and strokes. Br Med J 320:459-460, 2000.

22. Andrews TC, Raby K, Barry J, et al: Effect of cholesterol reduction on myocardial ischaemia in patients with coronary disease. Circulation 95:324-328, 1997.

23. O' Driscoll G, Green D, Taylor RR: Simvastatin, an HMG-coenzyme A reductase inhibitor, improves endothelial function within 1 month. Circulation 95:1126-1131, 1997.

24. Plehn JF, Davis BR, Sacks FM, et al: Reduction of stroke incidence after myocardial infarction with pravastatin: The cholesterol and recurrent event (CARE) study. Circulation 99:216-223, 1999.

25. White HD, Simes RJ, Anderson NE, et al: Pravastatin therapy and the risk of stroke. N Engl J Med 343:317-326, 2000.

26. Schwartz GG, Olsson AG, Ezekowitz ME, et al: Effects of atorvastatin on early recurrent ischemic events in acute coronary syndromes: The MIRACL study: A randomized, controlled trial. JAMA 285:1711-1718, 2001.

27. Heart Protection Study Collaborative Group: MRC/BHF Heart Protection Study of cholesterol lowering with simvastatin in 20,536 high-risk individuals: A randomised placebo-controlled trial. Lancet 360:7-22, 2002.

28. Multiple Risk Factor Interventional Trial Research Group: Multiple Risk Factor Interventional Trial: Risk factor changes and mortality results. JAMA 248:1465-1477, 1982.

29. Pooling Project Research Group: Relationship of blood pressure, serum cholesterol, smoking habit, relative weight and ECG abnormalities to incidence of major coronary events: Final report of the pooling project: The Pooling Project Research Group. J Chron Dis 31:201-306, 1978.

30. Multicentre Anti-Atheroma Study Investigators: Effect of simvastatin on coronary atheroma: The Mullticentre Anti-Atheroma Study (MAAS). Lancet 344:633-638, 1994.

31. Jukema JW, Bruschke AV, van Boven AJ, et al: Effects of lipid lowering by pravastatin on progression and regression of coronary

artery disease in symptomatic men with normal to moderately elevated serum cholesterol levels. The Regression Growth Evaluation Statin Study (REGRESS). Circulation 91:2528-2540, 1995.

32. Taylor A, Kent S, Flaherty P, et al: ARBITER: Arterial biology for the investigation of the treatment effects of reducing cholesterol: A randomized trial comparing the effects of atorvastatin and pravastatin on carotid intima medial thickness. Circulation 106:2055-2060, 2002.

33. Watts GF, Lewis B, Brunt JN, et al: Effects on coronary artery disease of lipid-lowering diet or diet plus cholestyramine in the St. Thomas' Atherosclerosis Regression Study (STARS). Lancet 339:563-569, 1992.

34. Schuler G, Hambrecht R, Schierf G, et al: Regular physical exercise and low-fat diet: Effects on progression of coronary artery disease. Circulation 86:1-11, 1992.

35. Law MR, Wald NJ, Thompson SG: By how much and how quickly does reduction in serum cholesterol concentration lower risk of ischaemic heart disease? Br Med J 308:367-372, 1994.

36. Law MR, Thompson SG, Wald NJ: Assessing possible hazards of reducing serum cholesterol. Br Med J 308:373-378, 1994.

37. Haskell WL, Alderman EL, Fair JM, et al: Effects of intensive multiple risk factor reduction on coronary atherosclerosis and clinical cardiac events in men and women with coronary artery disease. The Stanford Coronary Risk Intervention Project (SCRIP). Circulation 89:975-990, 1994.

38. Sachs FM, Pasternak RC, Gibson CM, et al: Effect on coronary atherosclerosis of decrease in plasma cholesterol concentrations in normocholesterolemic patients. Lancet 344:1182-1186, 1994.

39. Amsterdam E, Deedwanja P: A perspective on hyperlipidemia: Concepts of management in the prevention of coronary artery disease. Am J Med 105:69-74, 1998.

40. Rosseauw JE, Lewis B, Rifkind BM: The value of lowering cholesterol after myocardial infarction. N Engl J Med 323:1112-1119, 1990.

41. Di Napoli P, Taccardi AA, Oliver M, De Caterina R: Statins and stroke: Evidence for cholesterol-independent effects. Eur Heart J 23:1908-1921, 2002.

42. Downs JR, Clearfield M, Weis S, et al: Primary prevention of acute coronary events with lovastatin in men and woman with average cholesterol levels: Results of AFCAPS/TexCAPS. JAMA 279:1615-1622, 1998.

43. Colquhoun D, Hicks B, Glasziou P: Comparative meta-analysis of 6 statins and 9 non-statins coronary regression trials: Evidence that cholesterol lowering is the key to outcomes. Circulation 94:579, 1996.

44. ALLHAT Collaborative Research Group: Major outcomes in moderately hypercholesterolemic, hypertensive patients randomized to pravastatin vs usual care: The antihypertensive and lipid-lowering treatment to prevent heart attack trial (ALLHAT-LLT). JAMA 288:3042-3044, 2002.

45. Sever P, Dahlof B, Poulter N, et al: Prevention of coronary and stroke events with atorvastatin in hypertensive patients who have average or lower-than-average cholesterol concentrations, in the Anglo-Scandinavian Cardiac Outcomes Trial—Lipid-Lowering Arm (ASCOT-LLA): A multicentre randomised controlled trial. Lancet 361:1149-1158, 2003.

46. Ridker P, Rifa N, Clearfield M, et al: Measurement of C-reactive protein for the targeting of statin therapy in the primary prevention of acute coronary events. N Engl J Med 344:1959-1965, 2001.

47. Grundy S, Pasternak R, Greenland P, et al: Assessment of cardiovascular risk by use of multiple-risk-factor assessment equations: A statement for healthcare professionals from the American Heart Association and the American College of Cardiology. Circulation 100:1481-1492, 1999.

48. Kappagoda CT, Amsterdam EA: How much to lower serum cholesterol: Is it the wrong question? J Am Coll Cardiol 34:289-292, 1999.

49. Pekkanen J, Linn S, Heiss G, et al: Ten-year mortality from cardiovascular disease in relation to cholesterol level among men with and without pre-existing cardiovascular disease. N Engl J Med 332:1700-1707, 1990.

50. Fager G, Wiklund O: Cholesterol reduction and clinical benefit: Are there limits to our expectations? Arterioscler Thromb Vasc Biol 17:3527-3533, 1997

51. Jacobson TA: "The lower the better" in hypercholesterolemia therapy: A reliable clinical guideline? Ann Intern Med 133:549-554, 2000.

52. Shepherd J, Blauw G, Murphy M, et al: Prospective study of pravastatin in the elderly at risk. Lancet 360:1623-1630, 2002.

53. Postiglione A, Napoli C: Hyperlipidemia and atherosclerosis cerebrovascular disease. Curr Opin Lipidol 6:236-242, 1995.

54. Khaw KT: Epidemiology of stroke. J Neurol Neurosurg Psychiatr 661:333-338, 1996.

55. O'Leary DH, Polak JF, Kronmal RA, et al: Carotid-artery intima and media thickness as a risk factor for myocardial infarction and strokes in older adults. New Engl J Med 340:14-22, 1999.

56. Crouse JR 3rd, Byington RP, Bond MG, et al: Pravastatin, lipid and atherosclerosis in the carotid arteries (PLAC II). Am J Cardiol 76:54C-59C, 1995.

57. Menotti A, Blackburn H, Kromhout D, et al: The inverse relation of average population blood pressure and stroke mortality rates in the Seven Countries study: A paradox. Eur J Epidemiol 13:379-386, 1997.

58. Korne-Lubetzki I, Kleinman J, Eliashiv S, Eliakim M: Correlation between serum lipid and stroke in an Israeli population. Neurol Res 14(Suppl. 2):78-80, 1992.

59. Frick MH, Elo O, Haapa K, et al: Helsinki Heart Study: Primary prevention trial with gemfibrozil in middle-aged men with dyslipidemia. N Engl J Med 317:1237-1245, 1987.

60. Kagan A, McGee DL, Iano K, et al: Serum cholesterol and mortality in a Japanese-American population: The Honolulu Heart Program. Am J Epidemiol 114:11-20, 1981.

61. Iso H, Jacobs DJ, Wentworth D, et al, for, the MRFIT Research Group: Serum cholesterol levels and six-year mortality from stroke in 350,977 men screened for the Multiple Risk Factor Intervention Trial. N Engl J Med 320:904-910, 1989.

62. Prospective Studies Collaborators: Cholesterol, diastolic blood pressure, and stroke: 13,000 strokes in 450,000 people in 45 prospective cohorts. Lancet 346:1647-1653, 1995.

63. Committee of Principal Investigators: A co-operative trial in the primary prevention of ischemic heart disease using clofibrate—

6

Report from the Committee of Principal Investigators. Br Heart J 40:1069-1118, 1978.

64. Scandinavian Simvastatin Survival Study Group: Randomized trial of cholesterol lowering in 4444 patients with coronary artery disease: The Scandinavian Simvastatin Survival Study (4S). Lancet 344:1383-1389, 1994.

65. Waters D, Schwartz G, Olsson A, et al: Effects of atorvastatin on stroke in patients with unstable angina or non-Q-wave myocardial infarction. Circulation 106:1690-1695, 2002.

66. Alberts M: Suppression of recurrent transient ischemic attacks by a statin agent. Neurology 56:531-532, 2001.

67. Pasternak R: The ALLHAT lipid lowering trial—less is less. JAMA 288:3042-3044, 2002.

68. Blauw GJ, Lagaay AM, Smelt AH, Westendorp RG: Stroke, statins, and cholesterol: A meta-analysis of randomized placebo-controlled, double blind trials with HMG-CoA reductase inhibitors. Stroke 28:946-950, 1997.

69. Ross SD, Allen E, Connelly JE, et al: Clinical outcomes in statin treatment trials: A meta-analysis. Arch Intern Med 159:1793-1802, 1999.

70. Corvol J, Bouzamondo A, Sirol M, et al: Differential effects of lipid-lowering therapies on stroke prevention. Arch Intern Med 163:669-676, 2003.

71. Crouse JR, Byington RP, Hoen HM, Furberg CD: Reductase inhibitor monotherapy and stroke prevention. Arch Intern Med 157:1305-1310, 1997.

72. Warshafsky S, Packard D, Marks S, et al: Efficacy of 3-hydroxy-3-methylglutaryl coenzyme A reductase inhibitors for prevention of stroke. J Gen Intern Med 14:777-784, 1999.

73. Rubins H, Davenport J, Babikian V: Reduction in stroke with gemfibrozil in men with coronary heart disease and low HDL cholesterol: The Veterans Affairs HDL Intervention Trial (VA-HIT). Circulation 103:2828-2833, 2001.

74. Vaughan CJ, Murphy MB, Buckley BM: Statins do more than just lower cholesterol. Lancet 348:1079-1082, 1996.

75. Vaughan CJ, Delanty N: Neuroprotective properties of statins in cerebral ischemia and stroke. Stroke 30:1969-1973, 1999.

76. Delanty N, Vaughan CJ: Vascular effects of statins in stroke. Stroke 28:2315-2320, 1997.

77. Liao J: Statins and ischemic stroke. Atherosclerosis. 3:21-25, 2002.

78. Lefer AM, Scalia R, Lefer DJ: Vascular effects of HMG CoA-reductase inhibitors (statins) unrelated to cholesterol lowering: New concepts for cardiovascular disease. Cardiovasc Res 49:281-287, 2001.

79. Vaughan C, Delanty N: Neuroprotective properties of statins in cerebral ischemia and stroke. Stroke 31:889-890, 2000.

80. Zhang F, Iadecola C: Reduction of focal cerebral ischemic damage by delayed treatment with nitric oxide donors. J Cereb Blood Flow Metab 14:574-580, 1994.

81. Haller H: Endothelial function: General considerations. Drugs 53:1-10, 1997.

82. Rosenson RS, Tangney CC: Antiatherothrombotic properties of statins: Implications for cardiovascular event reduction. JAMA 279:1643-1650, 1998.

83. Morikawa E, Huang Z, Moskowitz M: L-arginine decreases infarct size

caused by middle cerebral arterial occlusion in SHR. Am J Physiol 263:H1632-H1635, 1992.

84. Hu SH, Sheng WS, Peterson PK, Chao CC: Differential regulation by cytokines of human astrocyte nitric oxide production. Glia 15:491-494, 1995.

85. Forster C, Clark HB, Ross NE, Iadecola C: Inducible nitric oxide synthase expression in human cerebral infarct. Acta Neuropathol 97:215-220, 1999.

86. Iadecola C, Zhang F, Casey R, et al: Delayed reduction of ischemic brain injury and neurologic deficit in mice lacking the inducible nitric oxide synthase gene. J Neurosci 17:9157-9164, 1997.

87. Ding M, St Pierre BA, Parkinson JF, et al: Inducible nitric-oxide synthase and nitric oxide production in human fetal astrocytes and microglia: A kinetic analysis. J Biol Chem 272:11327-11335, 1997.

88. Tung TJ, Bhardwaj A, Davson VL, et al: Neuroprotective FK506 does not alter in vivo nitric oxide production during ischemia and early reperfusion in rats. Stroke 30:1279-1285, 1999.

89. Pahan K, Sheikh FG, Namboodiri AMS, Singh I: Lovastatin and phenylacetate inhibit the induction on nitric oxide synthase and cytokines in rat primary astrocytes, microglia and macrophages. J Clin Invest 100:2671-2679, 1997.

90. Laufs U, La Fata V, Liao J: Inhibition of 3-hydroxy-3-methylglutaryl (HMG)-CoA reductase blocks hypoxia-mediated down-regulation of endothelial nitric oxide synthase. J Biol Chem 50:31725-31729, 1997.

91. Laufs U, La Fata V, Plutzky J, Liao JK: Upregulation of endothelial nitric oxide synthase by HMG CoA reductase inhibitors. Circulation 97:1129-1135, 1998.

92. Lefer AM, Cambpell B, Shin Y, et al: Simvastatin preserves the ischemic-reperfused myocardium in normocholesterolemic rat hearts. Circulation 100:178-184, 1999.

93. Di Napoli P, Di Muzio M, Maggi A, et al: Simvastatin reduces postischemic coronary dysfunction: Ultrastructural and functional findings after acute administration. Microvasc Res 59:181-185, 2000.

94. Jick H, Zornberg GL, Jick SS, et al: Statins and risk of dementia. Lancet 356:1627-1631, 2000.

95. Liu J, Garcia-Gardena G, Sessa WC: Palmitoylation of nitric oxide synthase is necessary for optimal stimulated release of nitric oxide: Implications for caveolae localization. Biochemistry 35:13277-13281, 1996.

96. Kohl NF, Mosser SD, deSolms SJ, et al: Selective inhibition of ras-dependent transformation by a farnesyltransferase inhibitor. Science 260:1934-1937, 1993.

97. Fukada J, Takao T, Ohguro H, et al: Farnesylated gamma-subunit photoreceptor G-protein indispensable for GTP-binding. Nature 346:658-660, 1990.

98. Lim L, Manser E, Leung T, Hall C: Regulation of phosphorylation pathways by p21 GTPases: The p21 Ras-related Rho subfamily and its role in phosphorylation signaling pathways. Eur J Biochem 242:171-185, 1996.

99. Aelst LW, D'Souza-Schorey C: Rho GTPases and signaling networks. Genes Dev 11:2295-2322, 1997.

100. Laufs U, Liao JK: Post-transcriptional regulation of endothelial nitric oxide synthase mRNA stability by Rho GTP-ase. J Biol Chem 273:24266-24271, 1998.

6

101. Laufs U, Liao JK: Targeting Rho in cardiovascular disease. Circ Res 87:526-528, 2000.
102. Shaw G, Kamen R: A conserved AU sequence from the 3' untranslated region of GM-CSF mRNA mediates selective mRNA degradation. Cell 46:659-667, 1986.
103. Boisvert WA, Santiago R, Curtiss LK, Terkeltaub RA: A leukocyte homologue of the IL-8 receptor CXCR-2 mediates the accumulation of macrophages in atherosclerotic lesions of LDL receptor-deficient mice. J Clin Invest 101:353-363, 1998.
104. Ridker PM, Glynn RJ, Hennekens CH: C-reactive protein adds to the predictive value of total and HDL cholesterol in determining risk of first myocardial infarction. Circulation 97:2007-2011, 1998.
105. Weber C, Erl W, Weber KS, Weber PC: Effects of oxidized low density lipoprotein, lipid mediators and statins on vascular cell interactions. Clin Chem Lab Med 37:243-251, 1999.
106. Prediman KS: Circulating markers of inflammation for vascular risk prediction. Circulation 105:1758-1759, 2000.
107. Rajavashisth T, Qiao JH, Tripathi S, et al: Heterozygous osteopetrotic (op) mutation reduces atherosclerosis in LDL receptor-deficient mice. J Clin Invest 101:2702-2710, 1998.
108. Weissberg P: Mechanisms modifying atherosclerotic disease: From lipids to vascular biology. Atherosclerosis 47(Suppl 1):S3-S10, 1999.
109. Amento EP, Ehsani N, Palmer H, Libby P: Cytokines and growth factors positively and negatively regulate interstitial collagen gene expression in human vascular smooth muscle cells. Arterioscler Thromb 11:1223-1230, 1991.
110. Sorlie PD, Nieto FJ, Adams E, et al: A prospective study of cytomegalovirus, herpes simplex virus 1, and coronary heart disease: The atherosclerosis risk in communities (ARIC) study. Arch Intern Med 10:2027-2032, 2000.
111. Gasbarrini A, Cremonini F, Armuzzi A, et al: The role of *Helicobacter pylori* in cardiovascular and cerebrovascular diseases. J Physiol Pharmacol 50:735-742, 1999.
112. Quinn TC, Gaydos CA: In vitro infection and pathogenesis of *Chlamydia pneumoniae* in endovascular cellls. Am Heart J 138:S507-S511, 1999.
113. Danesch J, Whincup P, Walker M, et al: *Chlamydia pneumoniae* IgG titres and coronary heart disease: Prospective study and meta-analysis. BMJ 321:208-213, 2000.
114. Danesch J, Whincup P, Walker M, et al: Low grade inflammation and coronary heart disease: Prospective study and updated meta-analysis. BMJ 321:199-204, 2000.
115. Libby P, Aikawa M, Kinlay S, et al: Lipid lowering improves endothelial functions. Int J Cardiol 74(Suppl 1):S3-S10, 2000.
116. Weber C, Erl W, Weber KSC, Weber P: HMG-CoA reductase inhibitors decrease CD11b expression and CD11b-dependent adhesion of monocyte to endothelium and reduce increased adhesiveness on monocytes isolated from patients with hypercholesterolemia. J Am Coll Cardiol 30:1212-1217, 1997.
117. Ridker P, Miles J, Downs J: Lovastatin 20-40 mg/day lowers high sensitivity C-reactive protein levels in AFCAPS/TexCAPS [abstract]. Circulation 102(Suppl):833, 2000.
118. Albert M, Danielson E, Rifai N, Ridker P: Effect of statin therapy on C-reactive protein levels: The pravastatin inflammation/CPR

6

evaluation (PRINCE): A randomised trial and cohort study. Am Med Assoc 286:64-70, 2001.

119. Liao J: Beyond lipid lowering: The role of statins in vascular protection. Int J Cardiol 86:5-18, 2002.

120. Kothe H, Dalhoff K, Rupp J, et al: Hydroxymethylglutaryl coenzyme A reductase inhibitors modify the inflammatory response of human macrophages and endothelial cells infected with *Chlamydia pneumoniae*. Circulation 101:1760-1763, 2000.

121. Lindgren A, Lindoff C, Norrving B, et al: Tissue plasminogen activator and plasminogen activator inhibitor-1 in stroke patients. Stroke 27:1066-1071, 1996.

122. Davì G, Averna M, Catalano I: Increased thromboxane biosynthesis in type IIa hypercholesterolemia: Circulation 85:1792-1798, 1992.

123. Libby P, Mach F, Schonbeck U, et al: Regulation of the thrombotic potential of atheroma. Thromb Haemost 82:736-741, 1999.

124. Fenton J, Shen G: Statins as cellular antithrombotics. Haemostasis 29:166-169, 1999.

125. Colli S, Eligini S, Lalli M, et al: Vastatins inhibit tissue factor in cultured human macrophages: A novel mechanism of protection against atherothrombosis. Arterioscler Thromb Vasc Biol 17:265-272, 1997.

126. Bourcier T, Libby P: HMG CoA reductase inhibitors reduce plasminogen activator inhibitor-1 expression by human vascular smooth muscle and endothelial cells. Arterioscler Thromb Vasc Biol 20:556-562, 2000.

127. Crisby M, Nordin-Fredriksson G, Shah P, et al: Pravastatin treatment increases collagen content and decreases lipid content, inflammation, metalloproteinases, and cell death in human carotid plaques: Implications for plaque stabilization. Circulation 103:926-933, 2001.

128. Steinberg D, Parthasarathy S, Carew TE, et al: Beyond cholesterol modifications of low-density lipoprotein that increase its atherogenicity. N Engl J Med 320:915-924, 1989.

129. Kita T, Yokode M, Iskii K, et al: The role of oxidized lipoproteins in the pathogenesis of atherosclerosis. Clin Exp Pharmacol Physiol Suppl 20:37-42, 1992.

130. Suzumura K, Yasuhara M, Tanaka K, et al: An in vivo study of the hydroxyl radical scavenging property of fluvastatin, an HMG-CoA reductase inhibitor. Chem Pharm Bull 47:1010-1012, 1999.

131. Youdim K, Martin A, Joseph J: Essential fatty acids and the brain: Possible health implications. Int J Dev Neurosci 18:383-389, 2000.

132. Jongkind JF, Verkerk A, Hoogerbrugge N: Monocytes from patients with combined hypercholesterolemia-hypertriglyceridemia and isolated hypercholesterolemia show increased adhesion to endothelial cell in vitro: Influence of intrinsic and extrinsic monocyte binding. Metabolism 44:374-378, 1995.

133. Ussein O, Schlezinger SA, Rosemblat M, et al: Reduced susceptibility of low density lipoprotein (LDL) to lipid peroxidation after fluvastatin therapy is associated with hypocholesterolemia effect of the drug and its binding to LDL. Atherosclerosis 128:11-18, 1997.

134. Tomas M, Senti M, Garcia-Faria F, et al: Effect of simvastatin therapy on paraoxonase activity and related lipoproteins in familial hypercholesterolemic patients. Arterioscler Thromb Vasc Biol 20:2113-2119, 2000.

6

135. Aviram M, Rosenblat M, Bisgaier CL, Newton RS: Atorvastatin and gemfibrozil metabolites, but not parent drugs, are potent antioxidants against lipoprotein oxidant. Atherosclerosis 138:271-280, 1998.
136. Chen L, Haught WH, Yang B, et al: Preservation of endogenous antioxidant activity and inhibition of lipid peroxidation as common mechanism of anti-atherosclerotic effects of vitamin E, lovastatin and amlodipine. J Am Coll Cardiol 30:569-575, 1997.
137. Hebert PR, Gaziano JM, Chan KS, Hennekens CH: Cholesterol lowering with statin drugs, risk of stroke, and total mortality: An overview of randomized trials. JAMA 278:313-321, 1997.

Statins and the Modulation of Cardiac Hypertrophy and Fibrosis: Implications in the Therapy of Heart Failure

Ali J. Marian

Cardiac hypertrophy and the accompanying fibrosis are the common intermediate- and long-term phenotypic responses of the heart to all forms of stress. The stimuli, whether internal, such as a genetic defect, or external, such as an increased load, induce a complex array of cellular and molecular changes that enhance protein synthesis and/or degradation, leading to cardiac hypertrophy and fibrosis. The histologic phenotype is characterized by myocyte enlargement, proliferation of fibroblasts, fibrosis, and cell death.[1] In the normal heart, approximately one third of the cells are cardiac myocytes, and the remainder are predominantly fibroblasts.[2] In the pathologic states, another cellular component, referred to as myofibroblasts, appears in the myocardium and plays a major role in evolving fibrosis, tissue repair, and inflammation.[3] As the name implies, myofibroblasts have phenotypic and functional similarities to both smooth muscle cells and fibroblasts. They express several molecular markers of smooth muscle (SM) cells, including SM α-actin and SM 22α genes but not SM myosin heavy chain, differentiating them from SM cells. Myofibroblasts also produce a variety of growth factors, cytokines, and chemokines, which also contribute to myocyte hypertrophy and interstitial fibrosis. The origin of myofibroblasts is largely unknown but may include interstitial and/or adventitial fibroblasts or progenitor stem cells.[3] Therefore, in response to stress, at least three major cellular components, namely myocytes, fibroblasts, and myofibroblasts, mediate the cardiac phenotypic response. Other cellular components, such as macrophages and plasma cells, also participate by

This work is supported in part by a grant from the National Heart, Lung, and Blood Institute, Specialized Centers of Research (P50-HL42267-01) and R01-HL68884.

143

producing a variety of autocrine and paracrine factors. Although all cellular components contribute to the expression of trophic and mitotic factors, their responses to stress digress with regard to cellular proliferation. The response of adult cardiac myocytes, which are considered terminally differentiated, is restricted predominantly to hypertrophy, whereas the responses of cardiac fibroblasts and myofibroblasts also include proliferation. The ensuing pathologic phenotype is increased production of trophic and mitotic factors leading to cardiac myocyte hypertrophy, myocyte death, reparative and replacement fibrosis, and increased extracellular matrix (ECM) protein content. Accordingly, the pathogenesis of cardiac hypertrophy and fibrosis in response to stress is closely but not completely linked. Nonetheless, these two phenotypes almost always coexist in the ensuing clinical phenotype of heart failure.

CLINICAL SIGNIFICANCE OF CARDIAC HYPERTROPHY AND FIBROSIS

Cardiac hypertrophy and fibrosis are the major determinants of morbidity and mortality in all forms of cardiovascular disease. Whereas hypertrophy is associated with a two- to fourfold increase in the overall mortality,[4] fibrosis plays a major role in the pathogenesis of cardiac arrhythmias and the risk of sudden cardiac death (SCD).[5] Cardiac hypertrophy is a strong and independent predictor of cardiovascular morbidity and mortality. Data from the Framingham Heart study, which consisted of a predominantly white population, showed that a 50-g/m^2 increase in left ventricular mass was associated with a relative risk of cardiovascular death of 1.73-fold in men and 2.12-fold in women.[6] The risk is similar or even greater in African Americans, in whom the presence of cardiac hypertrophy is associated with a twofold increase in overall cardiovascular mortality.[7] Cardiac hypertrophy is also associated with an increased risk of SCD, particularly in men.[4] In patients with hypertrophic cardiomyopathy (HCM), a genetic model of cardiac hypertrophy, there is a direct relationship between the extent of cardiac hypertrophy and the risk of SCD.[8] Even in asymptomatic patients, cardiac hypertrophy is considered a strong and independent predictor of a poor prognosis, whereas patients with minimal or mild hypertrophy are, in general, at low risk for premature death.[8] Cardiac hypertrophy is also a major cause of diastolic heart failure (heart failure with a normal ejection fraction), which may account for approximately half of all heart failure cases.[9] The annual mortality of patients with diastolic heart failure is approximately four times higher than that of a matched control group.[9] In addition, cardiac hypertrophy is also a major risk factor for atrial fibrillation, which is associated with a four- to fivefold increase in the risk of cerebrovascular stroke.[10]

7

Cardiac hypertrophy is commonly associated with interstitial fibrosis, which is considered a major determinant of susceptibility to cardiac arrhythmias and SCD.[11,12] Fibrosis impairs electrical coupling between the myocytes, reduces capillary density, induces myocyte hypoxia, and impairs myocyte metabolism.[1] Interstitial fibrosis also impedes uniform propagation of electrical activity in the myocardium and results in progressive increase of activation delay.[13] Patchy areas of fibrosis are often found at the site of focal reentry and ventricular tachycardia.[14] Interstitial fibrosis is also considered a major predictor of SCD in patients with HCM.[11]

Interstitial fibrosis is also a major determinant of myocardial stiffness and contributes significantly to diastolic heart failure.[15] Type I collagen, which is the predominant myocardial collagen, has a tensile strength close to that of steel. Myocardial stiffness is associated with interstitial collagen accumulation, content, and solubility.[16] Inversely, pharmacologic reversal of interstitial fibrosis is associated with improvement in diastolic function.[17] Collectively, the existing data strongly implicate cardiac hypertrophy and fibrosis as major determinants of mortality and morbidity from cardiovascular disease.

MOLECULAR BIOLOGY OF CARDIAC HYPERTROPHY

Cardiac myocytes lose their ability to proliferate during the postnatal period but preserve their capability to undergo growth in response to external and internal stimuli. Mechanical stress, or stretch, is the prototype stimulus for cardiac hypertrophic response, which involves multiple interacting mechanisms. It leads to the activation of stress sensors and the autocrine release of trophic and mitotic factors, including angiotensin II (Ang II).[18] In addition to mechanical stress, a large array of growth factors induce cardiac hypertrophic response, a process that is typically initiated by binding of the ligand to a series of cell surface or nuclear receptors, followed by activation of the intracytoplasmic signal transduction cascade, nuclear gene transcription, and protein synthesis. Growth factors can elicit their hypertrophic effects through endocrine, paracrine, or intracrine (autocrine) mechanisms or a combination thereof. In addition to intracellular interactions between signaling molecules, intercellular interactions also affect the phenotypic response. Cardiac myocytes, fibroblasts, and plasma cells produce trophic factors, mitogens, and cytokines that not only work in an autocrine fashion but also exert major paracrine effects on other cellular components. The initial hypertrophic response is marked by the expression of proto-oncogenes, such as c-*myc*, c-*jun*, and c-*fos*, and the subsequent induction of expression of a large number of genes, including atrial natriuretic peptide (ANP), brain natriuretic peptide (BNP), and skeletal

7

α-actin. In addition, expression of sarcoplasmic reticulum Ca^{2+}-ATPase 2a (SRECA2a) is suppressed, and the expressions of the α and β myosin heavy chain (MyHC) isoforms switch in response to hypertrophy. Alteration of gene expression occurs regardless of the etiology of the stimulus for hypertrophy, and thus, collectively, altered expressions of these genes are referred to as molecular markers of cardiac hypertrophy.

Transducers of Cardiac Myocyte Hypertrophy

Cardiac myocyte hypertrophy could occur as a result of extrinsic and intrinsic stimuli. External stimuli, such as growth factors, vasoactive peptides, cytokines, and adrenergic hormones exert their hypertrophic effects primarily through activation of cell surface (or nuclear) receptors and downstream signaling molecules. Intrinsic stimuli, such as genetic defects or increased intracellular calcium concentration, activate the intracellular signaling cascade, either directly or indirectly via cell surface receptors, and induce gene transcription and protein synthesis. Thus, regardless of the type of the stimulus, the key intermediary step in modulating the hypertrophic response is activation of the signal transducers, which link the stimuli to transcription factors, and induction of gene expression, ultimately inducing protein synthesis (Fig. 7-1).

A cadre of molecules carries the message from the extracellular stimuli to inside the nucleus and activates expression of

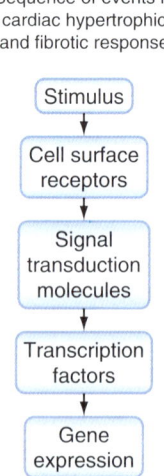

Sequence of events in
cardiac hypertrophic
and fibrotic response

Figure 7-1. Sequence of events in cardiac hypertrophic and fibrotic response.

Table 7–1	
Major Cell Surface Signal Receptors	
Cell Surface Receptors	Ligands
GPCRs	Mechanical stretch
	Vasoactive peptides (AT and ET-1)
	Adrenergic α agonist (Gαq)
	Adrenergic β₁ agonists (Gαs, cAMP/PKA)
RTKs	Transforming growth factor-β₁
	Insulin like growth factor-1
	Fibroblast growth factor-2
	Epidermal growth factor-1
	Platelet-derived growth factor
Integrins	Mechanical stretch, ECM proteins, AT
Cytokines	TNF-α and interleukins (JAK-STAT)

AT, angiotensin II; ECM, extracellular matrix; ET, endothelin; GPCRs, G-protein–coupled receptors; PKA, protein kinase A; RTKs, receptor tyrosine kinases.

the target genes (Table 7-1). The first step in the induction of the hypertrophic response is the binding of the ligands to their respective membrane or nuclear receptors. Several families of cell surface receptors (Fig. 7-2), intracellular signaling kinases, and phosphatases orchestrate the cardiac hypertrophic and fibrotic responses. The majority of growth factors and adrenergic hormones, such as Ang II and endothelin-1 (ET-1), activate the signal transduction molecules through binding to the seven-pass transmembrane G-protein–coupled receptors (GPCRs).[19,20] These receptors are composed of three subunits of α, β, and γ GTP-binding proteins, which form heterodimers and catalyze the exchange of GTP to GDP upon activation by cell surface receptors. In the resting state, the α subunit binds to GDP and forms a high-affinity complex with the βγ heterodimer. Upon activation by cell surface receptors, GDP is released from the α subunit, and the α subunit binds to GTP, dissociating it from the βγ heterodimer subunit. The α subunit–GTP complex comprises several sub-classes, including α_s and α_q, that are activated differentially by agonists, and each activates a different set of downstream effectors. The α_1 adrenergic, Ang II, and ET-1 receptors activate the Gα_q and its downstream effectors protein kinase C (PKC), small guanine nucleotide-binding proteins (small G proteins), mitogen-activated protein kinases (MAPKs), and extracellular signal-regulated kinases (ERK1/2). In contrast, the β₁-adrenergic receptors target the Gα_s subunit, which stimulates adenylate cyclase and activates protein kinase A (PKA). The latter in turn phosphorylates ryanodine receptor 2 (RyR2), the major calcium release channel in the sarcoplasmic reticulum. GPCRs return to the resting state

7

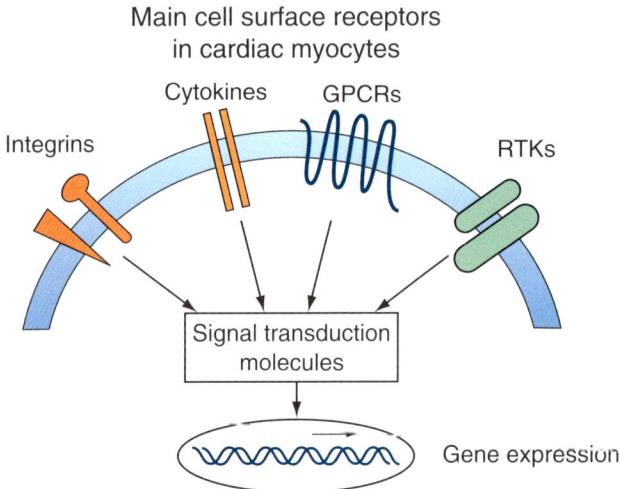

Figure 7-2 Main cell surface receptors in cardiac myocytes and fibroblasts. Transfer of messages from cell surface to nucleus involves intracellular signal transduction molecules. GPCRs, G-protein–coupled receptors; RTKs, receptor tyrosine kinases.

when the intrinsic GTPase activity of the α subunit hydrolyzes GTP to GDP. Subsequently, GDP binds to the α subunit and returns the receptor to the resting state.

A prototype of GPCR agonists is Ang II, which has a well-established role in cardiac hypertrophy and fibrosis. The downstream signaling pathways for Ang II are well characterized (Fig. 7-3). Ang II is known to activate $G\alpha_q$ and, subsequently, phospholipase C (PLC), which is responsible for the hydrolysis of phosphatidyl-inositol bisphosphate into diacylglycerol (DAG) and inositol trisphosphate (IP3). IP3 induces calcium release from the endoplasmic reticulum and, together with DAG, activates PKC. PKC and Ca^{+2} lie upstream of small G-protein Ras and a family of MAP kinases that include ERK1/2.[21] It is also important to note that the GPCR pathway is not restricted to activation of the classic Ras, Raf, MAPK, and ERK1/2 pathways but also activates and interacts with other signaling molecules, including Jun N-terminal kinase (JNK), p38, and other small G-protein–binding molecules RhoA, Rac1, and myosin light-chain kinase.[22-24] Furthermore, GPCRs, by activating PLC, could also activate the calcineurin-nuclear factor of activated T cells (NFAT) and Ca^{+2} calmodulin-dependent protein kinase pathways (CaMKII).[19,25-29] Thus, complex interactions between multiple signal transduction pathways exist and are involved in mediating the hypertrophic and profibrotic effects of GPCR agonists.

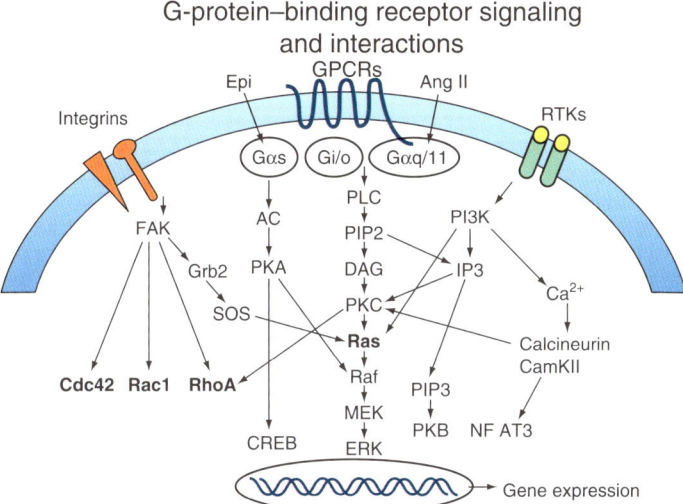

Figure 7-3. G-protein–binding receptor signaling and interactions with other signaling cascades leading to activation of Ras, RhoA, and Rac1. AC, adenylate cyclase; Ang II, angiotensin II; CREB, cyclic AMP response element binding protein; DAG, diacylglycerol; ERK, extracellular signal-regulated kinases; FAK, focal adhesion kinase; GPCRs, G-protein–coupled receptors; IP3, inositol triphosphate; MEK, mitogen activated protein kinase; NFAT, nuclear factor of activated T cells; PI3K, phosphatidylinositol-3-kinase; PIP, phosphatidylinositol phosphate; PKA, protein kinase A; PKB, protein kinase B; RTKs, receptor tyrosine kinases; SOS, son of sevenless.

Other major cell surface receptors involved in cardiac hypertrophic and fibrotic responses include the receptor tyrosine kinases (RTKs), cytokine receptor pathway, and integrins (see Table 7-1). RTKs comprise a series of heterodimeric receptors that modulate the signaling cascade for growth peptides, such as insulin-like growth factor-1 (IGF-1), fibroblast growth factors (FGFs), and transforming growth factor-β (TGF-β). There are also significant interactions between the RTK and the GPCR pathways. As such, Ras and its downstream targets *raf*, MAPKs, and ERK1/2 are also activated in response to RTK signaling. The primary mediators of signaling through TGF-β are Smad proteins, and those for the cytokine receptor pathway include activation of the JAK-STAT pathway. Another class of major cell surface receptors for hypertrophic stimuli is the integrins, which are heterodimeric transmembrane proteins that link the ECM to intracellular events.[30] Integrins are considered the main mediators of hypertrophic response to stretch.[31,32] The primary mediator of signaling through integrins include activation of focal adhesion kinase (FAK) and the

Rho family of small GTP-binding proteins Rho, Rac, and Cdc42. Rho-GTPases participate in a variety of cellular functions including actin cytoskeleton organization, cell polarity, gene transcription, microtubule dynamics, and the cell cycle.[33] There are also significant interactions between the integrin-signaling pathway and GPCR pathways. Activation of FAK by integrins recruits the Grb2 adapter molecule, which activates with the Ras guanine nucleotide exchange factor SOS and leads to activation of the MAPK pathway. Interaction between integrins and GPCR pathways is considered essential for the development of cardiac hypertrophy and fibrosis[24] in response to stress. Haploinsufficiency of Grb2 prevents the activation of p38 and JNK and the development of cardiac hypertrophy and fibrosis in response to pressure overload.[24]

MOLECULAR BIOLOGY OF CARDIAC FIBROSIS

Increased deposition of fibrillar collagen (i.e., fibrosis) is a common phenotype in all forms of cardiac injury and accompanies myocardial hypertrophy and remodeling. Accordingly, its molecular pathogenesis is closely but not exclusively linked to that of cardiac hypertrophy. Cardiac ECM is a dynamic and extensive connective tissue lattice that surrounds and provides support for cardiac myocytes and regulates their attachment and morphology. The main components of ECM are fibrillar collagen, fibronectins, glycosaminoglycans, proteoglycans, and a variety of trophic and mitotic factors. Fibrillar collagen is the predominant component of ECM in the heart and makes up approximately 2% to 3% of the normal myocardial mass. In pathologic states, fibrillar collagen could make up about 20% or more of the myocardium. Cardiac collagen exists in three levels: epimysium, perimysium, and endomysium. Epimysial collagen surrounds the boundaries of cardiac muscle, perimysial collagen connects groups of myocytes, and endomysium connects and supports the individual myocytes. Endomysial collagen, which is composed of struts that are 150 nm in diameter, prevents excessive elongation or shortening of the myocytes and couples contraction and relaxation of multiple myocytes. Approximately 85% of myocardial collagen is type I collagen, which is a heterotrimeric protein composed of two $\alpha_1(I)$ and one $\alpha_2(I)$ procollagen chains forming a triple helix. The two $\alpha_1(I)$ and one $\alpha_2(I)$ chains are transcribed as pre-procollagen in cardiac fibroblasts by genes located on chromosomes 17 and 7, respectively. After cleavage and posttranslation modifications, including hydroxylation and glycation, they assemble into procollagen triple-helix fibers in cardiac fibroblasts. Subsequently, N- and C-terminal domains are cleaved in the extracellular space and disulfide bonds are formed between the mature trimeric collagen chains, forming the fibrillar collagen.[34] The second most common collagen in the heart is type III collagen, which is approximately 11% of the total collagen content.[34] Other collagen types, such as IV, V, and VI, are also expressed in the heart but at very low levels. The fibrillar collagen network provides for the structural integrity of the myocardial architecture and transmission of the force generated by myocytes during contraction. It also prevents myocytes from excessive stretch by providing the necessary tensile strength. Finally, ECM proteins interact with integrins and cytoskeletal proteins and participate in maintaining the alignment of myofibrils with myocytes.

Collagen is synthesized by fibroblasts in response to growth factors and degraded by matrix metalloproteinases (MMPs) in the ECM. Excess production of collagen by fibroblasts or inhibition of its degradation by ECM proteins results in accumulation of collagen and fibrosis. A variety of autocrine and paracrine factors promote fibroblast proliferation and collagen synthesis including Ang II, TGF-β_1, FGF-2, and IGF-1.[3] Ang II, the best-characterized pro-fibrotic factor, not only promotes expression of collagen, fibronectin, and laminin but also stimulates fibroblast proliferation. The pro-fibrotic effect of Ang II is largely mediated through the Ang II type 1 receptor, which is a GPCR. Binding of Ang II to Ang II receptor-1 not only activates the classic pathway of PLC, PKC, and CaMKII but also activates a variety of other signaling molecules, including the RTK pathway in cardiac fibroblasts and myocytes (see Fig. 7-3). Activation of the signaling kinases RhoA and Rac1 requires isoprenylation and geranylation followed by association with the cell membrane. Selective blockade or deletion of Ang II receptor type 1 attenuates and reverses the pro-fibrotic effects of Ang II.[35,36] TGF-β and FGF-2 have emerged as major mediators of pro-fibrotic effects of Ang II. Mice deficient in TGF-β_1 or FGF-2 also show resistance to cardiac fibrosis and hypertrophy in response to pro-fibrotic and hypertrophic stimuli.[37,38] However, hypertrophic and pro-fibrotic responses, at least in response to pressure overload signaling through integrins, are dissociated, because inhibition of p38 prevents pressure overload–induced cardiac fibrosis but not hypertrophy.[24] Thus, it appears that activation of p38 is indispensable to pressure overload–induced cardiac fibrosis but is dispensable to pressure overload–induced cardiac hypertrophy. Furthermore, there is also significant cross-talk between Ang II and other trophic and mitotic factors, including TGF-β, ET-1, and cytokines.

Collagen is degraded in the ECM by a series of MMPs, which are also produced by cardiac fibroblasts. MMP-1, or interstitial collagenase, cleaves collagen at a single site and generates small and large gelatins, which subsequently become further degraded by MMP-2 (gelatinase A) into smaller fragments. Another set of ECM proteins, referred to as tissue inhibitors of MMPs (TIMPs) maintains ECM homeostasis. Cardiac-specific expression of MMP-1 leads to marked deterioration of cardiac systolic and diastolic functions.[39] In contrast, deletion of MMP-9 (gelatinase B) through gene targeting in mice leads to an accumulation of collagen following myocardial infarction.[40] Thus, a delicate balance between pro-fibrotic and antifibrotic factors maintains the integrity of the ECM in the myocardium, and its disturbance could lead to cardiac fibrosis and/or dilatation.

Central Role of Small GTPases in Cardiac Hypertrophy and Fibrosis

Small G proteins are molecular switches that regulate the growth and morphology of myocytes and fibroblasts. Over 60 small G proteins in mammals have been identified that generally fall into five categories—Ras, Rho, ADP ribosylation factors (ARFs), Rab, and Ran. Ras, RhoA, and Rac1 are considered the major mediators of hypertrophic response, expressed not only in response to GPCR agonists, such as Ang II and ET-1, but also in response to the activation of integrins and TRK pathways. The hypertrophic and fibrotic responses to Ang II are considered to occur primarily through activation of Ras, c-Raf, PI3K, MAPK. ERK1/2, and JNK, and to a smaller extent activation of RhoA and Rac1.[41] With regard to stress-induced hypertrophy and fibrosis, interactions between integrins and the Ras pathway are critical.[24,42] Similarly, the Rho family of small G proteins also activates ERK1/2 in response to stretch, induces expression of molecular markers of cardiac hypertrophy, and increases protein synthesis in cardiac myocytes.[42]

Small G proteins are bound to GTP in the active state and to GDP in the inactive state, a process that is regulated by guanine nucleotide exchange factors.[19] For the small G proteins to bind to the cell membrane and remain active, posttranslational lipidation, such as farnesylation or geranyl geranylation is essential. Lipidation of Ras, RhoA, and Rac1 occurs as a consequence of mevalonate metabolism during cholesterol biosynthesis and regulates their membrane association, GTPase activity, and thus activation of hypertrophic signaling pathways.

BIOLOGIC BASIS OF ANTIHYPERTROPHIC AND ANTIFIBROTIC EFFECTS OF STATINS

Signal transduction molecules are the key intermediary step in linking the external or internal stimuli to gene transcription and translation and thus to induction of hypertrophy and fibrosis. Accordingly, interventions to prevent, attenuate, or reverse hypertrophy or fibrosis are aimed at either removal of the stimulus or blockade of the intracellular processing of the stimuli by signaling molecules and/or blockade of gene transcription and translation. Although a diverse array of tools is available to achieve such goals, 3-hydroxy-3-methylglutaryl coenzyme A (HMG-CoA) reductase inhibitors (statins) have emerged as attractive drugs with pleiotropic effects on hypertrophic and fibrotic processes. By inhibiting the cholesterol biosynthetic pathway, statins also inhibit

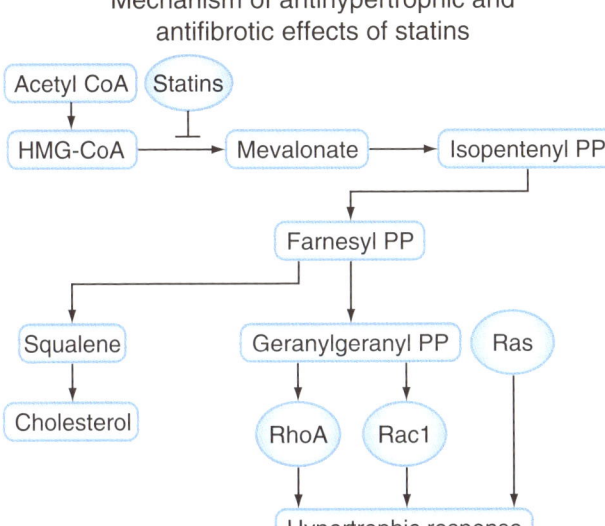

Mechanism of antihypertrophic and antifibrotic effects of statins

Figure 7-4. **Mechanism of antihypertrophic and antifibrotic effects of statins.** By blocking synthesis of mevalonate, statins not only prevent cholesterol biosynthesis but also inhibit farnesylation and geranyl geranylation of Ras, RhoA, and Rac1, which are major mediators of hypertrophy and fibrosis in the heart. Farnesylation and geranyl geranylation of Ras, RhoA, and Rac1 are necessary for their activation. HMG-CoA, 3-hydroxy-3-methylglutaryl coenzyme A; PP, pyrophosphate.

production of isoprenoid intermediates important to the activation of the small G proteins RhoA, Rac, and Ras. Specifically, HMG-CoA reductase inhibitors block conversion of HMG-CoA to L-mevalonate (Fig. 7-4), which ultimately, through a series of biochemical reactions, is converted to farnesyl pyrophosphate (FPP), squalene and cholesterol.[43] FPP is not only a precursor of squalene, but also an active regulator of cellular growth and proliferation through posttranslational modification of Ras.[44] In addition, FPP is also a precursor for geranylgeranyl pyrophosphate (GGPP), which is an important lipid attachment for RhoA, Rac1, and Cdc42. Isoprenylation of the small GTP-binding proteins Rho, Ras, and Rac is essential for their proper covalent attachment to the cell membrane, their subcellular localization, and the activation of their downstream signaling targets.[44,45] Statins, by inhibiting HMG-CoA reductase, also reduce levels of FPP and GGPP and thus prevent and attenuate isoprenylation and membrane association of small GTP-binding proteins. Thus, signaling through Rho, Ras, and Rac (and, consequently, hypertrophic and pro-fibrotic signals from external or internal stimuli) is blocked significantly.

7

One of the major downstream effectors for small GTP-binding proteins is the MAPK family, which is a major mediator of cardiac hypertrophic response. In addition to inhibition of the MAPK pathway, blockade of isoprenylation of small GTP-binding proteins produces a diverse array of antihypertrophic and antifibrotic effects. HMG-CoA reductase inhibitors reduce Ang II–induced production of reactive oxygen species, and thus the oxidative stress,[41,46,47] and decrease expression of pre-proendothelin-1.[48] The molecular bases of antihypertrophic and antifibrotic effects of statins are summarized in Table 7-2.

Reversal, Prevention, and Attenuation of Hypertrophy and Fibrosis in Experimental Animal Models

Observational studies in humans and experimental studies in animal models of cardiac hypertrophy, fibrosis, and failure suggest beneficial effects for HMG-CoA reductase inhibitors in the regression of cardiac hypertrophy and fibrosis, prevention of heart failure, and reduction of mortality. Some examples follow.

Table 7–2

Biologic Properties of HMG-CoA Reductase Inhibitors with Potential Antihypertrophic and Antifibrotic Effects

Blockade of isoprenylation of small GTPase-binding proteins[43-45]
Blockade of phosphatidylinositol-3-kinase (PI3K)/Akt pathway[71]
Reduction of oxidative stress[41,62]
Reduction of expression of cytokines and other inflammatory markers[72,73]
Reduced expression of growth factors, such as FGF2[63] and pre-proendothelin[48]
Reduced expression of ECM (thrombospondin-1, collagen I, and biglycan)[74]
Induction of apoptosis[75]
Down-regulation of Ang II receptor type 1,[47] inhibition of activity of angiotensin-1 converting enzyme 1[60]
Increased intracellular calcium concentration[76]
Increased expression of endothelial nitric oxide[77]
Restoration of autonomic balance[78]
Increased expression of integrins[79]
Inhibition of connective tissue growth factor[80] and FGF-2[63]
Reduced expression of matrix metalloproteinases-1, 3, and 9[81]
Immunosuppression through repression of MHC-II-mediated cell activation[82]
Modulation of homeostasis[56]

Ang II, angiotensin II; ECM, extracellular matrix; FGF, fibroblast growth factor; MHC, major histocompatibility complex.

HYPERTROPHIC CARDIOMYOPATHY

HCM is a genetic disease with an autosomal dominant mode of inheritance.[49] HCM is the most common cause of SCD in the young and a major cause of morbidity and mortality in older adults.[50,51] The clinical diagnosis of HCM is based on the presence of ventricular hypertrophy in the absence of other causes for hypertrophy. The pathologic phenotype comprises myocyte hypertrophy and disarray and interstitial fibrosis. Cardiac hypertrophy, myocyte disarray, and interstitial fibrosis are the major determinants of morbidity and mortality and the increased risk for SCD in HCM.[8,11,51,52] The estimated annual mortality of patients with HCM is approximately 1%.[51,53] However, patients with certain genetic mutations, a family history of SCD, or extensive ventricular hypertrophy are at a much higher risk.[54]

Current pharmacologic interventions in human patients are empirical and none have been shown to induce regression of cardiac hypertrophy, fibrosis, or disarray, the major predictors of mortality and morbidity in HCM.[8,11,52] Because the pathogenesis of HCM entails activation of signaling molecules, it is plausible that HMG-CoA reductase inhibitors, by blocking signaling kinases involved in cardiac hypertrophy and fibrosis, could attenuate cardiac hypertrophy and fibrosis in HCM. Experimental studies support the potential beneficial effects of statins in the prevention of agonist-mediated cardiac hypertrophy and fibrosis.[55-57] The impact of blockade of HMG-CoA reductase on cardiac phenotype was tested in a randomized study in the β-MyHC-Q403 transgenic rabbit model, which exhibits cardiac hypertrophy, interstitial fibrosis, and cardiac myocyte disarray and fully recapitulates the phenotype of human HCM.[58] Treatment with simvastatin resulted in a 37% reduction in left ventricular mass, a 20% reduction in septal and posterior wall thickness, and an approximately 50% reduction in collagen content.[59] Indeed, the collagen fraction was completely normalized in some animals with simvastatin therapy (Fig. 7-5). In addition, indices of left ventricular filling pressure were improved significantly. The molecular mechanism of regression of hypertrophy and fibrosis included inhibition of phosphorylation of ERK1/2, the downstream-signaling kinases in the MAPK pathway, regulated by small GTP-binding proteins. It remains to be tested whether treatment with HMG-CoA reductase inhibitors could also reverse, attenuate, or prevent evolving cardiac hypertrophy and fibrosis, major predictors of mortality and SCD in human patients with HCM.[8,11,52]

PRESSURE OVERLOAD– AND AGONIST-INDUCED HYPERTROPHY

Statins have been shown to prevent the development of cardiac hypertrophy in response to aortic banding and infusion of Ang II and norepinephrine in a cholesterol-independent manner.[41,55,60,61] In an experimental model of pressure overload–induced cardiac hypertrophy, generated by aortic banding, treatment with

7

Interstitial fibrosis with
statin therapy and placebo

Placebo   Simvastatin

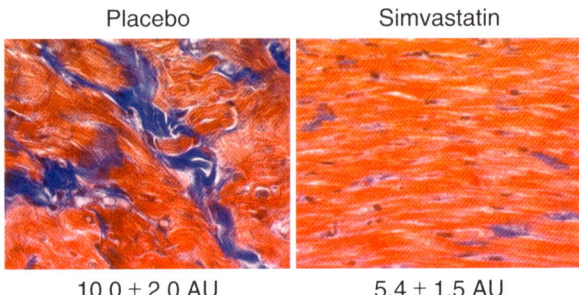

10.0 ± 2.0 AU   5.4 ± 1.5 AU

Figure 7-5. **Reversal of interstitial fibrosis with statin therapy in a transgenic rabbit model of human hypertrophic cardiomyopathy.** Means (and standards deviations) of the results in 12 animals in each group (treated and placebo) are shown. AU, arbitrary units.

simvastatin reduced cardiac hypertrophy and myocardial collagen content significantly and improved left ventricular diastolic performance.[60] Attenuation of hypertrophy and fibrosis was associated with reduced cardiac tissue angiotensin-converting enzyme (ACE) activity. This attenuation was greater than that observed with an ACE inhibitor, which was more effective in inhibiting cardiac ACE activity.[60] Thus, mechanisms in addition to the inhibition of ACE activity were probably involved. Subsequent studies in cultured neonatal rat cardiac myocytes and hypertensive rats provided additional mechanisms by showing that inhibition of hypertrophic response to norepinephrine, Ang II, or pressure overload was associated with reduced oxidative stress and inhibition of the geranyl geranylation of Rac1 and RhoA.[20,41,46,62] Other observed mechanisms included reduced expression of FGF-2 and interleukin (IL)-6, decreased activation of nuclear factor kappa B (NF-κB) and AP-1, and reduced deposition of collagen I, laminin, and fibronectin.[63] Furthermore, statins were also shown to attenuate pressure overload–induced cardiac hypertrophy via inhibition of membrane localization of Ras and the reduction of ERK2 phosphorylation and the cdk4/p27(kip1) ratio.[61] Moreover, treatment with statins has been associated with improved survival in animal models of hypertrophy.[63] Collectively, the results suggested multiple mechanisms by which statins result in anti-hypertrophic and antifibrotic effects.

Myocardial Infarction, Reperfusion Injury, and Heart Failure

Statins also have been shown to attenuate left ventricular remodeling, myocyte hypertrophy, and interstitial fibrosis, and to decrease left ventricular end-diastolic pressure in experimental models of myocardial infarction and reperfusion injury.[64-66] In rats with heart failure secondary to myocardial infarction, treatment with a statin improved systolic and diastolic function, attenuated expression of markers of cardiac hypertrophy and collagen I, increased expression of eNOS in the heart, and reduced levels of nitrotyrosine protein.[65] Statins also improved cardiac systolic function and survival in murine models of heart failure due to myocardial infarction and reduced expression of MMP-2 and MMP-13 in response to myocardial injury.[64,65] Thus HMG-CoA reductase inhibitors result in beneficial effects in experimental models of myocardial infarction and injury.

Human Studies

Despite the abundance of experimental data favoring the use of statins in prevention, attenuation, or reversal of cardiac hypertrophy, fibrosis, and heart failure, data in humans are restricted to observational studies and retrospective analyses. With regard to cardiac hypertrophy, the results of a small randomized study in hypertensive subjects showed treatment with pravastatin was associated with a significant reduction in left ventricular mass.[57] A previous study in heart transplant recipients showed no significant difference in the left ventricular mass between those who were on simvastatin and those who were not, but the left ventricular ejection fraction was increased modestly.[67] Post hoc data analyses from several clinical trials have suggested a beneficial effect for statins in preventing heart failure and in reducing mortality from heart failure. Analysis of data from the Scandinavian Simvastatin Survival Study (4S) showed that treatment with simvastatin was associated with a 20% reduction in the occurrence of heart failure.[68] Similarly, in an observational study of patients with prior myocardial infarction and elevated plasma low-density-lipoprotein levels, the use of statins was an independent predictor of heart failure.[69] The observed beneficial effect of statins in humans is likely to be the result of reduction of ischemic events, and whether HMG-CoA reductase inhibitors also result in beneficial effects on cardiac hypertrophy and fibrosis in humans requires additional investigation.

CONCLUSION

A plethora of in vitro and in vivo experimental data in conjunction with observational data in humans suggest an antihypertrophic and antifibrotic effect for statins independent of their effect on cholesterol. These benefits are mediated through a diverse array of biologic effects including an inhibition of the generation of isoprenylate intermediates by HMG-CoA reductase inhibitors. Collectively, these data demonstrate the need for prospective randomized clinical trials in humans with the phenotype of hypertrophy and fibrosis, major determinants of mortality and morbidity in a variety of cardiovascular diseases. A prototype of such a phenotype in humans is HCM, which has been modeled in animals and shown to be responsive to treatment with statins.[70] Whether the observed attenuation and reversal of hypertrophy, fibrosis, and myocardial dysfunction with statins in animal models are also relevant to humans requires proof through large-scale, prospectively designed, randomized studies.

References

1. Swynghedauw B: Molecular mechanisms of myocardial remodeling. Physiol Rev 79:215-262, 1999.
2. Powell DW, Mifflin RC, Valentich JD, et al: Myofibroblasts: I. Paracrine cells important in health and disease. Am J Physiol 277:C1-C9, 1999.
3. Manabe I, Shindo T, Nagai R: Gene expression in fibroblasts and fibrosis: Involvement in cardiac hypertrophy. Circ Res 91:1103-1113, 2002.
4. Haider AW, Larson MG, Benjamin EJ, Levy D. Increased left ventricular mass and hypertrophy are associated with increased risk for sudden death. J Am Coll Cardiol 32:1454-1459, 1998.
5. Assayag P, Carre F, Chevalier B, et al: Compensated cardiac hypertrophy: Arrhythmogenicity and the new myocardial phenotype: I. Fibrosis. Cardiovasc Res 34:439-444, 1997.
6. Levy D, Garrison RJ, Savage DD, et al: Prognostic implications of echocardiographically determined left ventricular mass in the Framingham Heart Study. N Engl J Med 322:1561-1566, 1990.
7. Benjamin EJ, Levy DD: Why is left ventricular hypertrophy so predictive of morbidity and mortality? Am J Med Sci 317:168-175, 1999.
8. Spirito P, Bellone P, Harris KM, et al: Magnitude of left ventricular hypertrophy and risk of sudden death in hypertrophic cardiomyopathy. N Engl J Med 342:1778-1785, 2000.
9. Vasan RS, Larson MG, Benjamin EJ, et al: Congestive heart failure in subjects with normal versus reduced left ventricular ejection fraction: Prevalence and mortality in a population-based cohort. J Am Coll Cardiol 33:1948-1955, 1999.
10. Kannel WB, Wolf PA, Benjamin EJ, Levy D: Prevalence, incidence, prognosis, and predisposing conditions for atrial fibrillation: Population-based estimates. Am J Cardiol 82:2N-9N, 1998.
11. Shirani J, Pick R, Roberts WC, Maron BJ: Morphology and significance of the left ventricular collagen network in young patients with hypertrophic cardiomyopathy and sudden cardiac death. J Am Coll Cardiol 35:36-44, 2000.
12. La Vecchia L, Ometto R, Centofante P, et al: Arrhythmic profile, ventricular function, and histomorphometric findings in patients with idiopathic ventricular tachycardia and mitral valve prolapse: Clinical and prognostic evaluation. Clin Cardiol 21:731-735, 1998.
13. Kawara T, Derksen R, de Groot JR, et al: Activation delay after premature stimulation in chronically diseased human myocardium relates to the architecture of interstitial fibrosis. Circulation 104:3069-3075, 2001.
14. Pogwizd SM, McKenzie JP, Cain ME: Mechanisms underlying spontaneous and induced ventricular arrhythmias in patients with idiopathic dilated cardiomyopathy. Circulation 98:2404-2414, 1998.

7

15. Burlew BS, Weber KT: Cardiac fibrosis as a cause of diastolic dysfunction. Herz 27:92-98, 2002.
16. Yamamoto K, Masuyama T, Sakata Y, et al: Myocardial stiffness is determined by ventricular fibrosis, but not by compensatory or excessive hypertrophy in hypertensive heart. Cardiovasc Res 55:76-82, 2002.
17. Matsumoto T, Wada A, Tsutamoto T, et al: Chymase inhibition prevents cardiac fibrosis and improves diastolic dysfunction in the progression of heart failure. Circulation 107:2555-2558, 2003.
18. Sadoshima J, Xu Y, Slayter HS, Izumo S: Autocrine release of angiotensin II mediates stretch-induced hypertrophy of cardiac myocytes in vitro. Cell 75:977-984, 1993.
19. Clerk A, Sugden PH: Small guanine nucleotide-binding proteins and myocardial hypertrophy. Circ Res 86:1019-1023, 2000.
20. Pierce KL, Premont RT, Lefkowitz RJ: Seven-transmembrane receptors. Nat Rev Mol Cell Biol 3:639-650, 2002.
21. Zou Y, Komuro I, Yamazaki T, et al: Protein kinase C, but not tyrosine kinases or Ras, plays a critical role in angiotensin II-induced activation of Raf-1 kinase and extracellular signal-regulated protein kinases in cardiac myocytes. J Biol Chem 271:33592-33597, 1996.
22. Kudoh S, Komuro I, Mizuno T, et al: Angiotensin II stimulates c-Jun NH2-terminal kinase in cultured cardiac myocytes of neonatal rats. Circ Res 80:139-146, 1997.
23. Ishizaki T, Morishima Y, Okamoto M, et al: Coordination of microtubules and the actin cytoskeleton by the Rho effector mDia1. Nat Cell Biol 3:8-14, 2001.
24. Zhang S, Weinheimer C, Courtois M, et al: The role of the Grb2-p38 MAPK signaling pathway in cardiac hypertrophy and fibrosis. J Clin Invest 111:833-841, 2003.
25. Zhu WZ, Wang SQ, Chakir K, et al: Linkage of beta1-adrenergic stimulation to apoptotic heart cell death through protein kinase A-independent activation of Ca2+/calmodulin kinase II. J Clin Invest 111:617-625, 2003.
26. Marks AR: Calcium and the heart: A question of life and death. J Clin Invest 2003 111:597-600.
27. Dorn GW, Brown JH. Gq signaling in cardiac adaptation and maladaptation. Trends Cardiovasc Med 9:26-34, 1999.
28. McKinsey TA, Olson EN: Cardiac hypertrophy: Sorting out the circuitry. Curr Opin Genet Dev 9:267-274, 1999.
29. Molkentin JD: Calcineurin and beyond: Cardiac hypertrophic signaling. Circ Res 87:731-738, 2000.
30. Ross RS, Borg TK: Integrins and the myocardium. Circ Res 88:1112-1119, 2001.
31. MacKenna DA, Dolfi F, Vuori K, Ruoslahti E: Extracellular signal-regulated kinase and c-Jun NH2-terminal kinase activation by mechanical stretch is integrin-dependent and matrix-specific in rat cardiac fibroblasts. J Clin Invest 101:301-310, 1998.
32. Geiger B, Bershadsky A: Exploring the neighborhood: Adhesion-coupled cell mechanosensors. Cell 110:139-142, 2002.
33. Etienne-Manneville S, Hall A: Rho GTPases in cell biology. Nature 420:629-635, 2002.
34. Swynghedauw B: Molecular Cardiology for the Cardiologist, 2nd ed. New York, Kluwer Academic, 1998, pp 131-138.
35. Harada K, Sugaya T, Murakami K, et al: Angiotensin II type 1A

7

receptor knockout mice display less left ventricular remodeling and improved survival after myocardial infarction. Circulation 100:2093-2099, 1999.

36. Schieffer B, Wirger A, Meybrunn M, et al: Comparative effects of chronic angiotensin-converting enzyme inhibition and angiotensin II type 1 receptor blockade on cardiac remodeling after myocardial infarction in the rat. Circulation 89:2273-2282, 1994.

37. Schultz JJ, Witt SA, Glascock BJ, et al: TGF-beta1 mediates the hypertrophic cardiomyocyte growth induced by angiotensin II. J Clin Invest 109:787-796, 2002.

38. Sano M, Fukuda K, Kodama H, et al: Interleukin-6 family of cytokines mediate angiotensin II-induced cardiac hypertrophy in rodent cardiomyocytes. J Biol Chem 275:29717-29723, 2000.

39. Kim HE, Dalal SS, Young E, et al: Disruption of the myocardial extracellular matrix leads to cardiac dysfunction. J Clin Invest 106:857-866, 2000.

40. Ducharme A, Frantz S, Aikawa M, et al: Targeted deletion of matrix metalloproteinase-9 attenuates left ventricular enlargement and collagen accumulation after experimental myocardial infarction. J Clin Invest 106:55-62, 2000.

41. Takemoto M, Node K, Nakagami H, et al: Statins as antioxidant therapy for preventing cardiac myocyte hypertrophy. J Clin Invest 108:1429-1437, 2001.

42. Aikawa R, Komuro I, Yamazaki T, et al: Rho family small G proteins play critical roles in mechanical stress-induced hypertrophic responses in cardiac myocytes. Circ Res 84:458-466, 1999.

43. Grunler J, Ericsson J, Dallner G: Branch-point reactions in the biosynthesis of cholesterol, dolichol, ubiquinone and prenylated proteins. Biochim Biophys Acta 1212:259-277, 1994.

44. Hori Y, Kikuchi A, Isomura M, et al: Post-translational modifications of the C-terminal region of the rho protein are important for its interaction with membranes and the stimulatory and inhibitory GDP/GTP exchange proteins. Oncogene 6:515-522, 1991.

45. Maltese WA, Robishaw JD: Isoprenylation of C-terminal cysteine in a G-protein gamma subunit. J Biol Chem 265:18071-18074, 1990.

46. Delbosc S, Cristol JP, Descomps B, et al: Simvastatin prevents angiotensin II-induced cardiac alteration and oxidative stress. Hypertension 40:142-147, 2002.
Wassmann S, Laufs U, Baumer AT, et al: HMG-CoA reductase inhibitors improve endothelial dysfunction in normocholesterolemic hypertension via reduced production of reactive oxygen species. Hypertension 37:1450-1457, 2001.

48. Hernandez-Perera O, Perez-Sala D, Soria E, Lamas S: Involvement of Rho GTPases in the transcriptional inhibition of preproendothelin-1 gene expression by simvastatin in vascular endothelial cells. Circ Res 87:616-622, 2000.

49. Marian AJ, Roberts R: The molecular genetic basis for hypertrophic cardiomyopathy. J Mol Cell Cardiol 33:655-670, 2001.

50. Maron BJ, Shirani J, Poliac LC, et al: Sudden death in young competitive athletes. Clinical, demographic, and pathological profiles. JAMA 276:199-204, 1996.

51. Maron BJ: Hypertrophic cardiomyopathy: A systematic review. JAMA 287:1308-1320, 2002.

52. Spirito P, Maron BJ: Relation between extent of left ventricular

hypertrophy and occurrence of sudden cardiac death in hypertrophic cardiomyopathy. J Am Coll Cardiol 15:1521-1526, 1990.

53. Cannan CR, Reeder GS, Bailey KR, et al: Natural history of hypertrophic cardiomyopathy: A population-based study, 1976 through 1990. Circulation 92:2488-2495, 1995.

54. Marian AJ: On predictors of sudden cardiac death in hypertrophic cardiomyopathy. J Am Coll Cardiol 41:994-996, 2003.

55. Oi S, Haneda T, Osaki J, et al: Lovastatin prevents angiotensin II-induced cardiac hypertrophy in cultured neonatal rat heart cells. Eur J Pharmacol 376:139-148, 1999.

56. Park HJ, Galper JB: 3-Hydroxy-3-methylglutaryl CoA reductase inhibitors up-regulate transforming growth factor-beta signaling in cultured heart cells via inhibition of geranylgeranylation of RhoA GTPase. Proc Natl Acad Sci USA 96:11525-11530, 1999.

57. Su SF, Hsiao CL, Chu CW, et al: Effects of pravastatin on left ventricular mass in patients with hyperlipidemia and essential hypertension. Am J Cardiol 86:514-518, 2000.

58. Marian AJ, Wu Y, Lim DS, et al: A transgenic rabbit model for human hypertrophic cardiomyopathy. J Clin Invest 104:1683-1692, 1999.

59. Patel R, Lim DS, Reddy D, et al: Variants of trophic factors and expression of cardiac hypertrophy in patients with hypertrophic cardiomyopathy. J Mol Cell Cardiol 32:2369-2377, 2000.

60. Luo JD, Zhang WW, Zhang GP, et al: Simvastatin inhibits cardiac hypertrophy and angiotensin-converting enzyme activity in rats with aortic stenosis. Clin Exp Pharmacol Physiol 26:903-908, 1999.

61. Indolfi C, Di Lorenzo E, Perrino C, et al: Hydroxymethylglutaryl coenzyme A reductase inhibitor simvastatin prevents cardiac hypertrophy induced by pressure overload and inhibits p21ras activation. Circulation 106:2118-2124, 2002.

62. Luo JD, Xie F, Zhang WW, Ma XD, et al: Simvastatin inhibits noradrenaline-induced hypertrophy of cultured neonatal rat cardiomyocytes. Br J Pharmacol 132:159-164, 2001.

63. Dechend R, Fiebeler A, Park JK, et al: Amelioration of angiotensin II-induced cardiac injury by a 3-hydroxy-3-methylglutaryl coenzyme a reductase inhibitor. Circulation 104:576-581, 2001.

64. Hayashidani S, Tsutsui H, Shiomi T, et al: Fluvastatin, a 3-hydroxy-3-methylglutaryl coenzyme a reductase inhibitor, attenuates left ventricular remodeling and failure after experimental myocardial infarction. Circulation 105:868-873, 2002.

65. Bauersachs J, Galuppo P, Fraccarollo D, et al: Improvement of left ventricular remodeling and function by hydroxymethylglutaryl coenzyme a reductase inhibition with cerivastatin in rats with heart failure after myocardial infarction. Circulation 104:982-985, 2001.

66. Bell RM, Yellon DM: Atorvastatin, administered at the onset of reperfusion, and independent of lipid lowering, protects the myocardium by up-regulating a pro-survival pathway. J Am Coll Cardiol 41:508-515, 2003.

67. Jenkins GH, Grieve LA, Yacoub MH, Singer DR: Effect of simvastatin on ejection fraction in cardiac transplant recipients. Am J Cardiol 78:1453-1456, 1996.

68. Kjekshus J, Pedersen TR, Olsson AG, et al: The effects of simvastatin on the incidence of heart failure in patients with coronary heart disease. J Card Fail 3:249-254, 1997.

69. Aronow WS, Ahn C: Frequency of congestive heart failure in older

persons with prior myocardial infarction and serum low-density lipoprotein cholesterol > or = 125 mg/dl treated with statins versus no lipid-lowering drug. Am J Cardiol 90:147-149, 2002.

70. Patel R, Nagueh SF, Tsybouleva N, et al: Simvastatin induces regression of cardiac hypertrophy and fibrosis and improves cardiac function in a transgenic rabbit model of human hypertrophic cardiomyopathy. Circulation 104:317-324, 2001.

71. Kureishi Y, Luo Z, Shiojima I, et al: The HMG-CoA reductase inhibitor simvastatin activates the protein kinase Akt and promotes angiogenesis in normocholesterolemic animals [see comments]. Nat Med 6:1004-1010, 2000.

72. von Haehling S, Anker SD, Bassenge E: Statins and the role of nitric oxide in chronic heart failure. Heart Fail Rev 8:99-106, 2003.

73. Weitz-Schmidt G, Welzenbach K, Brinkmann V, et al: Statins selectively inhibit leukocyte function antigen-1 by binding to a novel regulatory integrin site. Nat Med 7:687-692, 2001.

74. Riessen R, Axel DI, Fenchel M, et al: Effect of HMG-CoA reductase inhibitors on extracellular matrix expression in human vascular smooth muscle cells. Basic Res Cardiol 94:322-332, 1999.

75. Tan A, Levrey H, Dahm C, et al: Lovastatin induces fibroblast apoptosis in vitro and in vivo. A possible therapy for fibroproliferative disorders. Am J Respir Crit Care Med 159:220-227, 1999.

76. Veerkamp JH, Smit JW, Benders AA, Oosterhof A: Effects of HMG-CoA reductase inhibitors on growth and differentiation of cultured rat skeletal muscle cells. Biochim Biophys Acta 1315:217-222, 1996.

77. Endres M, Laufs U, Huang Z, et al: Stroke protection by 3-hydroxy-3-methylglutaryl (HMG)-CoA reductase inhibitors mediated by endothelial nitric oxide synthase. Proc Natl Acad Sci USA 95:8880-8885, 1998.

78. Pliquett RU, Cornish KG, Peuler JD, Zucker IH: Simvastatin normalizes autonomic neural control in experimental heart failure. Circulation 107:2493-2498, 2003.

79. Graf K, Kappert K, Stawowy P, et al: Statins regulate alpha2beta1-integrin expression and collagen I-dependent functions in human vascular smooth muscle cells. J Cardiovasc Pharmacol 41:89-96, 2003.

80. Eberlein M, Heusinger-Ribeiro J, Goppelt-Struebe M: Rho-dependent inhibition of the induction of connective tissue growth factor (CTGF) by HMG CoA reductase inhibitors (statins). Br J Pharmacol 133:1172-1180, 2001.

81. Fukumoto Y, Libby P, Rabkin E, et al: Statins alter smooth muscle cell accumulation and collagen content in established atheroma of Watanabe heritable hyperlipidemic rabbits. Circulation 103:993-999, 2001.

82. Kwak B, Mulhaupt F, Myit S, Mach F: Statins as a newly recognized type of immunomodulator. Nat Med 6:1399-1402, 2000.

7

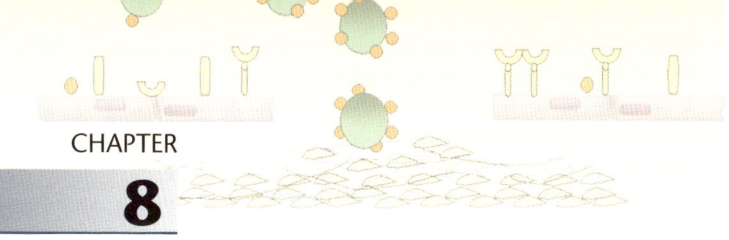

The Pleiotropic Effects of Statins: Relevance to Their Salutary Effects

Sebastian Wolfrum and James K. Liao

Elevated serum cholesterol levels are strongly associated with coronary atherosclerotic disease.[1] Atherosclerosis is mediated, in part, by the uptake of modified low-density lipoprotein (LDL) into the vascular wall.[2] Because the conversion of 3-hydroxy-3-methylglutaryl coenzyme A (HMG-CoA) to mevalonate is the early rate-limiting step in cholesterol biosynthesis, blocking the formation of mevalonate and subsequent cholesterol synthesis by statins has been proposed to be the predominant mechanism underlying the beneficial effects of statins. Indeed, therapeutic doses of statins potently reduce serum cholesterol levels in humans,[3] and a number of large clinical trials have demonstrated that statins markedly decrease the incidence of cardiovascular events in hypercholesterolemic individuals.[3-6]

Although the detrimental effects of high cholesterol levels are substantially reduced by statins, there is increasing evidence that statins may exert protective effects beyond cholesterol reduction.[7,8] This notion arises from subgroup analyses of the West of Scotland Coronary Prevention Study (WOSCOPS) and the Cholesterol and Recurrent Events (CARE) trial, which suggest that statin-treated subjects have a significantly lower risk for coronary heart disease than age-matched placebo-treated individuals, despite comparable serum cholesterol levels.[5,8,9] Meta-analyses of past clinical trials revealed that the risk of myocardial infarctions in individuals treated with statins is significantly lower than in individuals treated with other cholesterol-lowering agents or modalities, despite similar reduction in serum cholesterol levels in both groups.[10,11] In addition, experimental studies revealed that statin therapy not only is effective in hypercholesterolemia but also protects

The work described in this article was supported in part by the National Institutes of Health, the American Heart Association, and Deutsche Forschungsgemeinschaft.

normocholesterolemic animals against stroke,[12] myocardial infarction,[13-15] and vascular inflammatory responses.[16]

EVIDENCE FOR PLEIOTROPISM FROM IN VITRO DATA

Effects of Statins on the Endothelium

Many of the cholesterol-independent or "pleiotropic" effects of statins have been attributed to their ability to increase the bioavailability of nitric oxide (NO) in vascular endothelial cells. Indeed, statins have been shown to increase endothelial NO synthase (eNOS) expression and activity through two separate mechanisms. First, statins inhibit the Rho/Rho-kinase pathway, leading to the stabilization of eNOS mRNA (Fig. 8-1). Second, statins activate the phosphatidylinositol (PI) 3-kinase/protein kinase B (Akt) pathway, which leads to the phosphorylation and the subsequent activation of eNOS.

Inhibition of HMG-CoA reductase by statins

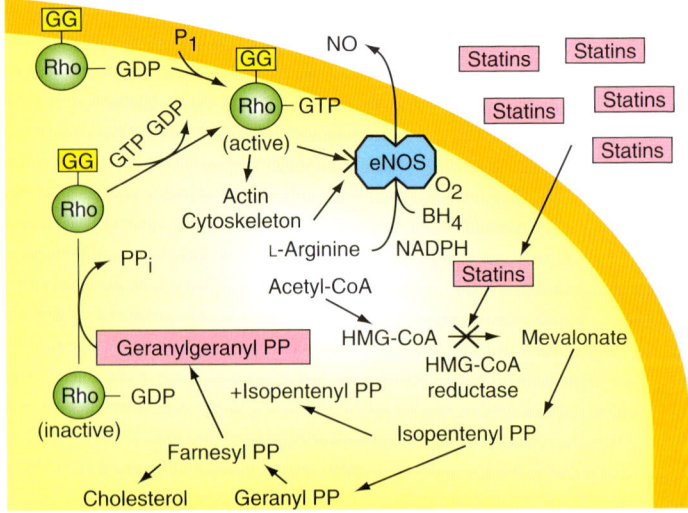

Figure 8-1. **Inhibition of HMG-CoA reductase by statins decreases the synthesis of isoprenoids and cholesterol.** The isoprenoid, geranylgeranyl (GG), is an important lipid attachment for Rho, which permits the subsequent membrane translocation and activation of Rho and Rho kinase. Inhibition of Rho/Rho-kinase activity by statins leads to an increase in eNOS expression and activity. (From Liao JK: Statins and ischemic stroke. Atheroscler Suppl 3:21, 2002; reproduced with the permission of the publisher.)

STATINS INHIBIT SYNTHESIS OF ISOPRENYLATED PROTEINS

Inhibition of HMG-CoA reductase by statins prevents the formation of various isoprenoid intermediates (see Fig. 8-1).[17] Farnesyl pyrophosphate (FPP) and geranylgeranyl pyrophosphate (GGPP), for example, serve as important lipid attachments for the posttranslational modification of a variety of proteins, including the subunit of heterotrimeric G proteins and the small GTP-binding protein Ras, and Ras-like proteins, such as Rho, Rab, Rac, Ra-1, and Rap.[18] Protein isoprenylation allows the covalent attachment, subcellular localization, and intracellular trafficking of several membrane-associated proteins. The small GTP-binding proteins Ras and Rho are major substrates for posttranslational modification by isoprenoids.[18-20] Posttranslational isoprenylation of these small GTP-binding proteins is required for their proper intracellular functions. Whereas translocation of Ras from the cytoplasm to the plasma membrane is dependent on farnesylation, geranyl geranylation contributes to the translocation of Rho in vascular endothelial cells.[21]

Rho is a major target of geranyl geranylation and there is increasing evidence that Rho negatively regulates eNOS expression and activity. For example, direct inhibition of Rho by *Clostridium botulinum* C3 transferase increases eNOS expression in a manner that is independent of isoprenylation.[21] The C3 transferase ADP ribosylates asparagine-41 of Rho and renders it biologically inactive in the GDP-bound state.[19] Furthermore, inhibition of Rho by overexpression of a dominant-negative mutant of RhoA also increases eNOS expression. In contrast, direct activation of Rho by *Escherichia coli* cytotoxic necrotizing factor (CNF)-1 leads to a decrease in eNOS expression.[19]

Treatment of endothelial cells with statins leads to accumulation of inactive Ras and Rho in the cytoplasm by inhibiting their isoprenylation. Inhibition of RhoA by statins up-regulates eNOS expression by prolonging the eNOS mRNA half-life. Although the effects of statins on Ras and Rho isoprenylation are reversed in the presence of FPP and GGPP, respectively, the effects of statins on eNOS expression are reversed only by GGPP and not by FPP or LDL cholesterol.[21] These findings are consistent with a cholesterol-independent effect of statins and suggest that inhibition of isoprenoid synthesis may contribute importantly to the restoration of endothelial function. Indeed, statins prevent the down-regulation of eNOS by oxidized LDL, tumor necrosis factor α (TNF-α), and hypoxia, conditions that are frequently associated with endothelial dysfunction.[21-24]

STATINS ACTIVATE THE PI 3-KINASE/AKT PATHWAY

The serine-threonine protein kinase Akt is an important regulator of various cellular processes, including cell metabolism and apoptosis.[25,26] Stimulation of receptor tyrosine kinases and G-protein–coupled receptors leads to activation PI 3-kinase, the products of which, such as phosphatidylinositol 3,4,5-triphosphate

(PIP$_3$), act as membrane-docking domains for plectrin–homology-containing proteins such as Akt.[27,28] Akt has been shown to phosphorylate and inhibit several downstream targets, such as glycogen synthase kinase-3, Bad, and caspase-9.[28,29] Interestingly, Akt also mediates insulin-stimulated activation of eNOS. Consequently, recent studies have focused on the activation of eNOS via the PI 3-kinase/Akt pathway and have demonstrated that eNOS is indeed a substrate of Akt that phosphorylates eNOS at Ser 1179 or 1177.[30-33] Indeed, statins can activate Akt, which leads to an increased NO production, a process that is inhibited by the PI 3-kinase inhibitor wortmannin. Furthermore, statins inhibit apoptosis of cultured endothelial cells, which could not be observed in cells that overexpress dominant-negative Akt.[34]

Therefore, there is increasing evidence that activation of the PI 3-kinase/Akt pathway may contribute to the endothelium-dependent effects of statins, in addition to stabilizing eNOS mRNA by inhibition of Rho. Activation of Akt might lead to eNOS activation even faster than the modulation of Rho proteins, although the precise mechanisms by which PI 3-kinase is activated by statins have not yet been identified.

STATINS MODULATE VASOCONSTRICTOR ACTIVITY

Because several vasoconstricting agents counteract the vasodilating effect of NO, endothelial dysfunction and development of atherosclerosis may also be attributed to the release of potent vasoconstrictors such as endothelin-1 (ET-1) or angiotensin II (Ang II). Indeed, circulating concentrations and tissue immunoreactivity of ET-1 are increased in patients with severe atherosclerosis.[35,36] ET-1 acts as a vasoconstrictive and mitogenic agent, and exposure to oxidized LDL (ox-LDL) leads to increased production and release of ET-1,[37] which promotes neointimal proliferation of atherosclerotic lesions.[38] Statins have been shown to inhibit pre-proET-1 mRNA expression and to reduce immunoreactive ET-1 in bovine endothelial cells, a phenomenon that is mediated by inhibition of Rho.[39,40] Through a similar mechanism, statins decrease the expression of angiotensin II type 1[41] and endothelin receptors (Fig. 8-2).[42]

STATINS DECREASE THE EXPRESSION OF LOX-1

Atherosclerosis is mediated, in part, by the uptake of modified LDL into the vascular wall.[2] Vascular endothelial cells internalize and degrade ox-LDL through a receptor-mediated pathway.[43] This lectin-like receptor for ox-LDL (LOX-1) is up-regulated in atherosclerotic tissues,[44] and increased expression of LOX-1 may promote some of the pathologic effects of ox-LDL, such as increased apoptosis, suppression of eNOS activity, and increased cell adhesion.[45] Li and co-workers recently reported that in human coronary artery endothelial cells, ox-LDL increased the expression of LOX-1 protein and mRNA, leading to an enhanced ox-LDL uptake. This effect was attenuated by co-treatment with statins.[46] Furthermore, the

Multiple effects of statins on circulating LDL levels

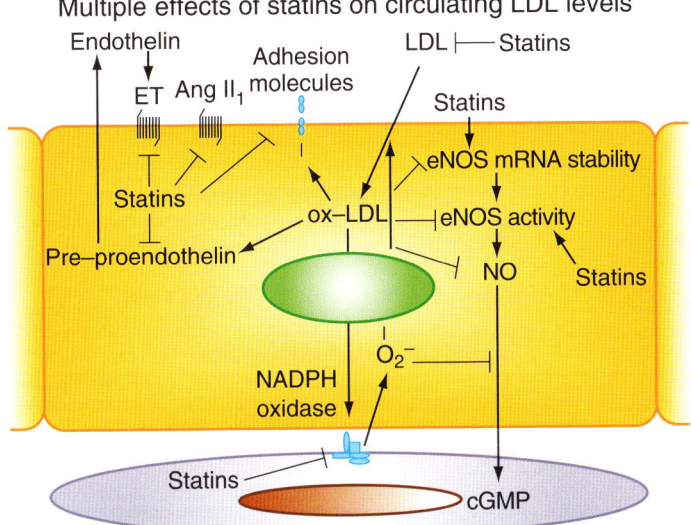

Figure 8-2. **Oxidized LDL (ox-LDL) impairs endothelial function and leads to endothelial cell activation.** Statins counteract these effects by reducing circulating LDL levels. Statins also act by enhancing the expression and activity of eNOS, reducing expression of vasoconstricting agents and adhesion molecules, and decreasing production of reactive oxygen species in endothelial cells (yellow). These effects collectively lead to an accumulation of cAMP in vascular smooth muscle cells (purple) followed by their relaxation. Ang II_1, angiotensin II type 1 receptor; ET, endothelin receptor; eNOS, endothelial nitric oxide synthase. (From Wolfrum S, Jensen KS, Liao JK: Endothelium-dependent effects of statins. Arterioscler Thromb Vasc Biol 23:729, 2003; reproduced with the permission of the publisher.)

decrease in eNOS activation after stimulation of LOX-1 could also be attenuated by statin therapy.[47] Mediation of LOX-1 expression by statins, leading to lower levels of ox-LDL within the vascular wall, may contribute to the beneficial effects of statins on atherosclerotic plaques.

STATINS EXERT FIBRINOLYTIC EFFECTS

Plasminogen activator inhibitor type-1 (PAI-1) is the major endogenous inhibitor of tissue type plasminogen activator (t-PA) and plays a pivotal role in the regulation of fibrinolysis.[48] High PAI-1 plasma levels and decreased levels of t-PA activity have been shown to be associated with coronary heart disease. Increased PAI-1 expression is observed in human atherosclerotic lesions, suggesting a putative role in atherosclerosis.[49]

There is increasing evidence from in vitro studies that statins positively affect the fibrinolytic system of cultured smooth muscle cells (SMCs) as well as endothelial cells. In these studies, a decrease in PAI-1 and an increase in t-PA were observed after co-treatment with statins in endothelial cells.[50-52] Several in vivo studies have also investigated the effect of statin therapy on the regulation of the fibrinolytic system, but the results are inconsistent. Whereas in some studies statins reportedly decreased PAI-1 plasma levels, other studies showed either minimal or no effect.[53-55] Nevertheless, statins may interfere with the progression of the atherosclerotic plaque and ensuing thrombosis after plaque rupture independent of their ability to reduce plasma cholesterol.[56]

Effects of Statins on Vascular Smooth Muscle Cells

STATINS INHIBIT SMOOTH MUSCLE CELL PROLIFERATION

In the pathogenesis of vascular lesions, including postangioplasty restenosis, transplant arteriosclerosis, and venous graft occlusion, proliferation of vascular SMCs (VSMCs) plays a key role.[57] Interestingly, statins attenuate vascular proliferative disease in transplant-associated arteriosclerosis, an immunologic rather than a lipid disorder, although hypercholesterolemia can also exacerbate the immunologic process.[57,58] In VSMCs, statin treatment leads to decreased DNA synthesis after stimulation with platelet-derived growth factor (PDGF).[59,60] Several findings indicate that statins inhibit VSMC proliferation by arresting the cell cycle during the G1-phase-to-S-phase transition. Specifically, statins decrease PDGF-induced retinoblastoma (Rb) gene product hyperphosphorylation and cyclin-dependent kinase (cdk)-2, cdk-4, and cdk-6 activities. This is correlated with increased levels of the cdk inhibitor p27(Kip1), without concomitant changes in levels of p16(INK4), p21(Waf1), or p53.

Because the small GTP-binding proteins Ras and Rho, which are modified under statin treatment, are implicated in cell cycle regulation, they are likely to be targets for the direct antiproliferative vascular effects of statins. Whereas Ras promotes cell cycle progression via activation of the mitogen-activated protein kinase pathway,[61] Rho causes cellular proliferation, possibly through destabilizing p27(Kip1) protein.[62] Interestingly, inhibition of VSMC proliferation by statins was reversed by GGPP, but not by FPP or LDL cholesterol, suggesting that Rho may play a greater role in SMC proliferation than Ras. Indeed, direct inhibition of Rho increases p27(Kip1) and decreases Rb hyperphosphorylation and SMC proliferation after PDGF stimulation.[59] Taken together, these findings indicate that Rho mediates PDGF-induced SMC proliferation and that inhibition of Rho by statins is the predominant mechanism by which statins inhibit vascular SMC proliferation.

STATINS DECREASE THE RELEASE OF REACTIVE OXYGEN SPECIES

Reactive oxygen species (ROS) directly affect endothelial function through scavenging and decreasing the bioavailability of NO.[63]

Because the amount of ROS generated in the endothelium is relatively low, most studies focus on other sources of ROS, such as SMCs and leukocytes.[64,65]

Statins attenuate Ang II-induced ROS production in vascular SMCs by inhibiting Rac1-mediated NADPH oxidase activity and down-regulating Ang II$_1$-receptor expression.[66] More recently, Wassmann and colleagues reported that atorvastatin reduced vascular mRNA expression of essential NADPH oxidase subunits p22phox and nox1 (gp91phox) by a mechanism that involves the translocation of Rac1 from the cytosol to the cell membrane.[64] Because NO is scavenged by ROS, these findings indicate that the antioxidant properties of statins may also contribute to their ability to improve endothelial function (see Fig. 8-2).[67,68] In addition, withdrawal of statin treatment in mice has been shown to impair endothelium-dependent relaxation by increasing vascular superoxide anion generation via a pathway involving the Rac-dependent activation of the gp91phox-containing vascular NADPH oxidase.[69]

Effects of Statins on Blood Cells

STATINS MODULATE ENDOTHELIUM-LEUKOCYTE INTERACTION

Atherosclerosis is a complex inflammatory process that is characterized by the presence of monocytes or macrophages and T lymphocytes in the atheroma.[2,70] Inflammatory cytokines secreted by these macrophages and T lymphocytes can modify endothelial function, SMC proliferation, collagen degradation, and thrombosis.[71] An early step in atherogenesis involves monocyte recruitment and adhesion to the endothelium.[70] Statins exert anti-inflammatory effects on the vascular wall by decreasing the number of inflammatory cells in atherosclerotic plaques.[72] The mechanism is unknown, but it may involve decreased expression of endothelial adhesion molecules (see Fig. 8-2) such as intercellular adhesion molecule-1 (ICAM-1) and cytokines such as interleukin-6 and -8, which are involved in the recruitment of inflammatory cells.[73,74]

Statins can also suppress the inflammatory response independent of HMG-CoA reductase inhibition by binding directly to a novel regulatory site of the β_2 integrin, leukocyte function antigen-1 (LFA-1). LFA-1 serves as a major counterreceptor for ICAM-1 on leukocytes.[75] The mechanism of the anti-inflammatory properties of statins was further elucidated by Yoshida and coworkers, who recently demonstrated that cerivastatin reduced monocyte adhesion to vascular endothelium by decreasing the expression of integrins and actin polymerization via inactivation of RhoA.[76]

STATINS MODULATE PLATELET FUNCTION

Platelets play a critical role in the development of acute coronary syndromes.[77] Acute thrombus formation at the site of plaque rupture and vascular injury is present in most episodes of acute coronary syndromes.[78-80] Hypercholesterolemia is associated with increases in platelet reactivity.[81,82] These abnormalities are linked to increases in the cholesterol-to-phospholipid ratio in platelets. Other potential mechanisms include increases in thromboxane A_2 biosynthesis,[83] platelet α_2-adrenergic receptor density,[84] and platelet cytosolic calcium.[85]

Statins have been shown to inhibit platelet function.[86-88] Potential mechanisms include a reduction in the production of thromboxane A_2 and modifications in the cholesterol content of platelet membranes.[72,89] The cholesterol content of platelet and erythrocyte membranes is reduced in patients undergoing statin therapy. This may lead to a decrease in the thrombogenic potential of these cells. Indeed, animal studies suggest that statin therapy inhibits platelet deposition on damaged vessels and reduces platelet thrombus formation.[79,90,91] Furthermore, in vitro experiments have demonstrated that statins inhibit tissue factor expression by macrophages, thereby potentially reducing the thrombotic potential of the vascular wall.[92]

In addition to reduction in platelet cholesterol content, the inhibition of Rho might be responsible for the reduced platelet activity under statin treatment. In their study, Kaneider and colleagues reported that statins inhibit platelet activation.[93] Therapeutic concentrations of statins inhibit ROS release and neutrophil-platelet interaction in a Rho-dependent manner. This might have implications for neutrophil-dependent endothelial dysfunction as seen in ischemia/reperfusion injury and atherosclerosis.

RELEVANCE OF PLEIOTROPIC EFFECTS IN CARDIOVASCULAR DISEASES

Endothelial Dysfunction

Endothelial dysfunction is usually defined as decreased bioavailability of vasodilators such as NO, or increased vasoconstrictors such as endothelin. Endothelial dysfunction is defined not only as impaired endothelium-dependent vasodilation but also as endothelial activation. Endothelial activation describes a proinflammatory, proliferative, and procoagulatory state that promotes atherogenesis and vascular inflammation. High cholesterol levels cause both endothelial dysfunction and endothelial activation, which are the earliest markers of atherosclerosis, occurring even in the absence of plaque formation.[94,95]

Plasma LDL apheresis rapidly improves endothelium-dependent vasodilation,[96] suggesting that statins could restore endothelial function by lowering serum cholesterol levels. However, in some studies using statins, restoration of endothelial function occurs before significant reduction in serum cholesterol levels,[97,98] suggesting that there are also cholesterol-independent effects of statins on endothelial function.

Because the synthesis, release, and activity of endothelium-derived NO are impaired in endothelial dysfunction, the ability of statins to increase the bioavailability of NO makes them desirable agents for improving endothelial function. As described earlier, statins exert many NO-dependent beneficial effects on the vascular wall, which include vasodilation, inhibition of platelet aggregation, leukocyte adhesion, and vascular smooth muscle proliferation. In addition, statins inhibit the generation of ROS, thereby preventing the inactivation of NO by superoxide anion (O_2^-). The increased release and production of ROS, produced by the NADPH oxidase system,[99] plays a pivotal role in the pathogenesis of endothelial dysfunction and atherosclerosis.

In animal models, the beneficial effect of increasing NO release with statins has been demonstrated by the regression of atherosclerosis, which was associated with up-regulation of eNOS mRNA and improvement of endothelial function.[100] Other studies tried to delineate the pleiotropic effects of statins by adjusting the cholesterol levels of statin-treated and placebo-treated animals with a cholesterol-rich diet. Because cholesterol levels were equal in statin-treated and placebo-treated animals, beneficial effects were regarded as cholesterol independent. Using this model, upregulation of eNOS and reduction in atherosclerosis were found in monkeys after treatment with statins.[101,102]

Because statins also increase NO production in humans at clinically relevant doses, this effect of statins on endothelial function has been studied in hyper- and normocholesterolemic individuals. In a randomized, placebo-controlled, double-blind study, statin therapy significantly increased the bioavailability of NO in hypercholesterolemic patients.[103] In another study, simvastatin augmented basal and acetylcholine-stimulated vasodilation and improved endothelial function within 1 month of treatment.[104]

Because improvement of endothelial function can also be attributed to a reduction in cholesterol levels, several studies focused on short-term effects of statins, where changes in LDL may play a lesser role. In these studies, cerivastatin and pravastatin rapidly improved endothelial function in normocholesterolemic and hypercholesterolemic individuals, respectively, within 2 weeks,[105,106] and in diabetic patients within 3 days.[107]

Blood Pressure Control

Because statins can increase eNOS activity and inhibit the expression of vasoconstrictive substances such as endothelin-1, it is likely that statins, either alone or given with another antihypertensive agent, will have some effect on systemic blood pressure. Indeed, in several animal models of hypertension, such as Dahl salt-sensitive rats and spontaneously hypertensive rats (SHR), statins reduce blood pressure and prevent hypertension-induced glomerular injury.[108-110] In contrast, Yamashita and co-workers did not find a decrease in blood pressure in stroke-prone, spontaneously hypertensive rats (SHR-SP) despite a marked reduction in proteinuria and renal fibrosis.[111] Thus, it is not entirely clear whether statins alone can decrease systemic blood pressure. Nevertheless, a reduction in cholesterol levels is correlated with a lower diastolic blood pressure.[112] Indeed, a small crossover study with 26 hypertensive and diabetic patients revealed that statin therapy reduced diastolic blood pressure, whereas another cholesterol-lowering agent, cholestyramine, had no effect, despite a reduction in cholesterol level similar to that of statins.[113] Finally, patients receiving statin therapy in addition to antihypertensive drugs have a more pronounced reduction in blood pressure, an effect that was independent of cholesterol lowering.[114] It is interesting to speculate that a reduction in blood pressure, and not cholesterol, by statins may explain some of their protective effects in ischemic stroke, a disease that is not generally associated with elevated cholesterol levels.

Plaque Stability

Plaque rupture is a major cause of acute coronary syndromes.[71,115-118] The stability of plaques depends on the integrity of their fibrous cap, which separates the highly thrombogenic materials within the lipid core from the bloodstream.[119] Fissuring, erosion, and ulceration of the fibrous cap eventually lead to plaque rupture and ensuing thrombosis.[117] The tensile strength of the fibrous cap is dependent on its collagen content. Because macrophages are capable of degrading the collagen-containing fibrous cap, they play an important role in the development and subsequent instability of atherosclerotic plaques.[120,121] Indeed, degradation of the plaque matrix appears to be most active in macrophage-rich regions.[116,117] Secretion of proteolytic enzymes, such as matrix metalloproteinases (MMPs), by activated macrophages may weaken the fibrous cap, particularly at the vulnerable shoulder region where the fibrous cap joins the arterial wall.[122,123]

Lipid lowering by statins may contribute to plaque stability by reducing plaque size or by modifying the physiochemical properties of the lipid core.[124,125] However, changes in plaque size by lipid lowering tend to occur over an extended time and are quite minimal, as assessed by angiography. The clinical benefits from lipid lowering are probably due to decreases in macrophage accumulation in atherosclerotic lesions and inhibition of MMP production by activated macrophages.[92] Indeed, statins inhibit the expression of MMPs and tissue factor by cholesterol-dependent and cholesterol-independent mechanisms,[51,92,124] with the cholesterol-independent or direct macrophage effects occurring much earlier. Whether MMPs are also influenced by statins in human plaques was investigated by Crisby and colleagues.[126] Patients received either pravastatin or placebo treatment 3 months before a scheduled carotid endarterectomy. MMP and oxidized LDL immunoreactivity were reduced, and interstitial collagen content was increased in pravastatin-treated patients. Therefore, the plaque-stabilizing properties of statins are mediated through a combined reduction in lipids, macrophages, and MMPs.[126] There is also evidence from clinical studies that statins can stabilize atherosclerotic plaques. Schartl and co-workers evaluated the density of plaques using intravascular ultrasound to estimate plaque stability.[127] Treatment with atorvastatin significantly increased the plaque density, compared to controls, after a 1-year treatment.

Ischemic Stroke

The correlation between ischemic stroke and serum cholesterol levels is weak.[128-130] Nevertheless, most of the clinical trials with statins demonstrated a large reduction in the incidence of ischemic stroke.[6,131] Thus, it appears likely that there are cholesterol-independent effects of statins that are beneficial for ischemic stroke.

Cerebral vascular tone and blood flow are regulated by endothelium-derived NO,[132] and eNOS knockout mice develop larger cerebral infarcts after cerebrovascular occlusion.[133] Furthermore, eNOS knockout mice tend to be relatively hypertensive and develop a greater proliferative and inflammatory response to vascular injury.[134] Thus, the beneficial effects of statins in ischemic stroke may be caused, in part, by their ability to up-regulate eNOS expression and activity. Indeed, pretreatment of mice with a statin, prior to experimental ischemic stroke, results in increases in cerebral blood flow and markedly reduces cerebral infarct sizes.[12] Because neither increase in cerebral blood flow nor neuro-protection was observed in eNOS knockout mice treated with statins, up-regulation of eNOS accounts for most, if not all, of the neuroprotective effects of these agents.

It has been reported that statins up-regulate t-PA and down-regulate PAI-1 expression through a mechanism that involves the inhibition of Rho geranyl geranylation.[50] In addition, as discussed later, Lefer and colleagues reported that statins attenuate P-selectin expression and leukocyte adhesion via increases in NO production in a model of cardiac ischemia and reperfusion.[13] Mechanisms of neuroprotection by statins might therefore include not only augmentation of cerebral blood flow but also, potentially, inhibition of platelet function and white blood cell accumulation.

The rapidity of statins' beneficial effect on ischemic stroke is quite remarkable. For example, in the Myocardial Ischemia Reduction with Aggressive Cholesterol Lowering (MIRACL) study, patients with acute coronary syndromes who were randomized to statin therapy had an almost 50% reduction in the incidence of ischemic strokes.[6] After a follow-up of 16 weeks, 24 strokes occurred in the placebo group compared to only 12 in the group treated with atorvastatin.[135] It is possible that statins have contributed to the decreased incidence of ischemic strokes in clinical trials, at least in part, by reducing the size of cerebral infarcts to a point where they are clinically unappreciated.

Myocardial Infarction and Reperfusion Injury

Results from recent studies suggest that statins not only reduce the incidence of cardiovascular events but also diminish the extent of ischemia/reperfusion injury.[14,15,136] These effects appear to be independent of cholesterol reduction and are associated with attenuated P-selectin expression and leukocyte adherence in an in vitro model of isolated rat hearts.[13,16] Using genetic and pharmacologic approaches, the role of eNOS in cardioprotection by statins was also delineated in in vivo models of myocardial infarction similar to those of ischemic stroke. Pretreatment with statins increased eNOS mRNA expression as well as eNOS activity, and cardioprotection by statins was completely abolished in eNOS knockout mice or after inhibition of eNOS with N(omega)-nitro-L-arginine methylester (L-NAME).[14,15] It appears that pretreatment with statins reduces ischemia/reperfusion injury in a NO-dependent manner.

Early statin therapy also appears to be of benefit in patients who have had myocardial infarction. In the MIRACL trial, patients with acute coronary syndrome showed a significant (16% relative risk) reduction in the combined endpoint (death, recurrent ischemia) in the statin group after only 4 months of treatment.[6] Furthermore, in animal studies, Bell and Yellon demonstrated that acute administration of statins at the onset of the reperfusion period reduced myocardial necrosis in isolated hearts.[178] These rapid effects of statins appear to be mediated via the PI 3-kinase/Akt pathway. Thus, statins not only reduce the incidence of myocardial infarction as shown in the large clinical trials but also reduce ischemia reperfusion injury. The cardiovascular protective effects appear to be mediated by a NO-dependent mechanism.

Inflammation

The presence of monocytes or macrophages and T lymphocytes in atheroma is characteristic for the complex inflammatory process in atherosclerosis.[70] These inflammatory cells secrete cytokines, thereby modifying endothelial function, SMC proliferation, collagen degradation, and thrombosis.[71] Statins possess anti-inflammatory properties because of their ability to reduce the number of inflammatory cells in atherosclerotic plaques.[70] Inhibition of adhesion molecules such as intercellular adhesion molecule-1 by statins is one mechanism, which leads to a reduced recruitment of inflammatory cells under statin treatment.[73,74] Interestingly, statins can also suppress the inflammatory response independent of HMG-CoA reductase inhibition by binding directly to a novel regulatory site of the β_2 integrin, leukocyte function antigen-1, which serves as a major counterreceptor for intercellular adhesion molecule-1 on leukocytes.[75]

High-sensitivity C-reactive protein (hs-CRP) is a clinical marker of inflammation[137] that is produced by the liver in response to proinflammatory cytokines, such as interleukin-6, and reflects low-grade systemic inflammation.[138] When compared with levels in normal individuals, hs-CRP is elevated in patients with coronary artery disease, coronary ischemia, and myocardial infarction.[139-141] Furthermore, elevated levels of hs-CRP are predictive of increased risk of coronary artery disease in apparently healthy men and women.[142,143] In hypercholesterolemic patients, statin therapy lowers hs-CRP levels.[137,144] Statins significantly decreased plasma hs-CRP levels over a 5-year period in patients who did not experience recurrent coronary events, as shown in the CARE trial.[145] Similarly, in a reanalysis of the Air Force/Texas Coronary Atherosclerosis Prevention Study (AFCAPS/TexCAPS), statin-treated patients who were free of acute major coronary events had reduced hs-CRP levels.[137]

Taken together, these studies indicate that statins are effective in decreasing systemic and vascular inflammation. However, any potential clinical benefits conferred by the lowering of hs-CRP are difficult to separate from the benefits of the lipid-lowering effects of statins without performing further clinical studies.

Neovascularization

An important therapeutic aim in reducing ischemia-induced tissue injury is to stimulate neovascularization.[146] Postnatal neovascularization is attributed mainly to the proliferation, migration, and remodeling of preexisting endothelial cells, a process termed angiogenesis.[147,148] However, bone marrow–derived circulating endothelial cells have also been demonstrated to be involved in this neovascularization process.[149,150] Indeed, transplantation of endothelial progenitor cells (EPCs) leads to postnatal neovascularization in the ischemic hind limb, augments ischemia-induced neovascularization in vivo,[151] and improves postischemic cardiac function.[152]

EPCs can be grown out of isolated CD133+ or CD34+ cell cultures.[149,153,154] Recent studies revealed that statins also promote vasculogenesis. Llevadot and co-workers demonstrated, in vitro, that the proliferation, migration, and cell survival of endothelial progenitor cells are enhanced by statin therapy.[155] Their experiments using overexpression of dominant-negative Akt to functionally block this pathway revealed that Akt mediates this pleiotropic effect of statins. In another study, statins not only increased the number of circulating EPCs but also induced their differentiation.[156] Interestingly, the induction of EPCs under statin therapy is associated with an accelerated reendothelialization after carotid balloon injury,[157] indicating that induction of EPCs may be of clinical relevance.

However, some studies report an antiangiogenic effect of statins,[158,159] which is mediated by inhibition of RhoA.[160] Thus, statins may exert opposing effects depending on the dose given. Low concentrations of statin may activate endothelial Ras and promote Akt and eNOS phosphorylation, leading to an angiogenic effect, whereas higher concentrations of statins are antiangiogenic despite promoting an increase in eNOS protein expression.[161] In some other studies, high concentrations of statins have also been shown to be angiogenic.[162] Further studies are necessary to elucidate the effects of statins on angiogenesis.

Restenosis

Prevention of restenosis after percutaneous transluminal coronary angioplasty (PTCA) remains one of the most challenging issues in the treatment of coronary artery disease, because restenosis limits the long-term beneficial effects of PTCA.[163] The development of restenosis after PTCA is a multifactorial event involving the proliferation of intimal SMCs, changes in extracellular matrix, and induction of proinflammatory and hemostatic factors.[164-166] In addition to exerting fibrinolytic and anti-inflammatory effects, statins reduce the PDGF-induced SMC proliferation through inhibition of Rho isoprenylation and up-regulation of p27(Kip1). Indeed, evidence from animal studies suggests that statins reduce the severity of restenosis after arterial injury by cholesterol-dependent[167] and cholesterol-independent mechanisms.[168]

The effect of statins on restenosis in patients after PTCA is controversial. In an earlier study, Sahni and colleagues observed a large decrease in the rate of restenosis in hypercholesterolemic patients receiving either lovastatin or placebo.[169] However, these findings should be interpreted cautiously, because the follow-up was incomplete and the study was not blinded. Another study, the Lovastatin Restenosis Trial (LRT), in which 404 patients were randomized to receive either lovastatin or placebo, also failed to show any beneficial effects of the statin on restenosis, despite substantial reduction in plasma cholesterol levels.[170,171] Similarly disappointing results were obtained in the Angioplasty Plus Probucol/Lovastatin Evaluation (APPLE), the Prevention of Restenosis by Elisor after Transluminal Coronary Angioplasty Trial (PREDICT), and the Fluvastatin Angioplasty Restenosis Trial (FLARE).[172-174] Finally, in a large prospective trial, statin therapy did not reduce restenosis after revascularization, although it significantly reduced fatalities during 6 months of follow-up.[175]

8

References

1. Klag MJ, Ford DE, Mead LA, et al: Serum cholesterol in young men and subsequent cardiovascular disease. N Engl J Med 328:5, 1993.
2. Ross R: The pathogenesis of atherosclerosis: A perspective for the 1990s. Nature 362:6423, 1993.
3. Scandinavian Simvastatin Survival Study Group: Randomised trial of cholesterol lowering in 4444 patients with coronary heart disease: The Scandinavian Simvastatin Survival Study (4S). Lancet 344:8934, 1994.
4. Packard CJ: Influence of pravastatin and plasma lipids on clinical events in the West of Scotland Coronary Prevention Study (WOSCOPS). Circulation 97:1440–1445, 1998.
5. Sacks FM, Pfeffer MA, Moye LA, et al: The effect of pravastatin on coronary events after myocardial infarction in patients with average cholesterol levels. Cholesterol and Recurrent Events Trial investigators. N Engl J Med 335:14, 1996.
6. Schwartz GG, Olsson AG, Ezekowitz MD, et al: Effects of atorvastatin on early recurrent ischemic events in acute coronary syndromes: The MIRACL study: A randomized controlled trial. JAMA 285:13, 2001.
7. Blum CB: Comparison of properties of four inhibitors of 3-hydroxy-3-methylglutaryl-coenzyme A reductase [published erratum appears in Am J Cardiol 74(6):639, 1994]. Am J Cardiol 73:14, 1994.
8. Massy ZA, Keane WF, Kasiske BL: Inhibition of the mevalonate pathway: Benefits beyond cholesterol reduction? Lancet 347:8994, 1996.
9. Shepherd J, Cobbe SM, Ford I, et al: Prevention of coronary heart disease with pravastatin in men with hypercholesterolemia. West of Scotland Coronary Prevention Study Group. N Engl J Med 333:20, 1995.
10. Brown BG, Zhao XQ, Sacco DE, et al: Lipid lowering and plaque regression: New insights into prevention of plaque disruption and clinical events in coronary disease. Circulation 87:6, 1993.
11. Pekkanen J, Linn S, Heiss G, et al: Ten-year mortality from cardiovascular disease in relation to cholesterol level among men with and without preexisting cardiovascular disease. N Engl J Med 322:24, 1990.
12. Endres M, Laufs U, Huang Z, et al: Stroke protection by 3-hydroxy-3-methylglutaryl (HMG)-CoA reductase inhibitors mediated by endothelial nitric oxide synthase. Proc Natl Acad Sci USA 95:15, 1998.
13. Lefer AM, Campbell B, Shin YK, et al: Simvastatin preserves the ischemic-reperfused myocardium in normocholesterolemic rat hearts. Circulation 100:2, 1999.
14. Lefer DJ, Scalia R, Jones SP, et al: HMG-CoA reductase inhibition protects the diabetic myocardium from ischemia-reperfusion injury. FASEB J 15:8, 2001.
15. Wolfrum S, Grimm M, Heidbreder M, et al: Acute reduction of myocardial infarct size by a hydroxymethyl glutaryl coenzyme a reductase inhibitor is mediated by endothelial nitric oxide synthase. J Cardiovasc Pharmacol 41:3, 2003.
16. Pruefer D, Scalia R, Lefer AM: Simvastatin inhibits leukocyte-endothelial cell interactions and protects against inflammatory processes in normocholesterolemic rats. Arterioscler Thromb Vasc Biol 19:12, 1999.

17. Goldstein JL, Brown MS: Regulation of the mevalonate pathway. Nature 343:6257, 1990.

18. Van Aelst L, D'Souza-Schorey C: Rho GTPases and signaling networks. Genes Dev 11:18, 1997.

19. Aktories K: Bacterial toxins that target Rho proteins. J Clin Invest 99:5, 1997.

20. Hall A: Small GTP-binding proteins and the regulation of the actin cytoskeleton. Annu Rev Cell Biol 10:31-54, 1994.

21. Laufs U, Liao JK: Post-transcriptional regulation of endothelial nitric oxide synthase mRNA stability by Rho GTPase. J Biol Chem 273:37, 1998.

22. Laufs U, Fata VL, Liao JK: Inhibition of 3-hydroxy-3-methylglutaryl (HMG)-CoA reductase blocks hypoxia-mediated down-regulation of endothelial nitric oxide synthase. J Biol Chem 272:50, 1997.

23. Laufs U, La Fata V, Plutzky J, et al: Upregulation of endothelial nitric oxide synthase by HMG CoA reductase inhibitors. Circulation 97:12, 1998.

24. Takemoto M, Sun J, Hiroki J, et al: Rho-kinase mediates hypoxia-induced downregulation of endothelial nitric oxide synthase. Circulation 106:1, 2002.

25. Franke TF, Kaplan DR, Cantley LC: PI3K: Downstream AKTion blocks apoptosis. Cell 88:4, 1997.

26. Coffer PJ, Jin J, Woodgett JR: Protein kinase B (c-Akt): A multifunctional mediator of phosphatidylinositol 3-kinase activation. Biochem J 335:Pt 1, 1998.

27. Downward J: Mechanisms and consequences of activation of protein kinase B/Akt. Curr Opin Cell Biol 10:2, 1998.

28. Murga C, Laguinge L, Wetzker R, et al: Activation of Akt/protein kinase B by G protein-coupled receptors: A role for alpha and beta gamma subunits of heterotrimeric G proteins acting through phosphatidylinositol-3-OH kinasegamma. J Biol Chem 273:30, 1998.

29. Cardone MH, Roy N, Stennicke HR, et al: Regulation of cell death protease caspase-9 by phosphorylation. Science 282:5392, 1998.

30. Fulton D, Gratton JP, McCabe TJ, et al: Regulation of endothelium-derived nitric oxide production by the protein kinase Akt. Nature 399:6736, 1999.

31. Dimmeler S, Fleming I, Fisslthaler B, et al: Activation of nitric oxide synthase in endothelial cells by Akt-dependent phosphorylation. Nature 399:6736, 1999.

32. Simoncini T, Hafezi-Moghadam A, Brazil DP, et al: Interaction of oestrogen receptor with the regulatory subunit of phosphatidylinositol-3-OH kinase. Nature 407:6803, 2000.

33. Haynes MP, Sinha D, Russell KS, et al: Membrane estrogen receptor engagement activates endothelial nitric oxide synthase via the PI3-kinase-Akt pathway in human endothelial cells. Circ Res 87:8, 2000.

34. Kureishi Y, Luo Z, Shiojima I, et al: The HMG-CoA reductase inhibitor simvastatin activates the protein kinase Akt and promotes angiogenesis in normocholesterolemic animals. Nat Med 6:9, 2000.

35. Lerman A, Edwards BS, Hallett JW, et al: Circulating and tissue endothelin immunoreactivity in advanced atherosclerosis. N Engl J Med 325:14, 1991.

36. Zeiher AM, Goebel H, Schachinger V, et al: Tissue endothelin-1 immunoreactivity in the active coronary atherosclerotic plaque: A

clue to the mechanism of increased vasoreactivity of the culprit lesion in unstable angina. Circulation 91:4, 1995.

37. Martin-Nizard F, Houssaini HS, Lestavel-Delattre S, et al: Modified low density lipoproteins activate human macrophages to secrete immunoreactive endothelin. FEBS Lett 293:1-2, 1991.

38. Weissberg PL, Witchell C, Davenport AP, et al: The endothelin peptides ET-1, ET-2, ET-3 and sarafotoxin S6b are co-mitogenic with platelet-derived growth factor for vascular smooth muscle cells. Atherosclerosis 85:2-3, 1990.

39. Hernandez-Perera O, Perez-Sala D, Navarro-Antolin J, et al: Effects of the 3-hydroxy-3-methylglutaryl-CoA reductase inhibitors, atorvastatin and simvastatin, on the expression of endothelin-1 and endothelial nitric oxide synthase in vascular endothelial cells. J Clin Invest 101:12, 1998.

40. Hernandez-Perera O, Perez-Sala D, Soria E, et al: Involvement of rho GTPases in the transcriptional inhibition of preproendothelin-1 gene expression by simvastatin in vascular endothelial cells. Circ Res 87:7, 2000.

41. Ichiki T, Takeda K, Tokunou T, et al: Downregulation of angiotensin II type 1 receptor by hydrophobic 3-hydroxy-3-methylglutaryl coenzyme A reductase inhibitors in vascular smooth muscle cells. Arterioscler Thromb Vasc Biol 21:12, 2001.

42. Xu CB, Stenman E, Edvinsson L: Reduction of bFGF-induced smooth muscle cell proliferation and endothelin receptor mRNA expression by mevastatin and atorvastatin. Biochem Pharmacol 64:3, 2002.

43. Kume N, Arai H, Kawai C, et al: Receptors for modified low-density lipoproteins on human endothelial cells: Different recognition for acetylated low-density lipoprotein and oxidized low-density lipoprotein. Biochim Biophys Acta 1091:1, 1991.

44. Kataoka H, Kume N, Miyamoto S, et al: Expression of lectinlike oxidized low-density lipoprotein receptor-1 in human atherosclerotic lesions. Circulation 99:24, 1999.

45. Li D, Mehta JL: Antisense to LOX-1 inhibits oxidized LDL-mediated upregulation of monocyte chemoattractant protein-1 and monocyte adhesion to human coronary artery endothelial cells. Circulation 101:25, 2000.

46. Li DY, Chen HJ, Mehta JL: Statins inhibit oxidized-LDL-mediated LOX-1 expression, uptake of oxidized-LDL and reduction in PKB phosphorylation. Cardiovasc Res 52:1, 2001.

47. Mehta JL, Li DY, Chen HJ, et al: Inhibition of LOX-1 by statins may relate to upregulation of eNOS. Biochem Biophys Res Commun 289:4, 2001.

48. Loskutoff DJ: A slice of PAI. J Clin Invest 92:6, 1993.

49. Aznar J, Estelles A: Role of plasminogen activator inhibitor type 1 in the pathogenesis of coronary artery diseases. Haemostasis 24:4, 1994.

50. Essig M, Nguyen G, Prie D, et al: 3-Hydroxy-3-methylglutaryl coenzyme A reductase inhibitors increase fibrinolytic activity in rat aortic endothelial cells: Role of geranylgeranylation and Rho proteins. Circ Res 83:7, 1998.

51. Bourcier T, Libby P: HMG CoA reductase inhibitors reduce plasminogen activator inhibitor-1 expression by human vascular smooth muscle and endothelial cells. Arterioscler Thromb Vasc Biol 20:2, 2000.

52. Wiesbauer F, Kaun C, Zorn G, et al: HMG CoA reductase inhibitors affect the fibrinolytic system of human vascular cells in vitro: A comparative study using different statins. Br J Pharmacol 135:1, 2002.

53. Dangas G, Smith DA, Unger AH, et al: Pravastatin: An antithrombotic effect independent of the cholesterol-lowering effect. Thromb Haemost 83:5, 2000.

54. Bevilacqua M, Bettica P, Milani M, et al: Effect of fluvastatin on lipids and fibrinolysis in coronary artery disease. Am J Cardiol 79:1, 1997.

55. Isaacsohn JL, Setaro JF, Nicholas C, et al: Effects of lovastatin therapy on plasminogen activator inhibitor-1 antigen levels. Am J Cardiol 74:7, 1994.

56. Maron DJ, Fazio S, Linton MF: Current perspectives on statins. Circulation 101:2, 2000.

57. Braun-Dullaeus RC, Mann MJ, Dzau VJ: Cell cycle progression: New therapeutic target for vascular proliferative disease. Circulation 98:1, 1998.

58. Kobashigawa JA, Katznelson S, Laks H, et al: Effect of pravastatin on outcomes after cardiac transplantation. N Engl J Med 333:10, 1995.

59. Laufs U, Marra D, Node K, et al: 3-Hydroxy-3-methylglutaryl-CoA reductase inhibitors attenuate vascular smooth muscle proliferation by preventing rho GTPase-induced down-regulation of p27(Kip1). J Biol Chem 274:31, 1999.

60. Yang Z, Kozai T, van der Loo B, et al: HMG-CoA reductase inhibition improves endothelial cell function and inhibits smooth muscle cell proliferation in human saphenous veins. J Am Coll Cardiol 36:5, 2000.

61. Hughes DA: Control of signal transduction and morphogenesis by Ras. Semin Cell Biol 6:2, 1995.

62. Hengst L, Reed SI: Translational control of p27Kip1 accumulation during the cell cycle. Science 271:5257, 1996.

63. Matsubara T, Ziff M: Increased superoxide anion release from human endothelial cells in response to cytokines. J Immunol 137:10, 1986.

64. Wassmann S, Laufs U, Muller K, et al: Cellular antioxidant effects of atorvastatin in vitro and in vivo. Arterioscler Thromb Vasc Biol 22:2, 2002.

65. Delbosc S, Morena M, Djouad F, et al: Statins, 3-hydroxy-3-methylglutaryl coenzyme A reductase inhibitors, are able to reduce superoxide anion production by NADPH oxidase in THP-1-derived monocytes. J Cardiovasc Pharmacol 40:4, 2002.

66. Wassmann S, Laufs U, Baumer AT, et al: Inhibition of geranylgeranylation reduces angiotensin II-mediated free radical production in vascular smooth muscle cells: Involvement of angiotensin AT1 receptor expression and Rac1 GTPase. Mol Pharmacol 59:3, 2001.

67. Harrison DG: Cellular and molecular mechanisms of endothelial cell dysfunction. J Clin Invest 100:9, 1997.

68. Munzel T, Sayegh H, Freeman BA, et al: Evidence for enhanced vascular superoxide anion production in nitrate tolerance: A novel mechanism underlying tolerance and cross-tolerance. J Clin Invest 95:1, 1995.

69. Vecchione C, Brandes RP: Withdrawal of 3-hydroxy-3-methylglutaryl coenzyme A reductase inhibitors elicits oxidative stress and induces endothelial dysfunction in mice. Circ Res 91:2, 2002.

70. Ross R: Atherosclerosis is an inflammatory disease. Am Heart J 138:5(Pt 2), 1999.

8

71. Libby P: Molecular bases of the acute coronary syndromes. Circulation 91:11, 1995.

72. Vaughan CJ, Gotto AM Jr, Basson CT: The evolving role of statins in the management of atherosclerosis. J Am Coll Cardiol 35:1, 2000.

73. Niwa S, Totsuka T, Hayashi S: Inhibitory effect of fluvastatin, an HMG-CoA reductase inhibitor, on the expression of adhesion molecules on human monocyte cell line. Int J Immunopharmacol 18:11, 1996.

74. Rezaie-Majd A, Maca T, Bucek RA, et al: Simvastatin reduces expression of cytokines interleukin-6, interleukin-8, and monocyte chemoattractant protein-1 in circulating monocytes from hypercholesterolemic patients. Arterioscler Thromb Vasc Biol 22:7, 2002.

75. Weitz-Schmidt G, Welzenbach K, Brinkmann V, et al: Statins selectively inhibit leukocyte function antigen-1 by binding to a novel regulatory integrin site. Nat Med 7:6, 2001.

76. Yoshida M, Sawada T, Ishii H, et al: HMG-CoA reductase inhibitor modulates monocyte-endothelial cell interaction under physiological flow conditions in vitro: Involvement of Rho GTPase-dependent mechanism. Arterioscler Thromb Vasc Biol 21:7, 2001.

77. Fitzgerald DJ, Roy L, Catella F, et al: Platelet activation in unstable coronary disease. N Engl J Med 315:16, 1986.

78. Fuster V, Badimon JJ, Badimon L: Clinical-pathological correlations of coronary disease progression and regression. Circulation 86(Suppl):6, 1992.

79. Lacoste L, Lam JY, Hung J, et al: Hyperlipidemia and coronary disease: Correction of the increased thrombogenic potential with cholesterol reduction. Circulation 92:11, 1995.

80. Willerson JT, Golino P, Eidt J, et al: Specific platelet mediators and unstable coronary artery lesions. Experimental evidence and potential clinical implications. Circulation 80:1, 1989.

81. Opper C, Clement C, Schwarz H, et al: Increased number of high sensitive platelets in hypercholesterolemia, cardiovascular diseases, and after incubation with cholesterol. Atherosclerosis 113:2, 1995.

82. Tremoli E, Colli S, Maderna P, et al: Hypercholesterolemia and platelets. Semin Thromb Hemost 19:2, 1993.

83. Notarbartolo A, Davi G, Averna M, et al: Inhibition of thromboxane biosynthesis and platelet function by simvastatin in type IIa hypercholesterolemia. Arterioscler Thromb Vasc Biol 15:2, 1995.

84. Baldassarre D, Mores N, Colli S, et al: Platelet alpha 2-adrenergic receptors in hypercholesterolemia: Relationship between binding studies and epinephrine-induced platelet aggregation. Clin Pharmacol Ther 61:6, 1997.

85. Le Quan Sang KH, Levenson J, Megnien JL, et al: Platelet cytosolic Ca2+ and membrane dynamics in patients with primary hypercholesterolemia: Effects of pravastatin. Arterioscler Thromb Vasc Biol 15:6, 1995.

86. Huhle G, Abletshauser C, Mayer N, et al: Reduction of platelet activity markers in type II hypercholesterolemic patients by a HMG-CoA-reductase inhibitor. Thromb Res 95:5, 1999.

87. Hale LP, Craver KT, Berrier AM, et al: Combination of fosinopril and pravastatin decreases platelet response to thrombin receptor agonist in monkeys. Arterioscler Thromb Vasc Biol 18:10, 1998.

88. Schror K: Platelet reactivity and arachidonic acid metabolism in type

II hyperlipoproteinaemia and its modification by cholesterol-lowering agents. Eicosanoids 3:2, 1990.

89. Lijnen P, Echevaria-Vazquez D, Petrov V: Influence of cholesterol-lowering on plasma membrane lipids and function. Methods Find Exp Clin Pharmacol 18:2, 1996.

90. Alfon J, Fernandez de Arriba A, Gomez-Casajus LA, et al: Alternative binding assay of GP IIb/IIIa antagonists with a nonradioactive labeling method of platelets. Thromb Res 102:3, 2001.

91. Alfon J, Royo T, Garcia-Moll X, et al: Platelet deposition on eroded vessel walls at a stenotic shear rate is inhibited by lipid-lowering treatment with atorvastatin. Arterioscler Thromb Vasc Biol 19:7, 1999.

92. Aikawa M, Rabkin E, Sugiyama S, et al: An HMG-CoA reductase inhibitor, cerivastatin, suppresses growth of macrophages expressing matrix metalloproteinases and tissue factor in vivo and in vitro. Circulation 103:2, 2001.

93. Kaneider NC, Egger P, Dunzendorfer S, et al: Rho-GTPase-dependent platelet-neutrophil interaction affected by HMG-CoA reductase inhibition with altered adenosine nucleotide release and function. Arterioscler Thromb Vasc Biol 22:6, 2002.

94. Osborne JA, Siegman MJ, Sedar AW, et al: Lack of endothelium-dependent relaxation in coronary resistance arteries of cholesterol-fed rabbits. Am J Physiol 256(Pt 1):3, 1989.

95. Liao JK: Endothelium and acute coronary syndromes. Clin Chem 44(Pt 2):8, 1998.

96. Tamai O, Matsuoka H, Itabe H, et al: Single LDL apheresis improves endothelium-dependent vasodilatation in hypercholesterolemic humans. Circulation 95:1, 1997.

97. Anderson TJ, Meredith IT, Yeung AC, et al: The effect of cholesterol-lowering and antioxidant therapy on endothelium-dependent coronary vasomotion. N Engl J Med 332:8, 1995.

98. Treasure CB, Klein JL, Weintraub WS, et al: Beneficial effects of cholesterol-lowering therapy on the coronary endothelium in patients with coronary artery disease. N Engl J Med 332:8, 1995.

99. Griendling KK, Sorescu D, Ushio-Fukai M: NAD(P)H oxidase: Role in cardiovascular biology and disease. Circ Res 86:5, 2000.

100. Kano H, Hayashi T, Sumi D, et al: A HMG-CoA reductase inhibitor improved regression of atherosclerosis in the rabbit aorta without affecting serum lipid levels: Possible relevance of up-regulation of endothelial NO synthase mRNA. Biochem Biophys Res Commun 259:2, 1999.

101. Williams JK, Sukhova GK, Herrington DM, et al: Pravastatin has cholesterol-lowering independent effects on the artery wall of atherosclerotic monkeys. J Am Coll Cardiol 31:3, 1998.

102. Sukhova GK, Williams JK, Libby P: Statins reduce inflammation in atheroma of nonhuman primates independent of effects on serum cholesterol. Arterioscler Thromb Vasc Biol 22:9, 2002.

103. John S, Schlaich M, Langenfeld M, et al: Increased bioavailability of nitric oxide after lipid-lowering therapy in hypercholesterolemic patients: A randomized, placebo-controlled, double-blind study. Circulation 98:3, 1998.

104. O'Driscoll G, Green D, Taylor RR: Simvastatin, an HMG-coenzyme A reductase inhibitor, improves endothelial function within 1 month. Circulation 95:1126, 1997.

105. Masumoto A, Hirooka Y, Hironaga K, et al: Effect of pravastatin on

endothelial function in patients with coronary artery disease (cholesterol-independent effect of pravastatin). Am J Cardiol 88:11, 2001.

106. John S, Delles C, Jacobi J, et al: Rapid improvement of nitric oxide bioavailability after lipid-lowering therapy with cerivastatin within two weeks. J Am Coll Cardiol 37:5, 2001.

107. Tsunekawa T, Hayashi T, Kano H, et al: Cerivastatin, a hydroxymethylglutaryl coenzyme A reductase inhibitor, improves endothelial function in elderly diabetic patients within 3 days. Circulation 104:4, 2001.

108. O'Donnell MP, Kasiske BL, Katz SA, et al: Lovastatin but not enalapril reduces glomerular injury in Dahl salt-sensitive rats. Hypertension 20:5, 1992.

109. Wilson TW, Alonso-Galicia M, Roman RJ: Effects of lipid-lowering agents in the Dahl salt-sensitive rat. Hypertension 31(Pt 2):1, 1998.

110. Jiang J, Sun CW, Alonso-Galicia M, et al: Lovastatin reduces renal vascular reactivity in spontaneously hypertensive rats. Am J Hypertens 11:10, 1998.

111. Yamashita T, Kawashima S, Miwa Y, et al: A 3-hydroxy-3-methylglutaryl co-enzyme A reductase inhibitor reduces hypertensive nephrosclerosis in stroke-prone spontaneously hypertensive rats. J Hypertens 20:12, 2002.

112. Goode GK, Miller JP, Heagerty AM: Hyperlipidaemia, hypertension, and coronary heart disease. Lancet 345:8946, 1995.

113. Tonolo G, Melis MG, Formato M, et al: Additive effects of simvastatin beyond its effects on LDL cholesterol in hypertensive type 2 diabetic patients. Eur J Clin Invest 30:11, 2000.

114. Borghi C, Prandin MG, Costa FV, et al: Use of statins and blood pressure control in treated hypertensive patients with hypercholesterolemia. J Cardiovasc Pharmacol 35:4, 2000.

115. Libby P, Sukhova G, Lee RT, Liao JK: Molecular biology of atherosclerosis. Int J Cardiol 62(Suppl 2):S23, 1997.

116. Fuster V: Elucidation of the role of plaque instability and rupture in acute coronary events. Am J Cardiol 76:9, 1995.

117. Fuster V, Stein B, Ambrose JA, et al: Atherosclerotic plaque rupture and thrombosis: Evolving concepts. Circulation 82(3 Suppl):II47, 1990.

118. Chesebro JH, Zoldhelyi P, Fuster V: Pathogenesis of thrombosis in unstable angina. Am J Cardiol 68:7, 1991.

119. Fernandez-Ortiz A, Badimon JJ, Falk E, et al: Characterization of the relative thrombogenicity of atherosclerotic plaque components: Implications for consequences of plaque rupture. J Am Coll Cardiol 23:7, 1994.

120. Moreno PR, Falk E, Palacios IF, et al: Macrophage infiltration in acute coronary syndromes: Implications for plaque rupture. Circulation 90:2, 1994.

121. Shah PK, Falk E, Badimon JJ, et al: Human monocyte-derived macrophages induce collagen breakdown in fibrous caps of atherosclerotic plaques: Potential role of matrix-degrading metalloproteinases and implications for plaque rupture. Circulation 92:6, 1995.

122. Henney AM, Wakeley PR, Davies MJ, et al: Localization of stromelysin gene expression in atherosclerotic plaques by in situ hybridization. Proc Natl Acad Sci USA 88:18, 1991.

123. Richardson PD, Davies MJ, Born GV: Influence of plaque configuration and stress distribution on fissuring of coronary atherosclerotic plaques. Lancet 2:8669, 1989.

124. Fukumoto Y, Libby P, Rabkin E, et al: Statins alter smooth muscle cell accumulation and collagen content in established atheroma of Watanabe heritable hyperlipidemic rabbits. Circulation 103:7, 2001.

125. Koh KK: Effects of statins on vascular wall: Vasomotor function, inflammation, and plaque stability. Cardiovasc Res 47:4, 2000.

126. Crisby M, Nordin-Fredriksson G, Shah PK, et al: Pravastatin treatment increases collagen content and decreases lipid content, inflammation, metalloproteinases, and cell death in human carotid plaques: Implications for plaque stabilization. Circulation 103:7, 2001.

127. Schartl M, Bocksch W, Koschyk DH, et al: Use of intravascular ultrasound to compare effects of different strategies of lipid-lowering therapy on plaque volume and composition in patients with coronary artery disease. Circulation 104:4, 2001.

128. Multiple Risk Factor Intervention Trial Research Group: Risk factor changes and mortality results. JAMA 248:12, 1982.

129. Sytkowski PA, Kannel WB, D'Agostino RB: Changes in risk factors and the decline in mortality from cardiovascular disease: The Framingham Heart Study. N Engl J Med 322:23, 1990.

130. Engstrom G, Lind P, Hedblad B, et al: Effects of cholesterol and inflammation-sensitive plasma proteins on incidence of myocardial infarction and stroke in men. Circulation 105:22, 2002.

131. Crouse JR, Byington RP, Furberg CD: HMG-CoA reductase inhibitor therapy and stroke risk reduction: An analysis of clinical trials data. Atherosclerosis 138:1, 1998.

132. Dalkara T, Yoshida T, Irikura K, et al: Dual role of nitric oxide in focal cerebral ischemia. Neuropharmacology 33:11, 1994.

133. Huang Z, Huang PL, Ma J, et al: Enlarged infarcts in endothelial nitric oxide synthase knockout mice are attenuated by nitro-L-arginine. J Cereb Blood Flow Metab 16:5, 1996.

134. Huang PL, Huang Z, Mashimo H, et al: Hypertension in mice lacking the gene for endothelial nitric oxide synthase. Nature 377:6546, 1995.

135. Waters DD, Schwartz GG, Olsson AG, et al: Effects of atorvastatin on stroke in patients with unstable angina or non-Q-wave myocardial infarction: A Myocardial Ischemia Reduction with Aggressive Cholesterol Lowering (MIRACL) substudy. Circulation 106:13, 2002.

136. Di Napoli P, Antonio Taccardi A, Grilli A, et al: Simvastatin reduces reperfusion injury by modulating nitric oxide synthase expression: An ex vivo study in isolated working rat hearts. Cardiovasc Res 51:2, 2001.

137. Ridker PM, Rifai N, Clearfield M, et al: Measurement of C-reactive protein for the targeting of statin therapy in the primary prevention of acute coronary events. N Engl J Med 344:26, 2001.

138. Baumann H, Gauldie J: The acute phase response. Immunol Today 15:2, 1994.

139. Liuzzo G, Biasucci LM, Gallimore JR, et al: The prognostic value of C-reactive protein and serum amyloid a protein in severe unstable angina. N Engl J Med 331:7, 1994.

140. Mendall MA, Patel P, Ballam L, et al: C reactive protein and its relation to cardiovascular risk factors: A population based cross sectional study. BMJ 312:7038, 1996.

8

141. Alderson LM, Endemann G, Lindsey S, et al: LDL enhances monocyte adhesion to endothelial cells in vitro. Am J Pathol 123:2, 1986.

142. Radomski MW, Rees DD, Dutra A, et al: S-nitroso-glutathione inhibits platelet activation in vitro and in vivo. Br J Pharmacol 107:3, 1992.

143. Ridker PM, Rifai N, Rose L, et al: Comparison of C-reactive protein and low-density lipoprotein cholesterol levels in the prediction of first cardiovascular events. N Engl J Med 347:20, 2002.

144. Musial J, Undas A, Gajewski P, et al: Anti-inflammatory effects of simvastatin in subjects with hypercholesterolemia. Int J Cardiol 77:2-3, 2001.

145. Ridker PM, Rifai N, Pfeffer MA, et al: Long-term effects of pravastatin on plasma concentration of C-reactive protein. The Cholesterol and Recurrent Events (CARE) Investigators. Circulation 100:3, 1999.

146. Isner JM, Asahara T: Angiogenesis and vasculogenesis as therapeutic strategies for postnatal neovascularization. J Clin Invest 103:9, 1999.

147. Risau W: Mechanisms of angiogenesis. Nature 386:6626, 1997.

148. Carmeliet P, Jain RK: Angiogenesis in cancer and other diseases. Nature 407:6801, 2000.

149. Asahara T, Murohara T, Sullivan A, et al: Isolation of putative progenitor endothelial cells for angiogenesis. Science 275:5302, 1997.

150. Asahara T, Masuda H, Takahashi T, et al: Bone marrow origin of endothelial progenitor cells responsible for postnatal vasculogenesis in physiological and pathological neovascularization. Circ Res 85:3, 1999.

151. Murohara T, Ikeda H, Duan J, et al: Transplanted cord blood-derived endothelial precursor cells augment postnatal neovascularization. J Clin Invest 105:11, 2000.

152. Kawamoto A, Gwon HC, Iwaguro H, et al: Therapeutic potential of ex vivo expanded endothelial progenitor cells for myocardial ischemia. Circulation 103:5, 2001.

153. Gehling UM, Ergun S, Schumacher U, et al: In vitro differentiation of endothelial cells from AC133-positive progenitor cells. Blood 95:10, 2000.

154. Bhattacharya V, McSweeney PA, Shi Q, et al: Enhanced endothelialization and microvessel formation in polyester grafts seeded with CD34(+) bone marrow cells. Blood 95:2, 2000.

155. Llevadot J, Murasawa S, Kureishi Y, et al: HMG-CoA reductase inhibitor mobilizes bone marrow–derived endothelial progenitor cells. J Clin Invest 108:3, 2001.

156. Dimmeler S, Aicher A, Vasa M, et al: HMG-CoA reductase inhibitors (statins) increase endothelial progenitor cells via the PI 3-kinase/Akt pathway. J Clin Invest 108:3, 2001.

157. Walter DH, Rittig K, Bahlmann FH, et al: Statin therapy accelerates reendothelialization: A novel effect involving mobilization and incorporation of bone marrow-derived endothelial progenitor cells. Circulation 105:25, 2002.

158. Vincent L, Soria C, Mirshahi F, et al: Cerivastatin, an inhibitor of 3-hydroxy-3-methylglutaryl coenzyme a reductase, inhibits endothelial cell proliferation induced by angiogenic factors in vitro and angiogenesis in in vivo models. Arterioscler Thromb Vasc Biol 22:4, 2002.

159. Vincent L, Chen W, Hong L, et al: Inhibition of endothelial cell migration by cerivastatin, an HMG-CoA reductase inhibitor: Contribution to its anti-angiogenic effect. FEBS Lett 495:3, 2001.

160. Park HJ, Kong D, Iruela-Arispe L, et al: 3-hydroxy-3-methylglutaryl coenzyme A reductase inhibitors interfere with angiogenesis by inhibiting the geranylgeranylation of RhoA. Circ Res 91:2, 2002.

161. Urbich C, Dernbach E, Zeiher AM, et al: Double-edged role of statins in angiogenesis signaling. Circ Res 90:6, 2002.

162. Sata M, Nishimatsu H, Suzuki E, et al: Endothelial nitric oxide synthase is essential for the HMG-CoA reductase inhibitor cerivastatin to promote collateral growth in response to ischemia. FASEB J 15:13, 2001.

163. Landau C, Faxon DP: Acronyms in angioplasty and restenosis: A summary of recent and ongoing clinical randomized trials. J Interv Cardiol 5:1, 1992.

164. Chesebro JH, Lam JY, Badimon L, et al: Restenosis after arterial angioplasty: A hemorrheologic response to injury. Am J Cardiol 60:3, 1987.

165. Welt FG, Rogers C: Inflammation and restenosis in the stent era. Arterioscler Thromb Vasc Biol 22:11, 2002.

166. Liu MW, Roubin GS, King SB 3rd: Restenosis after coronary angioplasty: Potential biologic determinants and role of intimal hyperplasia. Circulation 79:6, 1989.

167. Gellman J, Ezekowitz MD, Sarembock IJ, et al: Effect of lovastatin on intimal hyperplasia after balloon angioplasty: A study in an atherosclerotic hypercholesterolemic rabbit. J Am Coll Cardiol 17:1, 1991.

168. Soma MR, Donetti E, Parolini C, et al: HMG CoA reductase inhibitors: In vivo effects on carotid intimal thickening in normocholesterolemic rabbits. Arterioscler Thromb 13:4, 1993.

169. Sahni R, Maniet AR, Voci G, et al: Prevention of restenosis by lovastatin after successful coronary angioplasty. Am Heart J 121(Pt 1):6, 1991.

170. Weintraub WS, Boccuzzi SJ, Klein JL, et al: Lack of effect of lovastatin on restenosis after coronary angioplasty. Lovastatin Restenosis Trial Study Group. N Engl J Med 331:20, 1994.

171. Weintraub WS, Boccuzzi SJ, Brown CL 3rd, et al: Background and methods for the lovastatin restenosis trial after percutaneous transluminal coronary angioplasty. The Lovastatin Restenosis Trial Study Group. Am J Cardiol 70:3, 1992.

172. O'Keefe JH Jr, Stone GW, McCallister BD Jr, et al: Lovastatin plus probucol for prevention of restenosis after percutaneous transluminal coronary angioplasty. Am J Cardiol 77:8, 1996.

173. Bertrand ME, McFadden EP, Fruchart JC, et al: Effect of pravastatin on angiographic restenosis after coronary balloon angioplasty: Prevention of restenosis by elisor after transluminal coronary angioplasty. The PREDICT Trial Investigators. J Am Coll Cardiol 30:4, 1997.

174. Serruys PW, Foley DP, Jackson G, et al: A randomized placebo-controlled trial of fluvastatin for prevention of restenosis after successful coronary balloon angioplasty: Final results of the fluvastatin angiographic restenosis (FLARE) trial. Eur Heart J 20:1, 1999.

175. Bunch TJ, Muhlestein JB, Anderson JL, et al: Effects of statins on six-month survival and clinical restenosis frequency after coronary stent deployment. Am J Cardiol 90:3, 2002.
176. Liao JK: Statins and ischemic stroke. Atheroscler Suppl 3:21, 2002.
177. Wolfrum S, Jensen KS, Liao JK: Endothelium-dependent effects of statins. Arterioscler Thromb Vasc Biol 23:729, 2003.
178. Bell RM, Yellon DM: Atorvastatin, administered at the onset of reperfusion, and independent of lipid lowering, protects the myocardium by up-regulating a pro-survival pathway. J Am Coll Cardiol 41:508-515, 2003.

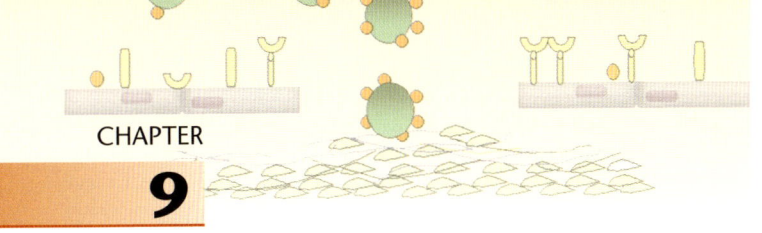

Effects of Statins on C-Reactive Protein: Are All Statins Similar?

Sridevi Devaraj and Ishwarlal Jialal

Atherosclerosis is the leading cause of morbidity and mortality in westernized populations. A strong and independent association has been established between elevated serum cholesterol levels and increased atherosclerotic disease.[1-3] Clinical and epidemiologic studies convincingly demonstrate that increased levels of low-density-lipoprotein (LDL) cholesterol promote premature athero-sclerosis. Several large clinical trials have demonstrated that statins (3-hydroxy-3-methylglutaryl coenzyme A [HMG-CoA] reductase inhibitors) decrease the incidence of cardiovascular events in both primary and secondary prevention.[4-8] Because serum LDL choles-terol levels are strongly associated with coronary artery disease, it has been generally assumed that cholesterol reduction by statins is the predominant mechanism underlying their beneficial effects on cardiovascular diseases. However, subgroup analyses of large clinical trials have suggested that the beneficial effects of statins may extend to mechanisms beyond cholesterol reduction. Subgroup analyses of the West of Scotland Coronary Prevention Study (WOSCOPS) and the Cholesterol and Recurrent Events (CARE) trial indicate that despite comparable serum cholesterol levels among the statin-treated and placebo groups, statin-treated subjects had a significantly lower risk of coronary artery disease (CAD) than age-matched, placebo-controlled subjects.[6,7,11,12] In the CARE study, greater reduction in cardiovascular events was observed in subjects with C-reactive protein levels in the highest quartile.[13] Furthermore, meta-analyses of cholesterol-lowering trials suggest that the risk of myocardial infarction in individuals treated with statins is significantly lower than that in individuals treated with other cholesterol-lowering agents or modalities, despite comparable reduction in serum cholesterol levels in both groups.[14,15] These findings suggest that statins may have beneficial effects beyond cholesterol lowering. Further evidence in support of the pleiotropic effects of statin therapy is provided by angiographic trials, which have demonstrated clinical improvements with statins that far exceed changes in the size of atherosclerotic lesions. In the

Familial Atherosclerosis Treatment Study (FATS) trial, statin therapy with bile acid resin decreased the incidence of coronary events by 70% despite producing only a 0.7% change in lesion regression.[14,16] Many of the beneficial effects of statins in the FATS trial were attributed to plaque stabilization. However, in the recent Myocardial Ischemia Reduction with Aggressive Cholesterol Lowering (MIRACL) trial, statins were found to be effective in reducing recurrent ischemic events as soon as 16 weeks after acute coronary ischemia.[17] Although the serum LDL cholesterol was reduced by 40%, this time frame was probably too short for appreciable changes in vascular remodeling. The clinical benefit of statin drugs used in these studies is manifested early in the course of lipid-lowering therapy, well before plaque regression could occur.

C-REACTIVE PROTEIN AND ATHEROSCLEROSIS

As discussed elsewhere in this book, there is growing evidence pointing to a pathogenic role of inflammation in atherosclerosis. Atherosclerosis is a complex inflammatory process that is characterized by the presence of monocytes, macrophages, and T lymphocytes in the atheroma.[18] Inflammatory cytokines and chemokines secreted by these macrophages and T lymphocytes can modify endothelial function, smooth muscle cell (SMC) proliferation, collagen degradation, and thrombosis. The earliest event in atherogenesis is endothelial cell dysfunction.[18] Various noxious insults, including hypertension, diabetes, dyslipidemia, smoking, and hyperhomocysteinemia, can result in endothelial cell dysfunction, which manifests primarily as a deficiency of nitric oxide (NO) and/or prostacyclin, among other aberrations. Following endothelial cell dysfunction, mononuclear cells such as monocytes and T lymphocytes attach to the endothelium; they initially roll loosely and thereafter adhere firmly to the endothelium, and then they migrate to the subendothelial space. Thereafter, they mature into macrophages, incorporate lipid from modified lipoproteins (e.g., oxidized LDL) via the scavenger receptor pathway, and become foam cells, the hallmark of the fatty streak lesion.

After the appearance of the early fatty streak lesion, SMCs migrate into the intima and form the fibrous cap. It is believed that the lipid-laden macrophage releases matrix metalloproteinases (MMPs), which cause a rent in the endothelium. Also, the lipid-laden macrophages are enriched in tissue factor. When tissue factor is released and comes in contact with the circulating blood, the result is thrombus formation and acute coronary syndromes (unstable angina and myocardial infarction). Thus, endothelial cell dysfunction, inflammation, smooth muscle cell proliferation, and thrombus formation culminate in acute coronary syndromes.

The prototypic marker of inflammation is C-reactive protein (CRP), a member of the pentraxin family.[19,20] CRP is characterized by a cyclic pentameric structure; it displays radial symmetry and has a molecular mass of 118,000 daltons.[19,20] CRP binds phospho-esters in the presence of calcium, and its synthesis in the liver is triggered by various proinflammatory cytokines derived from either monocytes, macrophages, or adipose tissue. The general consensus is that proinflammatory risk factors such as oxidized LDL and infectious agents trigger a proinflammatory response that results in the increased secretion of interleukin-1β (IL-1β) and tumor necrosis factor α (TNF-α), which then results in the release of the messenger cytokine interleukin-6 (IL-6). IL-6, following engagement of its receptor on the liver, causes the secretion and release of CRP and serum amyloid A (SAA).

Clinical studies have now confirmed that levels of high-sensitivity CRP (hsCRP) predict cardiovascular events in normal volunteers.[21] The consistency of these findings in these different populations is impressive. In both men and women, hsCRP as a risk factor for CAD appears to be additive to an elevated total cholesterol (>75th percentile) and a total cholesterol-to-HDL ratio.[22,23] Also, in a report from the Women's Health Study, the novel observation was made that in spite of these apparently healthy postmenopausal women having LDL cholesterol levels below 130 mg/dL, hsCRP continued to predict an approximately threefold increased risk for cardiovascular events in women in the fourth quartile compared to the first quartile. In addition, hsCRP has been shown to be a predictor for sudden death and peripheral vascular disease (PVD).[24]

STATINS AND C-REACTIVE PROTEIN

Several studies have shown that statin therapy lowers CRP levels independent of its lipid-lowering effects. In the CARE study,[25] which tested the effect of pravastatin on patients with a total cholesterol level lower than 6.2 mmol/L, it was shown that the greatest benefit was achieved in the group with the highest hsCRP levels (a 54% reduction in cardiovascular events compared to 25% in the lowest quartile for hsCRP). In addition to having a beneficial effect on the lipid profile, pravastatin may have its greatest benefit in patients with the highest hsCRP levels, suggesting an anti-inflammatory effect.

In the Air Force/Texas Coronary Atherosclerosis Prevention Study (AFCAPS/TexCAPS), a primary prevention trial with lovastatin, rates of coronary events increased significantly with increases in baseline CRP levels.[26] Lovastatin therapy (20 mg daily) decreased CRP levels 14% ($P < .001$), and this effect was independent of its lipid-lowering effects. If either the baseline LDL cholesterol or the baseline CRP were over the median, lovastatin decreased relative risk significantly; however, if *both* were over the median, then the effect failed to reach statistical significance. Thus, this study showed that in persons with LDL cholesterol below the median (149 mg/dL) and hsCRP levels over the median (1.6 mg/L), lovastatin conferred a benefit. On the other hand, if both were below the median, there was no benefit from statin therapy. This further underscores the usefulness of CRP measurement in deciding on drug therapy.

We showed in a prospective, randomized, double-blind, crossover study in patients with combined hyperlipidemia (LDL > 130 mg/dL, triglycerides 200-600 mg/dL) that a 6-week therapy of three commonly prescribed statins, simvastatin (20 mg/day), atorvastatin (10 mg/day) and pravastatin (40 mg/day) resulted in a significant reduction in hsCRP levels.[27] There was no significant difference in the magnitude of reduction in hsCRP with the three statins, suggesting a class effect (Fig. 9-1). In this study, we failed to show a significant correlation with regard to LDL cholesterol reduction and hsCRP reduction. This agreed with results of the CARE study, suggesting that the effects of statins might be

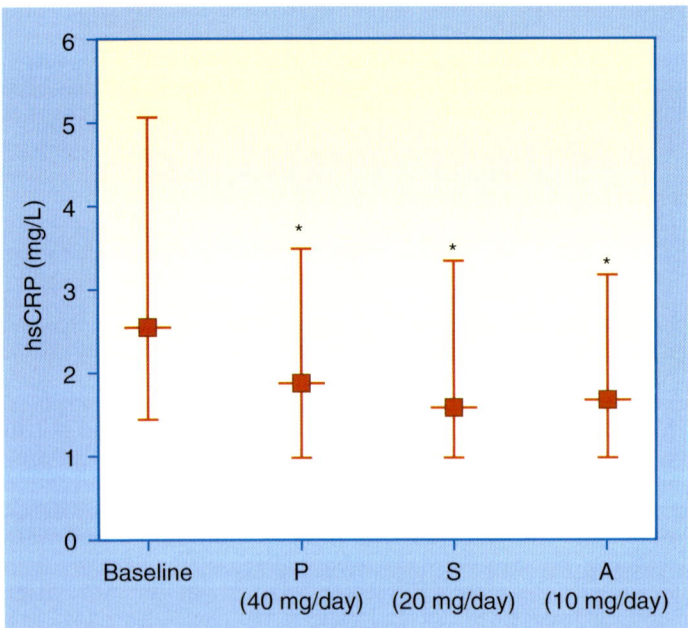

Effect of statin therapy on hsCRP levels

Figure 9-1.   Effect of statin therapy on hsCRP levels. Data are presented as 25th percentile, median, and 75th percentile. *P < .025 compared with baseline. A, atorvastatin; P, pravastatin; S, simvastatin. (From Jialal I, Stein D, Balis D, et al: Effect of hydroxymethyl glutaryl coenzyme A reductase inhibitor therapy on high sensitive C-reactive protein levels. Circulation 103(15):1933-1935, 2001.)

pleiotropic. This is the only study that could determine responders, because two blood samples were obtained a week apart, both before and after therapy with statins. Also, 79% of patients responded with a reduction in CRP levels. Furthermore, we failed to show an effect on serum IL-6 levels or levels of soluble IL-6 receptor. However, we are reporting for the first time that the three statins were equipotent in lowering levels of soluble P selectin (Fig. 9-2). Simvastatin, 40 or 80 mg/day, has also been shown to reduce hsCRP levels in patients with combined hyperlipidemia; there does not appear to be a dose-response relationship, and the effect of the two different doses of statin was independent of LDL cholesterol lowering.[28]

Strandberg and co-workers compared the effects of statin therapy on CRP levels in 60 hypercholesterolemic patients with coronary disease who participated in the Treat to Target study comparing atorvastatin and simvastatin.[29] CRP levels fell significantly after statin therapy, and this reduction was independent of changes in LDL cholesterol or triglycerides.

Two recent studies have confirmed that simvastatin (40 and 80 mg/day) and atorvastatin (40 mg/day) decreased hsCRP levels.[28,30] However, simvastatin therapy (20-40 mg/day for 1 year) was ineffective in reducing CRP levels in 129 patients with familial

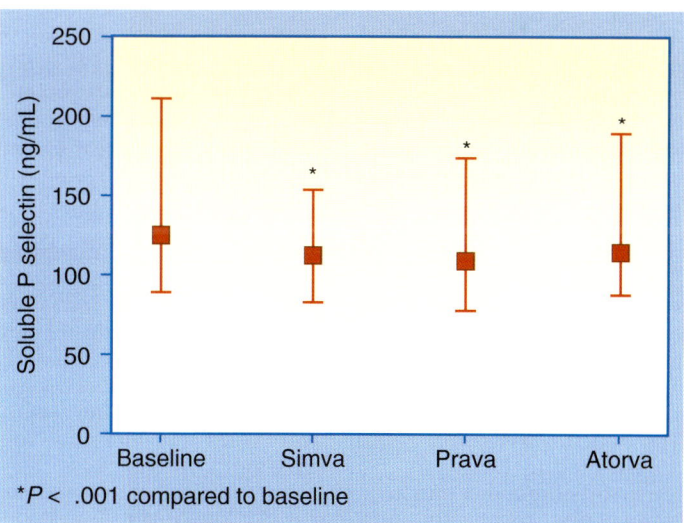

Figure 9-2. Effect of statin therapy on P-selectin levels. Data are presented as 25th percentile, median, and 75th percentile. Atorva, atorvastatin; Prava, pravastatin; Simva, simvastatin.

hypercholesterolemia. Thus, CRP levels may not be a marker for atherosclerosis in patients with familial hypercholesterolemia and without cardiovascular disease. However, these findings need to be confirmed.

Cerivastatin (0.4 and 0.8 mg/day for 8 weeks) has also been shown to be effective in lowering CRP levels in patients with primary hypercholesterolemia (13% median reduction).[31] Although LDL cholesterol decreased in a dose-dependent manner in that study, there was no clear dose-response effect of cerivastatin on CRP levels.

In the Pravastatin Inflammation/CRP Evaluation trial (PRINCE),[32] which was a double-blind, primary prevention prospective trial and an open-label secondary prevention trial, participants received 40 mg/day pravastatin or placebo for 24 weeks. Reduction in CRP (17% in the primary prevention group and 13% in the secondary prevention group) was observed that was independent of LDL cholesterol levels. This prospective study thus provides further evidence for the anti-inflammatory effects of statins and confirms the findings of Jialal and colleagues.[27]

Tan and co-workers studied the effect of atorvastatin on CRP and endothelial-dependent vasodilation in type 2 diabetes mellitus.[33] They showed that although atorvastatin therapy, 10 mg/day for 3 months, did not lower CRP levels significantly, 20 mg/day for an additional 3 months resulted in a significant reduction from baseline in the CRP levels compared to placebo. Interestingly, they also showed a correlation between the improvement in endothelial-dependent vasodilation and CRP levels in the diabetic group. A recent study in type 2 diabetic subjects reported that atorvastatin (10 and 80 mg) for 30 weeks resulted in a strong and significant reduction in, hsCRP levels compared to placebo (15% and 47%, respectively; $P < .001$), and this reduction in CRP was independent of effects on lipid lowering or changes in IL-6 levels.[34] Thus, these two studies further advance our understanding of statins in a model of increased inflammation (i.e., type 2 diabetes mellitus).

Horne and colleagues prospectively studied the combined predictive value of lipid and CRP levels on survival among patients with angiographically defined severe coronary artery disease (>70% stenoses).[35] A second objective was to determine if statin therapy affected the survival of patients with and without elevated CRP. The distribution of statins in the 985 patients was 63% simvastatin, 15% atorvastatin, 13% pravastatin, 5% lovastatin, and 4% fluvastatin. The patients were followed up for 3 years and mortality was documented in 11% of the cohort. Although, in this study, lipid levels did not predict survival, subjects on statin therapy, whether simvastatin, atorvastatin, pravastatin, lovastatin, or fluvastatin, had a significantly decreased risk of mortality of 0.049 ($P < .05$). This benefit could be attributed to an elimination of increased mortality across increasing hsCRP tertiles. Adding lipid levels to

CRP levels was not prognostically useful for secondary risk assessment. Furthermore, this study showed that a clinical benefit with statin therapy was primarily in patients with elevated CRP.

Recently, the effect of statin therapy on hsCRP levels was examined in the Swiss Intervention Trial for Lowering Cholesterol (SWITCH). In this trial, Reisen and colleagues showed that in 150 patients with or at risk for CAD, treatment with atorvastatin (20 mg/day) for 1 month decreased CRP levels in those patients with a baseline median CRP higher than 1.35 mg/L by 22% to 40% ($P < .05$) and by 32% to 36% after 3 months compared to baseline.[36] Furthermore, this short-term effect of atorvastatin on CRP lowering was independent of its effects on lipids. These results may be important with respect to the early benefit of statin therapy, especially in acute coronary syndromes.

The Atorvastatin versus Simvastatin on Atherosclerosis Progression (ASAP) study was a 2-year randomized double-blind trial with 325 hypercholesterolemic patients treated with atorvastatin 80 mg/day or simvastatin 40 mg/day, respectively. Both statins reduced hsCRP levels, with atorvastatin being significantly better than simvastatin at the doses employed. No correlations were observed between hsCRP levels and change in lipids; however, significant associations were seen in changes in carotid intima-media thickness progression and the extent of CRP reduction.[37]

The Arterial Biology for the Investigation of Treatment Effects of Reducing Cholesterol (ARBITER) trial was a randomized clinical trial of 161 patients at intermediate risk for CAD.[38] The patients were administered either pravastatin (40 mg/day) or atorvastatin (80 mg/day). Long-term treatment with atorvastatin resulted in significant lowering of hsCRP compared with pravastatin (12 months, $P < .005$).

Another study examined the effect of fluvastatin alone and in combination with bezafibrate on CRP levels in CAD patients with mixed hyperlipidemia.[39] Fluvastatin therapy failed to significantly reduce levels of CRP, arguing against a class effect of the statin drugs on CRP. However, this needs to be confirmed in other studies.

Randomized trials of statin therapy in individuals without overt dyslipidemia but with high hsCRP levels are needed to establish if this is an additional indicator for statin therapy.

OTHER ANTI-INFLAMMATORY EFFECTS OF STATINS

Statins and Endothelial Function

Acute plasma LDL apheresis improves endothelium-dependent vasodilation,[40] suggesting that statins could restore endothelial function, in part by lowering serum cholesterol levels. However, in some studies with statins, restoration of endothelial function occurs before significant reduction in serum cholesterol levels has occurred,[41-49] suggesting that statins may exert additional effects on endothelial function beyond that of cholesterol reduction.

Statins and Monocyte-Macrophage Function

Recent studies suggest that statins possess anti-inflammatory properties by virtue of their ability to reduce the number of inflammatory cells in atherosclerotic plaques.[50] Studies performed in primary cultures of mouse peritoneal macrophages showed that fluvastatin significantly decreases cholesterol esterification in macrophages. Statin therapy results in inhibition of adhesion molecules, such as intercellular adhesion molecule-1, which are involved in the recruitment of inflammatory cells.[51] A recent study has shown that statins can suppress the inflammatory response independent of HMG-CoA reductase inhibition by binding directly to a novel regulatory site of the β_2 integrin, leukocyte function antigen-1, which serves as a major counterreceptor for intercellular adhesion molecule-1 on leukocytes.[52] Subjects with hypercholesterolemia exhibit increased adhesion of monocytes to endothelial cells in vitro, and this response is diminished with lovastatin and simvastatin.[53] Weber and co-workers have shown that these statins significantly decrease CD11b expression on monocytes.[54]

Statins also cause decreased lipopolysaccharide-induced secretion of IL-6 and TNF-α. Simvastatin reduces monocyte expression of TNF-α and IL-1β in patients with hypercholesterolemia,[55] whereas atorvastatin reduces monocyte chemoattractant protein-1 (MCP-1) levels in the intima and media of hypercholesterolemic rabbits.[56] This effect is related to a reduction in activation of nuclear factor B, a transcription factor involved in the induction of other proinflammatory cytokines, such as IL-1 and TNF-α, and the regulation of E-selectin expression.[57,58] Simvastatin has also been shown to reduce expression of IL-6 and the chemokines IL-8 and MCP-1 in circulating monocytes from hypercholesterolemic patients.[59] Lipophilic statins have also been shown to decrease tissue factor expression and activity in cultured human monocyte-derived macrophages.[60] Expression of MCP-1, an important chemokine responsible for monocyte chemotaxis and transmigration, is also significantly reduced with statin therapy via the inhibition of mevalonate-derived products.

RECOMMENDATIONS FOR THE USE OF CRP IN CLINICAL PRACTICE

Recently, a consensus document from the American Heart Association (AHA) and the Centers for Disease Control (CDC) was released with regard to the measurement of CRP.[61] To reduce interindividual variability, the assay should be performed in a metabolically stable state without obvious inflammatory or infectious conditions. They recommend that two measurements be taken, fasting or nonfasting and optimally 2 weeks apart, and averaged. If a level higher than 10 mg/L is identified, any obvious source of inflammation or infection should be examined, because this could obscure prediction of coronary risk. The suggested cut-points of coronary risk are CRP levels lower than 1, 1 to 3, and higher than 3.0 mg/L to denote low-, moderate-, and high-risk groups; these correspond to approximate tertiles of hsCRP in the adult population.

CRP is an independent predictor of future cardiovascular events that adds prognostic information to lipid screening, to the metabolic syndrome, and to the Framingham Risk Score. Specifically, patients at intermediate risk (Framingham risk 10% to 20%) may benefit most from the measurement of hsCRP.

CONCLUSIONS

Thus, statins exert beneficial pleiotropic effects on cells of the vascular wall. The development of statin drugs has been one of the most exciting advances in the prevention and treatment of atherosclerosis. The cardiovascular benefits of statin therapy extend beyond their effects on plasma lipids. Combining CRP measurements with lipid screening may improve targeting of statin therapy in primary prevention. Furthermore, it appears that the anti-inflammatory properties of statins are a class effect. Ongoing studies will establish if certain statins at high doses demonstrate greater anti-inflammatory effects.

References

1. Gordon T, Kannel WB: Premature mortality from coronary heart disease: The Framingham Study. JAMA 215:1617-1625, 1971.
2. Kannel WB, Castelli WP, Gordon T, et al: Serum cholesterol, lipoproteins, and the risk of coronary heart disease: The Framingham Study. Ann Intern Med 74:1-12, 1971.
3. Iso H, Jacobs DR Jr, Wentworth D, et al: Serum cholesterol levels and six-year mortality from stroke in 350,977 men screened for the multiple risk factor intervention trial. N Engl J Med 320:904-910, 1989.
5. Randomised trial of cholesterol lowering in 4444 patients with coronary heart disease: The Scandinavian Simvastatin Survival Study (4S). Lancet 344:1383-1389, 1994.
6. Prevention of cardiovascular events and death with pravastatin in patients with coronary heart disease and a broad range of initial cholesterol levels: The Long-Term Intervention with Pravastatin in Ischaemic Disease (LIPID) Study Group. N Engl J Med 339:1349-1357, 1998.
7. Sacks FM, Pfeffer MA, Moye LA, et al: The effect of pravastatin on coronary events after myocardial infarction in patients with average cholesterol levels: Cholesterol and Recurrent Events Trial investigators. N Engl J Med 335:1001-1009, 1996.

8. Shepherd J, Cobbe SM, Ford I, et al: Prevention of coronary heart disease with pravastatin in men with hypercholesterolemia: West of Scotland Coronary Prevention Study Group. N Engl J Med 333:1301-1307, 1995.
9. Downs JR, Clearfield M, Weis S, et al: Primary prevention of acute coronary events with lovastatin in men and women with average cholesterol levels: Results of AFCAPS/TexCAPS: Air Force/Texas Coronary Atherosclerosis Prevention Study. JAMA 279:1615-1622, 1998.
11. Massy ZA, Keane WF, Kasiske BL: Inhibition of the mevalonate pathway: Benefits beyond cholesterol reduction? Lancet 347:102-103, 1996.
12. Packard CJ: Influence of pravastatin and plasma lipids on clinical events in the West of Scotland Coronary Prevention Study (WOSCOPS). Circulation 97:1440-1445, 1998.
13. Ridker PM, Rifai N, Pfefffer MA: Long-term effects of pravastatin on plasma concentration of C-reactive protein. The Cholesterol and Recurrent Events (CARE) Investigators. Circulation 100:230-235, 1999.
14. Brown BG, Zhao XQ, Sacco DE, et al: Lipid lowering and plaque regression: New insights into prevention of plaque disruption and clinical events in coronary disease. Circulation 87:1781-1791, 1993.
15. Pekkanen J, Linn S, Heiss G, et al: Ten-year mortality from cardiovascular disease in relation to cholesterol level among men with and without preexisting cardiovascular disease. N Engl J Med 322:1700-1707, 1990.
16. Brown BG, Hillger L, Zhao XQ, et al: Types of change in coronary stenosis severity and their relative importance in overall progression and regression of coronary disease: Observations from the FATS Trial: Familial Atherosclerosis Treatment Study. Ann N Y Acad Sci 748:407-418, 1995.
17. Schwartz GG, Olsson AG, Ezekowitz MD, et al: Effects of atorvastatin on early recurrent ischemic events in acute coronary syndromes: The MIRACL Study: A randomized controlled trial. JAMA 285:1711-1718, 2001.
18. Ross R. Atherosclerosis—an inflammatory disease. N Engl J Med. 340:115-126, 1999.
19. Jialal I, Devaraj S: Inflammation and atherosclerosis: The value of the high-sensitivity C-reactive protein assay as a risk marker. Am J Clin Pathol 116(Suppl):S108-S115, 2001.
20. Jialal I, Devaraj S: Role of C-reactive protein in the assessment of cardiovascular risk. Am J Cardiol 91:200-202, 2003.
21. Rifai N, Ridker PM: High-sensitivity C-reactive protein: A novel and promising marker of coronary heart disease. Clin Chem 47:403-411, 2001.
22. Ridker PM, Glynn RJ, Hennekens CH: CRP adds to the predictive value of total and HDL cholesterol in determining risk of first MI. Circulation 97:2007-2011, 1998.
23. Ridker PM, Hennekens CH, Buring JE, et al: CRP and other markers of inflammation in the prediction of CAD in women. N Engl J Med 342:836-843, 2000.
24. Ridker PM, Cushman M, Stampfer MJ, et al: Plasma concentration of C-reactive protein and risk of developing peripheral vascular disease. Circulation 97:425-428, 1998.
25. Ridker PM, Rifai N, Pfeffer MA, et al: Long-term effects of pravastatin on plasma concentration of C-reactive protein. Circulation 100:230-235, 1999.

26. Ridker PM, Rifai N, Clearfield M, et al: Measurement of C-reactive protein for the targeting of statin therapy in the primary prevention of acute coronary events. N Engl J Med 344:1959-1965, 2001.

27. Jialal I, Stein D, Balis D, et al: Effect of hydroxymethyl glutaryl coenzyme A reductase inhibitor therapy on high sensitive C-reactive protein levels. Circulation 103:1933-1935, 2001.

28. Miller M, Jialal I: Effects of simvastatin (40 and 80 mg) on highly sensitive C-reactive protein in patients with combined hyperlipidemia. Am J Cardiol 89:468-469, 2001.

29. Strandberg TE, Vanhanen H, Tikkanen MJ: Associations between change in C-reactive protein and serum lipids during statin treatment. Ann Med 32:579-583, 2000.

30. Gomez-Gerique JA, Ros E, Olivan J, et al: Effect of atorvastatin and bezafibrate on plasma levels of C-reactive protein in combined (mixed) hyperlipidemia. Atherosclerosis 162:245-51; 2002.

31. Ridker PM, Rifai N, Lowenthal SP: Rapid reduction in C-reactive protein with cerivastatin among 785 patients with primary hypercholesterolemia. Circulation 103:1191-1193, 2001.

32. Albert MA, Danielson E, Rifai N, et al: Effect of statin therapy on C-reactive protein levels: The pravastatin inflammation/CRP evaluation (PRINCE): A randomized trial and cohort study. JAMA 286:64-70, 2001.

33. Tan KCB, Chow WS, Tam SCF, et al: Atorvastatin lowers C-reactive protein and improves endothelium-dependent vasodilation in type 2 diabetes mellitus. J Clin Endocrinol Metab 87:563-568, 2002.

34. Van de Ree MS, Huisman MV, Princen HMG, et al: Strong decrease of hsCRP with high dose atorvastatin in patients with type 2 diabetes mellitus. Atherosclerosis 166:129-135, 2003.

35. Horne BD, Muhlestein JB, Carlquist JF, et al: Statin therapy, lipid levels, C-reactive protein and the survival of patients with angiographically severe CAD. J Am Coll Cardiol 36:1774-1780, 2000.

36. Reisen WF, Engler H, Risch M, et al: Short term effects of atorvastatin on CRP. Eur Heart J 23:794-799, 2002.

37. van Wissen S, Trip MD, Smilde TJ, et al: Differential hsCRP reduction in patients with familial hypercholesterolemia treated with aggressive or conventional statin therapy. Atherosclerosis 165:361-366, 2002.

38. Taylor AJ, Kent SM, Flaherty PJ, et al: ARBITER: Arterial Biology for the Investigation of Treatment Effects of Reducing Cholesterol. Circulation 106:2055-2060, 2002.

39. Cortellaro M, Cofrancesco E, Boschetti C, et al: Effects of fluvastatin and bezafibrate combination on plasma fibrinogen, tPA and CRP in CAD patients with mixed hyperlipidemia (FACT Study). Thromb Hemost 83:549-553, 2000.

40. Kinlay S, Libby P, Ganz P: Endothelial function and coronary artery disease. Curr Opin Lipidol 12:383-389, 2001.

41. Egashira K, Hirooka Y, Kai H, et al: Reduction in serum cholesterol with pravastatin improves endothelium-dependent coronary vasomotion in patients with hypercholesterolemia. Circulation 89:2519-2524, 1994.

42. Treasure CB, Klein JL, Weintraub WS, et al: Beneficial effects of cholesterol-lowering therapy on the coronary endothelium in patients with coronary artery disease. N Engl J Med 332:481-487, 1995.

43. Anderson TJ, Meredith IT, Yeung AC, et al: The effect of cholesterol-lowering and antioxidant therapy on endothelium-dependent coronary vasomotion. N Engl J Med 332:488-493, 1995.

44. Omori H, Nagashima H, Tsurumi Y, et al: Direct in vivo evidence of a vascular statin: A single dose of cerivastatin rapidly increases vascular endothelial responsiveness in healthy normocholesterolaemic subjects. Br J Clin Pharmacol 54:395-399, 2002.

45. Fabian E, Varga A: Effect of simvastatin therapy on endothelial function of hypercholesteremic patients with syndrome X. Orv Hetil 143:2067-2071, 2002.

46. Asberg A, Hartmann A, Fjeldsa E, et al: Atorvastatin improves endothelial function in renal-transplant recipients. Nephrol Dial Transplant 16:1920-1924, 2001.

47. Liao JK: Beyond lipid lowering: The role of statins in vascular protection. Int J Cardiol 86:5-18, 2002.

48. Tamai O, Matsuoka H, Itabe H, et al: Single LDL apheresis improves endothelium-dependent vasodilatation in hypercholesterolemic humans. Circulation 95:76-82, 1997.

49. O'Driscoll G, Green D, Taylor RR: Simvastatin, an HMG-coenzyme A reductase inhibitor, improves endothelial function within 1 month. Circulation 95:1126-1131, 1997.

50. Koh KK: Effects of statins on vascular wall: Vasomotor function, inflammation, and plaque stability. Cardiovasc Res 47:648-657, 2000.

51. Niwa S, Totsuka T, Hayashi S: Inhibitory effect of fluvastatin, an HMG-CoA reductase inhibitor, on the expression of adhesion molecules on human monocyte cell line. Int J Immunopharmacol 18:669-675, 1996.

52. Weitz-Schmidt G, Welzenbach K, Brinkmann V, et al: Statins selectively inhibit leukocyte function antigen-1 by binding to a novel regulatory integrin site. Nat Med 7:687-692, 2001.

53. Serrano CV, Yoshida VM, Venturinelli ML, et al: Effect of simvastatin on monocyte adhesion molecule expression in patients with hypercholesterolemia. Atheroscler 157:505-512, 2001.

54. Weber C, Erl W, Weber K, Weber PC: HMG-CoA reductase inhibitors decrease CD11b expression and reduce increased adhesiveness of monocytes isolated from patients with hypercholesterolemia. J Am Coll Cardiol 30:1212-1217, 1997.

55. Ferro D, Parrotto S, Basili S, et al: Simvastatin inhibits the monocyte expression of proinflammatory cytokines in patients with hypercholesterolemia. J Am Coll Cardiol 36:427-431, 2000.

56. Bustos C, Hernandez-Presa MA, Ortego M, et al: HMG-CoA reductase inhibition by atorvastatin reduces neointimal inflammation in a rabbit model of atherosclerosis. J Am Coll Cardiol 32:2057-2064, 1998.

57. Hatada EN, Krappmann D, Scheidereit C: NF-B, and the innate immune response. Curr Opin Immunol 12:52-58, 2000.

58. Boyle EM Jr, Kovacich JC, Canty TG Jr, et al: Inhibition of nuclear factor-B nuclear localization reduces human E-selectin expression and the systemic inflammatory response. Circulation 98(Suppl II):II282-288, 1998.

59. Rezai Majd A, Maca T, Bucek RA, et al: Simvastatin reduces expression of cytokines IL-6, IL-8 and MCP-1 in circulating monocytes from hypercholesterolemic patients. Arterioscler Thromb Vasc Biol 22:1194-1199, 2002.

60. Colli S, Eligini S, Lalli M, et al: Vastatins inhibit tissue factor in cultured human macrophages: A novel mechanism of protection against atherothrombosis. Arterioscler Thromb Vasc Biol 17:265-272, 1997.

61. Pearson TA, Mensah GA, Alexander RW, et al: Markers of inflammation and cardiovascular disease: Application to clinical and public health practice: A statement for healthcare professionals from the Centers for Disease Control and Prevention and the American Heart Association. Circulation 107:499-511, 2003.

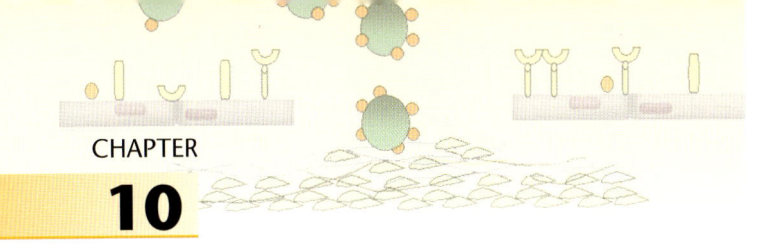

CHAPTER

10

Actions of Statins on Ox-LDL–Mediated Signaling and Inflammation

Dayuan Li and Jawahar L. Mehta

Increasing evidence indicates that oxidized low-density lipoprotein (ox-LDL) plays a more important role in atherosclerosis than does native LDL. The atherosclerotic regions, particularly those prone to rupture, exhibit the accumulation of ox-LDL and large numbers of macrophages and inflammatory cells.[1-3] Recent studies show that 3-hydroxy-3-methylglutaryl coenzyme A (HMG-CoA) reductase inhibitors (statins) not only decrease the plasma level of LDL but also have other unique effects on ox-LDL–mediated injuries.

The development of statins has been a major milestone in the primary and secondary prevention of coronary heart disease. In a variety of animal models, these agents decrease the extent of atherosclerosis.[4] Proposed mechanisms include favorable effects on plasma lipoproteins, endothelial function, plaque architecture and stability, thrombosis, and oxidation. Mechanisms independent of LDL cholesterol lowering may play an important role in the clinical benefits conferred by these drugs and may ultimately broaden their indication from lipid-lowering to antiatherogenic agents.[5]

This chapter specifically emphasizes the effects of statins on ox-LDL–induced inflammation and activation of signaling pathways.

OXIDATIVELY MODIFIED LDL IN ATHEROSCLEROSIS

A high serum level of LDL cholesterol is one of the most prominent risk factors for atherosclerosis. The current knowledge of atherogenesis includes a critical role of oxidation of native LDL (n-LDL).[1,2] Ox-LDL causes endothelial dysfunction, an early event in atherogenesis.[6] Ox-LDL is taken up by the recently described lectin-like receptor for ox-LDL (LOX-1) on endothelial cells, resulting in the expression of inflammatory mediators and cell activation followed by cell injury.[7,8] Ox-LDL is taken up by scavenger receptors on macrophages, resulting in the formation of cholesterol-loaded foam cells.[3] Ox-LDL causes lipid peroxidation, expression of leukocyte adhesion molecules, release of vascular smooth muscle growth factors, and impairment of endothelial nitric oxide synthase (eNOS) expression and activity.[2,6,9] It triggers activation of inflammatory signaling pathways such as CD40/CD40L.[10] Ox-LDL also facilitates thrombus formation by reducing fibrinolysis and by promoting procoagulant activity via induction of tissue factor expression[11] and alterations in tissue plasminogen activator (t-PA) and its inhibitor (PAI-1).[12] Loss of eNOS activity, expression of adhesion molecules and CD40, leukocyte adhesion to endothelium, and platelet aggregation all contribute to the adverse role of ox-LDL in the development of atherosclerosis.

OX-LDL, ITS RECEPTORS, AND THEIR PATHOPHYSIOLOGIC ACTIONS

Traditionally, it has been believed that the biologic effects of ox-LDL are exerted via activation of scavenger receptors on the surfaces of macrophages and smooth muscle cells.[13] Scavenger receptors for ox-LDL (types I and II macrophage scavenger receptors, CD36 and CD68) are mainly expressed on macrophages and smooth muscle cells. Scavenger receptors were originally implicated in the uptake of cholesterol in atherosclerotic tissues.[14,15] Multiple functions of scavenger receptors, including endocytosis, phagocytosis, and monocyte adhesion and signal transduction triggered by the binding and uptake of modified LDL cholesterol, may also be involved in this process. However, experimental studies have shown that endothelial cells express only a very small amount of scavenger receptors.[16] LOX-1, a receptor specific for ox-LDL, found predominantly on endothelial cells, has a biochemical structure different from that of the scavenger receptors.[17] Several studies have demonstrated that the uptake of ox-LDL by endothelial cells is mediated by LOX-1.[17-20] Whereas the uptake of ox-LDL by endothelial cells does not result in foam cell formation, ox-LDL uptake in vascular endothelium causes endothelial activation and/or dysfunction. Ox-LDL induces loss of endothelial integrity, and alterations in cell secretory function.[19,21,22] Studies have shown that LOX-1 mediates ox-LDL–induced apoptosis in human coronary artery endothelial cells.[23] These changes in endothelial biology provide a basis for leukocyte, monocyte, and platelet deposition on the vascular intima, which is an early event in atherosclerosis.

STATINS AND OX-LDL FORMATION

There is increasing evidence that the clinical benefits obtained with statins cannot be solely attributed to a decrease in native LDL cholesterol.[5,24-26] These drugs may also have beneficial effects on endothelial dysfunction, LDL oxidation, thrombogenic factors, cellular inflammation, and plaque formation and stability. There is evidence that ox-LDL formation is associated with atherosclerosis, myocardial ischemia/reperfusion injury, and heart failure.[27-29] Girona and colleagues showed that the formation of ox-LDL and oxidized-HDL particles is significantly decreased in patients treated with simvastatin.[30] Crisby and co-workers reported that pravastatin markedly reduces ox-LDL formation in atherosclerotic plaques, determined by immunoreactivity.[27] In vitro studies have confirmed that statins inhibit ox-LDL–induced vascular endothelial cell injury by inhibiting the uptake of ox-LDL and monocyte adhesion.[8,31] These observations taken together indicate that inhibition of ox-LDL formation may be an important mechanism of the benefits of statins in the treatment of cardiovascular disease, beyond the lowering of cholesterol.

STATINS AND OX-LDL UPTAKE

As mentioned earlier, the pathologic effects of ox-LDL are mainly mediated by its receptors, including (1) scavenger receptors in macrophages and smooth muscle cells and (2) LOX-1 in endothelial cells.[16-20,32] A recent study by our group showed that statins inhibit ox-LDL uptake in endothelial cells.[31] This study showed that incubation of human coronary artery endothelial cells with ox-LDL markedly increased the binding of iodine-125(^{125}I)–ox-LDL to human endothelial cells. To determine if statins influence ox-LDL binding, endothelial cells were treated with statins followed by incubation with ox-LDL. Pretreatment of endothelial cells with two different statins, simvastatin and atorvastatin, significantly decreased ox-LDL binding to endothelial cells compared with ox-LDL alone. A high concentration of statins (10 μM) had a more potent inhibitory effect on ox-LDL binding than the low concentration (1 μM). These results are consistent with the effects of statins on the inhibition of ox-LDL–mediated LOX-1 expression (mRNA and protein) on endothelial cells, as previous studies showed that ox-LDL per se up-regulates the expression of LOX-1. These results are summarized in Figure 10-1. Inhibitory effects of statins on ox-LDL uptake have major clinical significance in designing therapy for patients with atherosclerosis.

STATINS AND EXPRESSION OF OX-LDL RECEPTORS

Ox-LDL receptors mediate ox-LDL uptake by endothelial cells and macrophages and facilitate ox-LDL–induced pathophysiologic changes. It has been speculated that inhibition of the expression of these receptors would prevent the effects of ox-LDL in these cells.

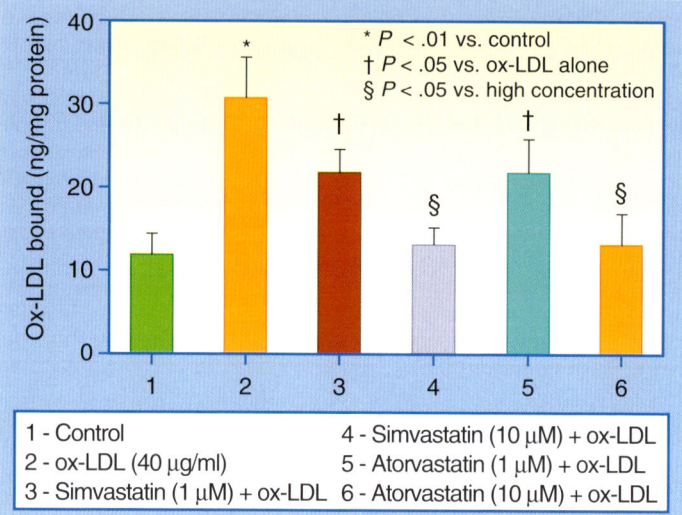

Figure 10-1 Statins and endothelial cell-bound iodine-125 (^{125}I)-ox-LDL. Incubation of human coronary artery endothelial cells with ox-LDL increased the amount of ^{125}I-ox-LDL on endothelial cells. Pretreatment of endothelial cells with simvastatin or atorvastatin (1 and 10 μM) decreased ^{125}I-ox-LDL binding to human endothelial cells. High concentrations of statins had a more potent effect than low concentrations. The data (mean ± SD) are based on six independent experiments.

In fact, this concept has been supported by several studies.[8,23,28,31,33] LOX-1 mediates ox-LDL–induced expression of adhesion molecules, monocyte adhesion to endothelial cells, and endothelial apoptosis.[31,34,35] LOX-1 mediates the inhibitory effect of ox-LDL on the expression and activity of eNOS.[36]

Recent studies have shown that overexpression of LOX-1 in cardiac myocytes markedly increases apoptosis by activation of the p38 mitogen-activated protein kinase (MAPK) signaling pathway.[37] Up-regulation of LOX-1 increases myocardial ischemia/reperfusion injury by increasing myocardial apoptosis and lipid peroxidation.[28] These effects of ox-LDL mediated through LOX-1 expression can be inhibited by reduction of LOX-1 gene expression. In one study, two different commonly used statins, simvastatin and atorvastatin, were shown to inhibit the expression of LOX-1 gene elicited by ox-LDL in human endothelial cells.[8] Decrease in LOX-1 expression results in a reduction in binding (uptake) of ^{125}I-ox-LDL and ox-LDL–induced monocyte adhesion and apoptosis in human endothelial cells. A high concentration of statins (10 μM) has a more powerful effect

Role of LOX-1 in the actions of ox-LDL

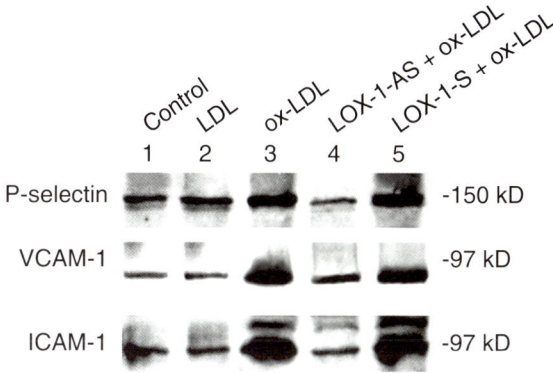

Figure 10-2 Role of lectin-like receptor for ox-LDL (LOX-1) in the actions of ox-LDL. Incubation of human coronary artery endothelial cells with ox-LDL (40 µg/mL) markedly increased the expression of adhesion molecules determined by Western blot. In contrast, native LDL (40 µg/mL) did not affect the expression of these adhesion molecules. Pretreatment of endothelial cells with an antisense to LOX-1 mRNA (LOX-1-AS, 0.5 µM) completely blocked the effects of ox-LDL on the expression of these adhesion molecules. Note that LOX-1-sense (LOX-1-S, 0.5 µM) had no effect. This figure represents six independent experiments. ICAM-1, intercellular adhesion molecule-1; VCAM-1, vascular cell adhesion molecule-1.

than a low concentration of statins (1 µM). These results are shown in Figures 10-2 and 10-3.

STATINS AND OX-LDL–INDUCED INFLAMMATION

Evidence from many studies suggests that atherosclerosis is a complex inflammatory disease that, from its origin to ultimate clinical endpoint, involves inflammatory cells (T cells, monocytes, macrophages), inflammatory factors (cytokines, chemokines), and inflammatory responses from vascular cells (endothelial expression of adhesion molecules).[38,39] Many of the beneficial effects of statins have been ascribed to their anti-inflammatory effects. The anti-inflammatory mechanisms have yet to be fully elucidated but may involve inhibition of adhesion molecules, such as intercellular adhesion molecule-1, which are involved in the recruitment of inflammatory cells.[40] A recent study showed that simvastatin markedly reduces the expression of IL-6, IL-8, and monocyte chemoattractant protein-1 (MCP-1) mRNA in cultured human umbilical vein endothelial cells.[41] Weitz-Schmidt and colleagues reported that statins could suppress the inflammatory response by

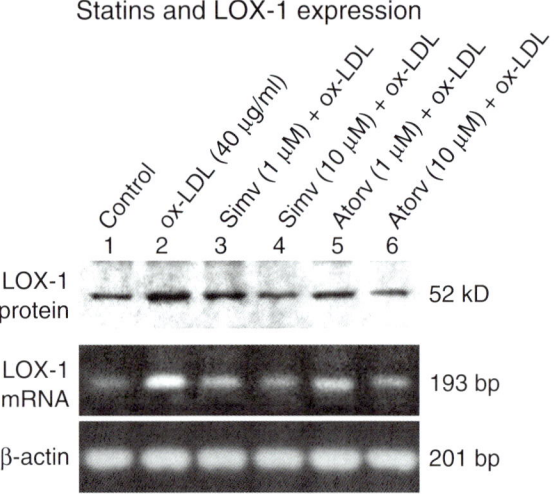

Figure 10-3 **Statins and LOX-1 expression.** Ox-LDL (40 µg/mL) increased the expression of LOX-1 mRNA and protein. Pretreatment of human coronary artery endothelial cells with simvastatin or atorvastatin (1 and 10 µM) decreased ox-LDL–induced up-regulation of LOX-1. A high concentration (10 µM) of simvastatin (Simv) or atorvastatin (Atorv) had a more powerful effect than the low concentration (1 µM). This figure represents six independent experiments.

binding directly to a novel regulatory site of the β_2 integrin, leukocyte function antigen-1, which serves as a major counter-receptor for intercellular adhesion molecule-1 on leukocytes (reviewed in Chapter 15).[42]

A recent study from our group demonstrated that ox-LDL induces a 2.5-fold increase in MCP-1 mRNA and protein expression in human coronary artery endothelial cells.[33] A specific antisense directed at LOX-1 mRNA completely blocked ox-LDL–mediated up-regulation of MCP-1 expression in human coronary artery endothelial cells. In another study, we observed that ox-LDL up-regulates the expression of ox-LDL–induced P selectin, inter-cellular adhesion molecule-1 (ICAM-1), and vascular cell adhesion molecule-1 (VCAM-1) in human endothelial cells.[8] The effects of ox-LDL appear to be mediated by its receptor LOX-1, because the use of an antisense directed at LOX-1 mRNA decreases LOX-1 expression and subsequently inhibits the gene expression of these adhesion molecules. Furthermore, the pretreatment of human endothelial cells with statins blocks ox-LDL–induced gene expression of adhesion molecules and adhesion of monocyte to endothelial cells. These results are shown in Figures 10-4 and 10-5.

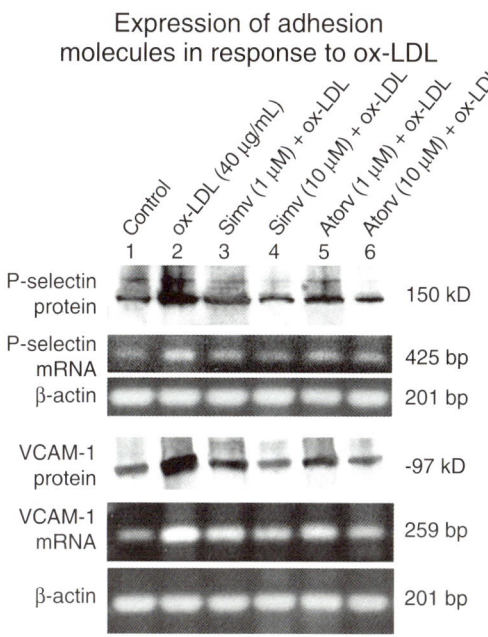

Expression of adhesion
molecules in response to ox-LDL

Figure 10-4 **Expression of adhesion molecules in response to ox-LDL.**
Incubation of endothelial cells with ox-LDL (40 μg/mL) for 24 hours
increased the expression of P-selectin and vascular cell adhesion molecule-
1 (VCAM-1) mRNA and protein. Pretreatment of endothelial cells with
simvastatin (Simv) or atorvastatin (Atorv) (1 and 10 μM) for 30 minutes
decreased ox-LDL–induced expression of these adhesion molecules. A high
concentration (10 μM) of Simv or Atorv had a greater effect than the low
concentration (1 μM). Adhesion molecule mRNA was determined by
semiquantitative reverse transcription–polymerase chain reaction (RT-
PCR). Each band density of adhesion molecules was normalized by internal
reference β-actin and expressed as a ratio of adhesion molecule mRNA to β-
actin mRNA. Adhesion molecule protein was determined by Western blot
analysis. This figure represents six independent experiments.

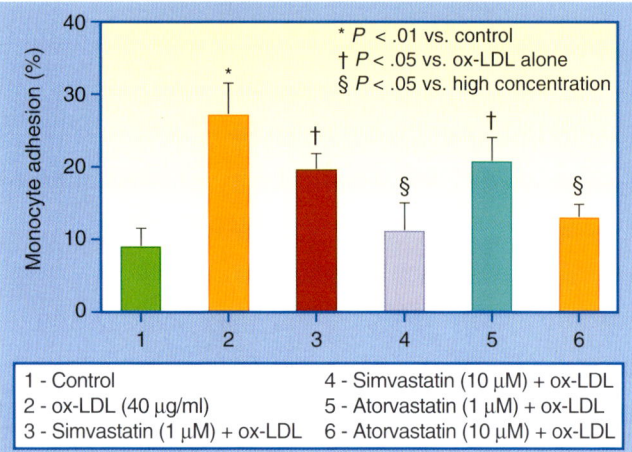

Figure 10-5 Statins and monocyte adhesion. Ox-LDL promotes monocyte adhesion to endothelial cells. Pretreatment of endothelial cells with
simvastatin or atorvastatin (1 and 10 μM, respectively) reduced ox-LDL–
induced monocyte adhesion. A high concentration of statins had a more
pronounced effect than the low concentration. These data are a summary
(mean ± SD) of six independent experiments.

Inflammation elicited by ox-LDL and its inhibition by
statins have been further studied by the CD40/CD40L signaling
pathway.[10,43] It is widely recognized that the activation of
CD40/CD40L signaling plays a critical role in atherosclerosis.[44,45] We
recently reported that ox-LDL induces gene expression of CD40
and CD40L in a concentration- and time-dependent manner.[10]
This effect of ox-LDL on CD40/CD40L signaling is mediated by its
receptor LOX-1 through protein kinase C activation in endothelial
cells. Wagner and co-workers have demonstrated that statins
reduce cytokine-induced up-regulation of CD40 expression in
endothelial cells and monocytes by interfering with the de novo
synthesis of the transcription factor IRF-1.[43] This effect takes place
independently of the blockade of HMG-CoA reductase and results
in an attenuation of CD40-mediated gene expression, exemplified
by the Th1 cytokine interleukin-12 (IL-12) (Figs. 10-6 and 10-7).

Ox-LDL may also affect the stability of atherosclerotic plaques,
which is determined in part by expression of a family of enzymes,
the matrix metalloproteinases (MMPs). Li and colleagues showed
that ox-LDL induces gene expression of MMPs in human endothelial cells.[46] These observations taken together suggest that
ox-LDL accumulation may play a critical role in the rupture of

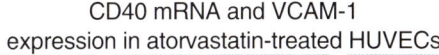

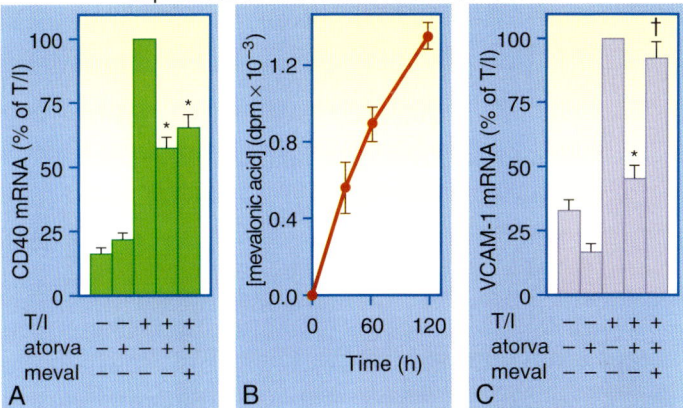

Figure 10-6 Effect of 400 μmol/L mevalonic acid (meval) on atorvastatin (atorva) inhibition of cytokine-stimulated CD40 and vascular cell adhesion molecule-1 (VCAM-1) mRNA expression in cultured human umbilical vein endothelial cells (HUVECs). Statistical summary ($N = 3$ to 10) of CD40 mRNA **(A)** and VCAM-1 **(C)** expression in atorvastatin-treated HUVECs after 9 hours of exposure to 100 U/mL TNF-α plus 1000 U/mL IFN-γ (T/I). *$P < .05$ versus T/I; $P < .05$ versus T/I + atorva. **B,** Time-dependent uptake of ^{14}C-mevalonic acid (exogenous concentration of 400 μmol/L) by the cultured HUVECs. Assuming an endothelial cell volume of 0.5 pL, the intracellular concentration of mevalonic acid after 30, 60, and 120 minutes corresponded to 355, 563, and 856 μmol/L, respectively.

fibrin-poor atherosclerotic plaques. Experimental studies have shown that statins can reduce MMP secretion and activity, which serves to stabilize the rupture-prone plaque.[47]

STATINS AND OX-LDL–INDUCED ACTIVATION OF SIGNALING PATHWAYS

Recent experimental and clinical evidence indicate that some of the cholesterol-independent, or pleiotropic, effects of statins involve improving or restoring endothelial function, enhancing the stability of atherosclerotic plaques, and decreasing oxidative stress and vascular inflammation. Many of these pleiotropic effects of statins are mediated by their ability to block the synthesis of important isoprenoid intermediates that serve as lipid attachments for a variety of intracellular signaling molecules. In particular, the inhibition of the small GTP-binding proteins Rho, Ras, and Rac, whose proper membrane localization and function are dependent on isoprenylation, may play an important role in mediating the

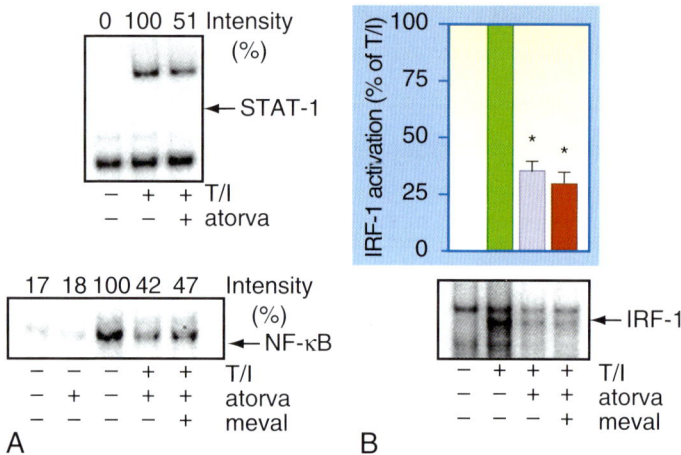

Figure 10-7 **Effects of atorvastatin (atorva) on transcription factor activation and lack of effect of exogenous mevalonic acid (meval). A,** Effects of 1-hour preincubation with 10 µmol/L atorva on the nuclear translocation of signal transducer and activator of transcription-1 (STAT-1) and nuclear factor kappa B (NF-κB) (specific DNA-protein complexes are designated by *arrows*) in cultured human umbilical vein endothelial cells (HUVECs) stimulated for 3 hours with T/I. Typical electrophoretic mobility shift assay (EMSA) is shown; qualitatively identical results were obtained for each transcription factor with at least three further batches of HUVECs. **B,** Statistical summary ($N = 3$ or 4, with typical EMSA at the bottom) of cytokine-stimulated nuclear translocation of interferon regulatory factor-1 (IRF-1) in atorvastatin-treated HUVECs and lack of effect of co-treatment with 400 µmol/L mevalonic acid. *$P < .05$ versus T/I. The identity of IRF-1 binding to the labeled oligonucleotides was confirmed by supershift analysis with an appropriate antibody.

Statins and activation of MAPKs

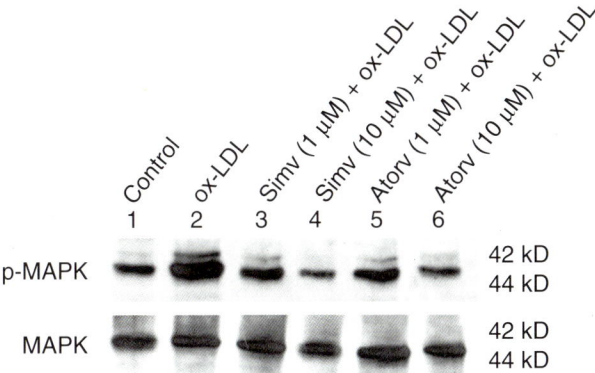

Figure 10-8 Statins and activation of mitogen-activated protein kinase (MAPK). Incubation of endothelial cells with ox-LDL did not change MAPK protein but activated MAPK. Pretreatment of endothelial cells with simvastatin or atorvastatin (1 and 10 μM) attenuated ox-LDL–induced activation of MAPK. The high concentration of statins had a more pronounced effect than the low concentration. This is representative of six independent experiments.

direct cellular effects of statins on the vascular wall.[48-50] Recent studies have shown that statins modulate intracellular signaling pathways to generate their biologic effects. (See Chapters 8, 10, 13).

It is clear that statins increase the expression and activity of eNOS by the activation of the phosphatidylinositol (PI) 3-kinase (PKB)/Akt pathway.[31,51] Skaletz-Rorowski and colleagues reported that lovastatin blocks basic fibroblast growth factor–induced MAPK signaling in coronary smooth muscle cells via phosphatase inhibition.[52] Pretreatment of human endothelial cells with simvastatin and atorvastatin were shown to increase PKB activity and decrease MAPK activity, which may be the basis of the up-regulation of eNOS and down-regulation of adhesion molecules. Furthermore, we have shown that both simvastatin and atorvastatin inhibit ox-LDL–induced transcription factor nuclear factor kappa B (NF-κB) activation in endothelial cells. These observations suggest that statins modulate intracellular signal pathways (Figs. 10-8 and 10-9).

CONCLUSION

Statins exert many protective effects on the vessel wall. These include beneficial effects on endothelial function, LDL oxidation, the stability of atherosclerotic plaques, vascular smooth muscle cell proliferation and platelet aggregation, and reduction of vascular

10

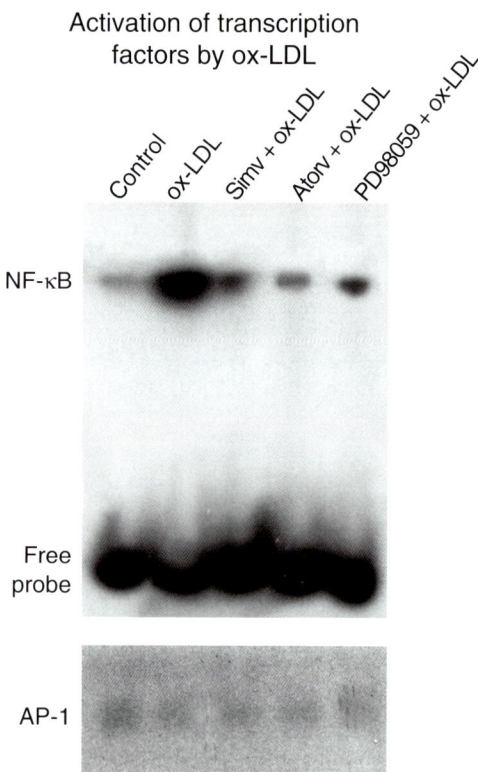

Figure 10-9 Activation of transcription factors by ox-LDL. Incubation of endothelial cells with ox-LDL induced activation of nuclear factor-kappa B (NF-κB) but not activator protein-1 (AP-1). Both simvastatin and atorvastatin (10 μM each) attenuated this effect of ox-LDL on NF-κB activity. Pretreatment of endothelial cells with mitogen-activated protein kinase (MAPK) inhibitor PD98059 also prevented ox-LDL–induced NF-κB activation, which is consistent with the concept that statins inhibit MAPK activation and subsequently inhibit NF-κB activation. These gels are representative of six independent experiments.

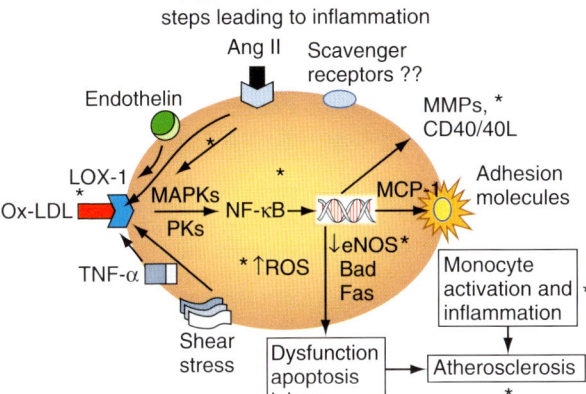

Figure 10-10 Sites of actions of statins in the proinflammatory cascade in the endothelial cells exposed to oxidized-LDL, angiotensin (Ang) II, endothelin, tumor necrosis factor-alpha (TNF-α), and shear stress. These different mediators of inflammation may be working at least in part by activating the lectin-like receptor for ox-LDL (LOX-1). Activation of LOX-1 via mitogen-activated protein kinase (MAPK) and protein kinase signaling activates nuclear factor-kappa B (NF-κB), with subsequent alteration in the transcription of several genes involved in monocyte activation and inflammation, endothelial dysfunction, and injury (including apoptosis). These steps may be collectively involved in atherosclerosis. Activation of metalloproteinases and CD40/CD40L signaling may be relevant in precipitation of acute coronary syndromes. The sites of actions of statins are multiple (*asterisk*).

inflammation. In particular, inhibition of ox-LDL effects by statins may lead to restoration of endothelial function, inhibition of inflammation, and decrease in atherosclerosis, which may act as a brake on the progression of atherosclerosis. These effects of statins on vascular biology are summarized in Figure 10-10.

References

1. Steinberg D, Witztum JL: Lipoproteins and atherogenesis. JAMA 264:3047-3052, 1990.
2. Jialal I, Devaraj S: The role of ox-LDL in atherogenesis. J Nutr 126:1053S-1057S, 1996.
3. Gerrity RG: The role of the monocyte in atherogenesis: I. Transition of blood-borne monocytes into foam cells in fatty lesions. Am J Pathol 103:181-190, 1981.
4. Alfon J, Guasch JF, Berrozpe M, Badimon L: Nitric oxide synthase II (NOS II) gene expression correlates with atherosclerotic intimal thickening: Preventive effects of HMG-CoA reductase inhibitors. Atherosclerosis 145:325-331, 1999.

5. Luscher TF, Tanner FC, Noll G: Lipids and endothelial function: Effects of lipid lowering and other therapeutic interventions. Curr Opin Lipidol 7:234-240, 1996.

6. Kugiyama K, Kerns SA, Morrisett JD, et al: Impairment of endothelium dependent arterial relaxation by lysolecithin in modified low density lipoproteins. Nature 344:160-162, 1990.

7. Sawamura T, Kume N, Aoyama T, et al: An endothelial receptor for oxidized low-density lipoprotein. Nature 386:73-77, 1997.

8. Li DY, Chen HJ, Romeo F, et al: Statins modulate ox-LDL-mediated adhesion molecule expression in human coronary artery endothelial cells: Role of LOX-1. J Pharmacol Exp Ther 302:1-5, 2002.

9. Drake TA, Hanani K, Fei H, et al: Minimally oxidized low density lipoprotein induces tissue factor expression in cultured human endothelial cells. Am J Pathol 138:601-607, 1991.

10. Li D, Liu L, Chen H, et al: LOX-1, an oxidized LDL endothelial receptor, induces CD40/CD40L signaling in human coronary artery endothelial cells. Arterioscler Thromb Vasc Biol 23:816-821, 2003.

11. Keidar S, Attias J: Angiotensin II injection into mice increases the uptake of oxidized LDL by their macrophages via a proteoglycan-mediated pathway. Biochem Biophys Res Commun 239:63-67, 1997.

12. Rahman MM, Varghe Z, Fuller BJ, et al: Renal vasoconstriction induced by oxidized LDL is inhibited by scavengers of reactive oxygen species. Clin Nephrol 51:98-107, 1999.

13. Amberger A, Maczek C, Jurgens G, et al: Co-expression of ICAM-1, VCAM-1, ELAM-1 and Hsp60 in human arterial and venous endothelial cells in response to cytokines and oxidized low-density lipoproteins. Cell Stress Chaperones 2:94-103, 1997.

14. Witztum JL, Steinberg D: Role of oxidized low-density lipoprotein in atherogenesis. J Clin Invest 88:1785-1792, 1991.

15. Erl W, Weber PC, Weber C: Monocytic cell adhesion to endothelial cells stimulated by oxidized low-density lipoprotein is mediated by distinct endothelial ligands. Atherosclerosis 136:297-303, 1998.

16. Bickel PE, Freeman MW: Rabbit aortic smooth muscle cells express inducible macrophage scavenger receptor messenger RNA that is absent from endothelial cells. J Clin Invest 90:1450-1457, 1992.

17. Sawamura T, Kume N, Aoyama T, et al: An endothelial receptor for oxidized low-density lipoprotein. Nature 386:73-77, 1997.

18. Mehta JL, Li DY: Identification and autoregulation of receptor for OX-LDL in cultured human coronary artery endothelial cells. Biochem Biophys Res Commun 248:511-514, 1998.

19. Li DY, Zhang YC, Philips MI, et al: Upregulation of endothelial receptor for oxidized low-density lipoprotein (LOX-1) in cultured human coronary artery endothelial cells by angiotensin II type 1 receptor activation. Circ Res 84:1043-1049, 1999.

20. Kume N, Murase T, Moriwaki H, et al: Inducible expression of lectin-like oxidized LDL receptor-1 in vascular endothelial cells. Circ Res 83:322-327, 1998.

21. Mehta A, Yang B, Khan S, et al: Oxidized low-density lipoproteins facilitate leukocyte adhesion to aortic intima without affecting endothelium-dependent relaxation: Role of P-selectin. Arterioscler Thromb Vasc Biol 15:2076-2083, 1995.

22. Li DY, Tomson K, Yang BC, et al: Modulation of constitutive nitric oxide synthase, Bcl-2 and Fas expression in cultured human coronary

endothelial cells exposed to anoxia-reoxygenation and angiotensin II: Role of AT1 receptor activation. Cardiovasc Res 41:109-115, 1999.

23. Li D, Mehta JL: Upregulation of endothelial receptor for oxidized LDL (LOX-1) by oxidized LDL and implications in apoptosis of human coronary artery endothelial cells: Evidence from use of antisense LOX-1 mRNA and chemical inhibitors. Arterioscler Thromb Vasc Biol 20:1116-1122, 2000.

24. Scandinavian Simvastatin Survival Study Group: Randomised trial of cholesterol lowering in 4444 patients with coronary heart disease: The Scandinavian Simvastatin Survival Study (4S). Lancet 344:1383-1389, 1994.

25. Sacks FM, Pfeffer MA, Moye LA, et al: The effect of pravastatin on coronary events after myocardial infarction in patients with average cholesterol levels. Cholesterol and Recurrent Events Trial investigators. N Engl J Med 335:1001-1009, 1996.

26. The Long-Term Intervention with Pravastatin in Ischemic Disease (LIPID) Study Group: Prevention of cardiovascular events and death with pravastatin in patients with coronary heart disease and a broad range of initial cholesterol levels. N Engl J Med 339:1349-1357, 1998.

27. Crisby M, Nordin-Fredriksson G, Shah PK, et al: Pravastatin treatment increases collagen content and decreases lipid content, inflammation, metalloproteinases, and cell death in human carotid plaques: Implications for plaque stabilization. Circulation 103:926-933, 2001.

28. Li DY, Williams V, Liu L, et al: LOX-1 inhibition in myocardial ischemia-reperfusion injury: Modulation of MMP-1 and inflammation. Am J Physiol 283:H1795-H1801, 2002.

29. Tsutsui T, Tsutamoto T, Wada A, et al: Plasma oxidized low-density lipoprotein as a prognostic predictor in patients with chronic congestive heart failure. J Am Coll Cardiol 39:957-962, 2002.

30. Girona J, La Ville AE, Sola R, et al: Simvastatin decreases aldehyde production derived from lipoprotein oxidation. Am J Cardiol 83:846-851, 1999.

31. Li DY, Chen HJ, Mehta JL. Statins inhibit oxidized-LDL-mediated LOX-1 expression, uptake of oxidized-LDL and reduction in PKB phosphorylation. Cardiovasc Res 52:130-135, 2001.

32. Zhou YF, Guetta E, Yu ZX, et al: Human cytomegalovirus increases modified low-density lipoprotein uptake and scavenger receptor mRNA expression in vascular smooth muscle cells. J Clin Invest 98:2129-2138, 1996.

33. Li DY, Mehta JL: Antisense to LOX-1 inhibits oxidized LDL-mediated upregulation of monocyte chemoattractant protein-1 and monocyte adhesion to human coronary artery endothelial cells. Circulation 101:2889-2895, 2000.

34. Keaney JF Jr, Guo Y, Cunningham D, et al: Vascular incorporation of alpha-tocopherol prevents endothelial dysfunction due to oxidized LDL by inhibiting protein kinase C stimulation. J Clin Invest 98:386-394, 1996.

35. Waters D, Higginson L, Gladstone P, et al: Effects of monotherapy with an HMG-CoA reductase inhibitor on the progression of coronary atherosclerosis as assessed by serial quantitative arteriography. The Canadian Coronary Atherosclerosis Intervention Trial. Circulation 89:959-968, 1994.

36. Mehta JL, Li DY, Chen HJ, et al: Inhibition of LOX-1 by statins may

relate to upregulation of eNOS. Biochem Biophys Res Commun 289:857-861, 2001.

37. Iwai-Kanai E, Hasegawa K, Sawamura T, et al: Activation of lectin-like oxidized low-density lipoprotein receptor-1 induces apoptosis in cultured neonatal rat cardiac myocytes. Circulation 104:2948-2954, 2001.

38. Ross R: The pathogenesis of atherosclerosis: A perspective for the 1990s. Nature 362:801-809, 1993.

39. Ross R: Atherosclerosis is an inflammatory disease. Am Heart J 138:S419-420, 1999.

40. Niwa S, Totsuka T, Hayashi S: Inhibitory effect of fluvastatin, an HMG-CoA reductase inhibitor, on the expression of adhesion molecules on human monocyte cell line. Int J Immunopharmacol 18:669-675, 1996.

41. Rezaie-Majd A, Maca T, Bucek RA, et al: Simvastatin reduces expression of cytokines interleukin-6, interleukin-8, and monocyte chemoattractant protein-1 in circulating monocytes from hypercholesterolemic patients. Arterioscler Thromb Vasc Biol 22:1194-1199, 2002.

42. Weitz-Schmidt G, Welzenbach K, Brinkmann V, et al: Statins selectively inhibit leukocyte function antigen-1 by binding to a novel regulatory integrin site. Nat Med 7:687-692, 2001.

43. Wagner AH, Gebauer M, Guldenzoph B, Hecker M: 3-hydroxy-3-methylglutaryl coenzyme A reductase-independent inhibition of CD40 expression by atorvastatin in human endothelial cells. Arterioscler Thromb Vasc Biol 22:1784-1789, 2002.

44. Lutgens E, Gorelik L, Daemen MJ, et al: Requirement for CD154 in the progression of atherosclerosis. Nat Med 5:1313-1316, 1999.

45. Mach F, Schonbeck U, Sukhova GK, et al: Reduction of atherosclerosis in mice by inhibition of CD40 signaling. Nature 394:200-203, 1998.

46. Li D, Liu L, Chen H, et al: LOX-1 mediates oxidized low-density lipoprotein-induced expression of matrix metalloproteinases in human coronary artery endothelial cells. Circulation 107:612-617, 2003.

47. Sukhova GK, Schonbeck U, Rabkin E, et al: Evidence for increased collagenolysis by interstitial collagenases-1 and -3 in vulnerable human atheromatous plaques. Circulation 99:2503-2509, 1999.

48. Kaneider NC, Egger P, Dunzendorfer S, et al: Reversal of thrombin-induced deactivation of CD39/ATPDase in endothelial cells by HMG-CoA reductase inhibition: Effects on Rho-GTPase and adenosine nucleotide metabolism. Arterioscler Thromb Vasc Biol 22:894-900, 2002.

49. Takemoto M, Liao JK: Pleiotropic effects of 3-hydroxy-3-methylglutaryl coenzyme A reductase inhibitors. Arterioscler Thromb Vasc Biol 21:1712, 2001.

50. Eto M, Kozai T, Cosentino F, et al: Statin prevents tissue factor expression in human endothelial cells: Role of Rho/Rho-kinase and Akt pathways. Circulation 105:1756-1759, 2002.

51. Kureishi Y, Luo Z, Shiojima I, et al: The HMG-CoA reductase inhibitor simvastatin activates the protein kinase Akt and promotes angiogenesis in normocholesterolemic animals. Nat Med 6:1004-1010, 2000.

52. Skaletz-Rorowski A, Muller JG, Kroke A, et al: Lovastatin blocks basic fibroblast growth factor-induced mitogen-activated protein kinase signaling in coronary smooth muscle cells via phosphatase inhibition. Eur J Cell Biol 80:207-212, 2001.

Statins, Inflammation, and C-Reactive Protein

Gavin J. Blake and Paul M. Ridker

Hyperlipidemia is a central risk factor for atherothrombosis. Many large-scale clinical trials have demonstrated that cholesterol lowering with statin therapy reduces cardiac event rates in both primary and secondary prevention.[1-8] These trials, however, have raised further debate, suggesting that the benefits of statin therapy may extend beyond lipid lowering alone.

First, statin therapy appears to be effective irrespective of baseline lipid values. For example, in the Heart Protection study, patients with low-density-lipoprotein cholesterol (LDL-C) levels lower than 100 mg/dL gained a benefit with simvastatin therapy that was similar to that obtained by those with higher LDL-C values.[6] Similarly, in the Myocardial Ischemia Reduction with Aggressive Cholesterol Lowering (MIRACL) study of patients with acute coronary syndromes, atorvastatin was as effective among those with LDL-C lower than 121 mg/dL, the study median, as it was among those with LDL-C higher than 121 mg/dL.[7]

Second, despite substantial reductions in cardiac event rates with statin therapy, the absolute angiographic reductions in percentage stenosis have been trivial.[9] Third, the observed clinical benefit with statin therapy may be greater than that expected on the basis of lipid changes alone. For example, although the Framingham risk model predicted a 24% reduction in event rates on the basis of cholesterol reduction, the observed risk reduction with pravastatin was 36% in the West of Scotland Coronary Prevention Study (WOSCOPS).[10] Fourth, the benefits of statin therapy appear to occur earlier than those observed with other lipid-lowering therapies such as cholestyramine and ileal bypass.[11,12] Finally, statins protect against stroke and yet LDL-C level is not an important risk factor for cerebrovascular events.[13]

THE ROLE OF INFLAMMATION IN ATHEROTHROMBOSIS

Recent advances in basic science have illuminated the pivotal role that inflammatory processes play in multiple stages of atherothrombosis.[14] From the initial recruitment of circulating inflammatory cells to the diseased endothelium, to eventual rupture of a vulnerable plaque, inflammation and hyperlipidemia work in tandem to promote atherosclerosis. Indeed, in this regard, plasma levels of several markers of inflammation have been found to predict incident cardiovascular events, including C-reactive protein (CRP), CD40 ligand, interleukin-6 (IL-6), and cell adhesion molecules such as soluble intercellular adhesion molecule-1 (sICAM-1) and soluble vascular cell adhesion molecule-1 (sVCAM-1).[15]

The vulnerable plaque is characterized by abundant inflammation that overwhelms the plaque's capacity for repair.[16] Smooth muscle cells predominate in stable plaques, with few inflammatory cells. In contrast, macrophages and T cells predominate in regions of plaque rupture or fissuring, with relatively few smooth muscle cells. Macrophages can secrete matrix metalloproteinases (MMPs), which, by breaking down interstitial collagen, weaken the fibrous cap, predisposing it to rupture.

ANTI-INFLAMMATORY EFFECTS OF STATINS— LABORATORY EVIDENCE

One potential mechanism through which statin therapy may afford atheroprotection may relate to potential anti-inflammatory effects of these agents. Several studies have suggested important effects of statin therapy on macrophage function. Fluvastatin and simvastatin have been shown to inhibit MMP-9 (gelatinase B) activity and secretion by macrophages.[17] Fluvastatin decreases MMP-1 expression in endothelial cells in a time- and dose-dependent manner.[18] These effects are reversed by the addition of mevalonate, suggesting that they are mediated by 3-hydroxy-3-methylglutaryl coenzyme A (HMG-CoA) reductase inhibition.

Statin therapy has been shown to favorably alter the composition of atheromatous plaque, independent of lipid-lowering effects. Pravastatin has been shown to decrease macrophage content, lipid oxidation, inflammation, MMP-2, and cell death while increasing collagen content in human carotid plaques.[19] Despite similar changes in lipid profile caused by diet alone, pravastatin-treated monkeys had better vasodilator function, with fewer macrophages in the intima and media, and less neovascularization in the intima.[20] Recent data confirm that statin therapy alters the composition of atheromatous plaque without significant changes in the burden of atherosclerosis. Although the intima-to-media ratios in the abdominal aortas of monkeys did not differ, treatment with pravastatin or simvastatin reduced inflammation and features of plaque vulnerability compared with control animals with similar lipid levels.[21] Macrophage content was lowered 2.4-fold with pravastatin and 1.3-fold with simvastatin (both $P < .001$ compared with control), whereas statin-treated animals had approximately twofold lower VCAM-1, IL-1β, and tissue factor expression. On the other hand, smooth muscle cell and collagen content, features of stable plaque, were significantly higher in statin treated animals.[21]

Oxidized LDL is an important component of the atherogenic pathway. Macrophages take up oxidized LDL to form foam cells. Oxidized LDL also stimulates monocyte tissue factor expression and inhibits endothelial nitric oxide synthase (eNOS), thus impairing endothelium-dependent vasodilation.[22,23] Statins may inhibit the oxidation of LDL by a variety of mechanisms. Through their lipid-lowering effects, statins reduce the amount of LDL available for oxidation. Fluvastatin and lovastatin have been shown to bind to phospholipids on the surface of LDL and thus prevent the diffusion of free radicals, generated under oxidative stress, into the lipoprotein core.[24] Simvastatin reduces macrophage superoxide formation, thereby decreasing cell oxygen production.[25] Atorvastatin and fluvastatin have also been shown to have direct antioxidant effects.[26,27]

The ligation of CD40 and its receptor has been found to mediate multiple pathways central to atherogenesis,[28] and interruption of the binding of the CD40 ligand with its receptor has been found to prevent atheroma formation in atherosclerosis-prone mice.[29] Treatment of human vascular endothelial cells and mononuclear phagocytes with oxidized LDL augments the basal expression of CD40 and CD40 ligand mRNA and protein.[30] Statin therapy with either cerivastatin, atorvastatin, or simvastatin reduced the expression of the CD40 receptor-ligand dyad. Patients treated with statins were also noted to have lower CD40 ligand levels than controls.[30] Thus, statin therapy may limit the expression of CD40 ligand in two ways, directly as well as via lower lipoprotein levels. This effect may have clinical relevance, because plasma levels of CD40 ligand have been found to predict future cardiovascular events in apparently healthy women and in those with acute coronary syndromes.[31,32] Furthermore, levels of CD40 ligand were found to be elevated in patients with evidence of lipid pooling in carotid atheroma on high-resolution magnetic resonance imaging (MRI).[33]

Statins also up-regulate eNOs expression in vitro under cholesterol-clamped conditions.[23] Statin therapy up-regulated eNOS expression almost fourfold and completely prevented its down-regulation by oxidized LDL. Furthermore, 4 weeks of simvastatin therapy produced a significant increase in endothelium-dependent vasodilation in patients with moderate hypercholesterolemia.[34]

Endotoxemia is a potent stimulus for vascular inflammation characterized by enhanced leukocyte recruitment to the vascular endothelium. Pretreatment with simvastatin attenuated endotoxin-induced leukocyte rolling and transmigration in rat mesenteric arteries.[35] Simvastatin also caused a 50% up-regulation of eNOS expression and a 50% decrease in P-selectin expression.

Statin treatment also reduces the prenylation of the Rho protein, thereby reducing its biologic activity.[36] The reduction of Rho prenylation may attenuate vascular inflammation through a combination of actions, including reduction of nuclear factor kappa B (NF-κB) activation, restoration of nitric oxide (NO) production, and reduction of monocyte adhesion to the cell wall. NF-κB is a transcription factor involved in the induction of monocyte chemoattractant protein-1 (MCP-1) and other inflammatory cytokines such as IL-1b and tumor necrosis factor α (TNF-α). Atorvastatin has been found to reduce levels of MCP-1 in the intima and media of hyper-cholesterolemic rabbits, an effect that was related to a reduction in NF-κB activation.[37]

Statin therapy decreases macrophage expression of sICAM-1 and lipopolysaccharide-induced secretion of IL-6 and TNF-α by monocytes and macrophages.[38-40] Simvastatin reduces monocyte expression of TNF-α and IL-1b.[41] Simvastatin has also been shown to inhibit expression of plasminogen activator inhibitor-1 (PAI-1) in human endothelial and vascular smooth muscle cells.[42]

Further anti-inflammatory actions of statins may be independent of HMG-CoA reductase inhibition. Statins inhibit lymphocyte adhesion to ICAM-1 and can impair T-cell activation by binding to the lymphocyte function-associated antigen-1 on leucocytes.[43] Thus via multiple mechanisms, statins have anti-inflammatory properties that may potentially contribute to their atheroprotective effects.

C-REACTIVE PROTEIN: AN INFLAMMATORY MARKER FOR CARDIOVASCULAR RISK PREDICTION

The burgeoning evidence that vascular inflammation plays a central role in atherothrombosis has led to intense interest in whether plasma levels of markers of inflammation can help better predict cardiovascular events. In this regard, plasma levels of a variety of inflammatory mediators have been found to predict cardiovascular risk, including cytokines such as IL-6, IL-1β, and TNF-α; cell adhesion molecules such as sICAM-1 and sVCAM-1; proatherogenic enzymes such as MMP-9 and lipoprotein-associated phospholipase A2; and chemokines such as MCP-1.[15] The inflammatory marker that has attracted the greatest interest for clinical use is C-reactive protein (CRP).[44]

Produced largely in the liver in response to stimulation by IL-6, CRP has been thought of as a downsteam marker of the inflammatory cascade. Plasma levels of CRP have been found to predict future cardiovascular events in a wide variety of clinical settings, including apparently healthy men and women, women with the metabolic syndrome, patients with stable and unstable coronary artery disease, and patients undergoing percutaneous coronary intervention (PCI).[45-51] Furthermore, baseline levels of

CRP predict not only risk for myocardial infarction but also risk for stroke, cardiovascular death, sudden cardiac death, peripheral vascular disease, and restenosis after PCI.[46-64] Importantly, the predictive values of CRP and LDL cholesterol are additive, with CRP improving risk prediction at all levels of LDL cholesterol and Framingham risk scores.[46]

The robust link between CRP and atherosclerotic risk has led to a reexamination of the role of CRP in atherothrombosis. Emerging data suggest that CRP may play a more direct role in atherogenesis. CRP localizes with the complement membrane attack complex in early atherosclerotic tissue,[65] and CRP opsonization of LDL mediates LDL uptake by macrophages.[66] Furthermore, CRP stimulates monocyte release of IL-1, IL-6, and TNF-α, causes ICAM-1 and VCAM-1 expression by endothelial cells, and mediates MCP-1 induction.[67-69] Thus, CRP may mediate several important steps in the recruitment of inflammatory cells to the subendothelial space and in the formation of foam cells.

Recent data suggest that CRP may have other proinflammatory properties. The proinflammatory effects of CRP may be mediated via increased secretion of IL-6 and endothelin-1, a potent vasoconstrictor.[70] Further research has shown that CRP may directly quench the production of NO by endothelial cells[71,72] and may induce PAI-1 expression and activity in human endothelial cells.[73]

CLINICAL EVIDENCE FOR ANTI-INFLAMMATORY ACTIONS OF STATINS—THE LINK TO CRP

As outlined, CRP appears to activate many of the inflammatory pathways that statin therapy has been found to inhibit. To assess the potential clinical relevance of this interaction, two key questions need to be considered. First, does statin therapy directly lower CRP levels? And second, could CRP be used to target statin therapy for the prevention of cardiovascular events in clinical practice?

The first data to suggest that statin therapy might lower CRP levels came from the Cholesterol and Recurrent Events (CARE) study. Compared with placebo, pravastatin resulted in a 22% reduction in median CRP levels over a 5-year period, an effect that was independent of statin-induced changes in LDL cholesterol.[74] Further post hoc data suggested that atorvastatin, simvastatin, and cerivastatin each lowered CRP levels, suggesting that statin-induced lowering of CRP is a class effect (Fig. 11-1).[75-78] Statin therapy has also been reported to attenuate the increase in CRP observed with hormone replacement therapy.[79]

The Pravastatin Inflammation/CRP Evaluation (PRINCE) trial was specifically designed to address the direct effect of statin therapy on CRP levels, randomizing 1702 patients without overt cardiovascular disease to pravastatin or placebo.[80] After 24 weeks of therapy, pravastatin caused a 16.9% decrease in CRP levels.

11

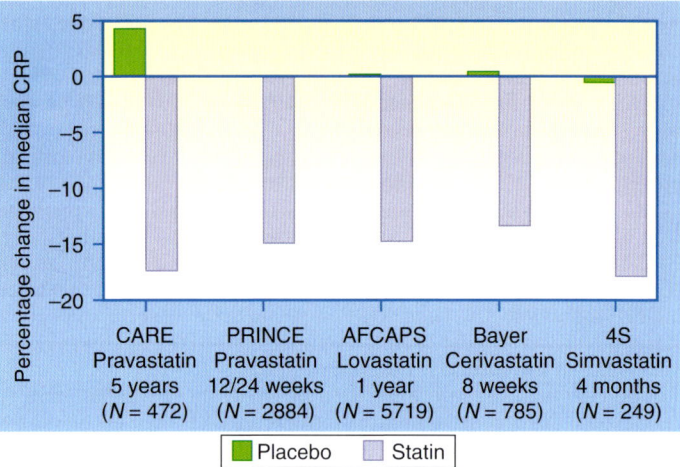

Figure 11-1. **Effect of statin therapy on C-reactive protein levels.** 4S, Scandinavian Simvastatin Survival study; AFCAPS, Air Force/Texas Coronary Atherosclerosis Prevention study; CARE, Cholesterol and Recurrent Events; PRINCE, Pravastatin Inflammation/CRP Evaluation.

Importantly, the reduction in CRP did not correlate with reduction in LDL cholesterol.

Initial data suggesting that the benefits of statin therapy might be greatest among those with heightened vascular inflammation also came from the CARE study.[81] In this randomized study of pravastatin versus placebo among patients with prior myocardial infarction, those with elevated levels of CRP and serum amyloid A (SAA) who were assigned to placebo were at highest risk. Randomization to pravastatin therapy was most effective among those with heightened vascular inflammation, preventing 54% of recurrent events compared with 25% among those without evidence of persistent inflammation (Fig. 11-2). This difference was observed despite identical baseline LDL cholesterol levels in these two groups.

Similar post hoc data have since been reported among patients undergoing PCI. Baseline levels of CRP were a robust independent predictor of adverse outcome among those not taking statin therapy, but the increased risk associated with elevated CRP levels was markedly attenuated among those taking statin therapy.[82-84] These data raise the hypothesis that a CRP-guided strategy may improve targeting of statin therapy among those undergoing PCI.

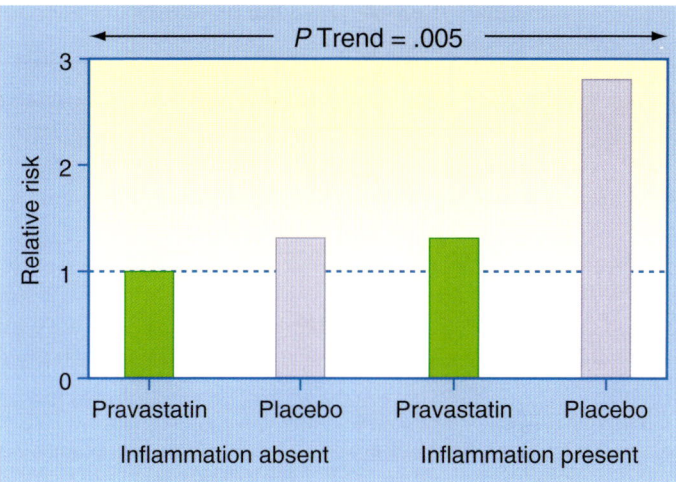

Figure 11-2. Relative risks of recurrent coronary events among patients who have had myocardial infarction, according to the presence or absence of ongoing inflammation and according to placebo or pravastatin therapy. (Adapted from Ridker PM, Rifai N, Pfeffer MA, et al: Inflammation, pravastatin, and the risk of coronary events after myocardial infarction in patients with average cholesterol levels. Cholesterol and Recurrent Events (CARE) Investigators. Circulation 98:839-844, 1998.)

Perhaps the greatest impact of CRP testing to target statin therapy is in the primary prevention setting, where the majority of cardiovascular events occur among individuals without overtly elevated lipid levels who are currently not identified by lipid testing. A recent analysis from the Air Force/Texas Coronary Atherosclerosis Prevention Study (AFCAPS/TexCAPS) sought to test the hypothesis that the benefits of statin therapy in the primary prevention setting might be greatest among those with elevated CRP.[78] Individuals were divided into four groups on the basis of median LDL cholesterol and CRP levels. Those with elevated LDL cholesterol (>149 mg/dL) were at elevated risk and benefited from randomization to lovastatin irrespective of CRP levels. Those with low LDL cholesterol and low CRP were at low risk and did not benefit from randomization to lovastatin compared with placebo. In contrast, those with low LDL cholesterol but high CRP were at high risk and derived benefit from lovastatin therapy similar to that seen among those with elevated LDL cholesterol (Fig. 11-3). Similar data were observed if the ratio of total cholesterol to high-density-lipoprotein (HDL) cholesterol was considered. These post hoc data have potentially far-reaching implications for the targeting of statin therapy for prevention of cardiovascular disease and need to be directly tested in randomized trials.[85]

Relative risks with lovastatin therapy

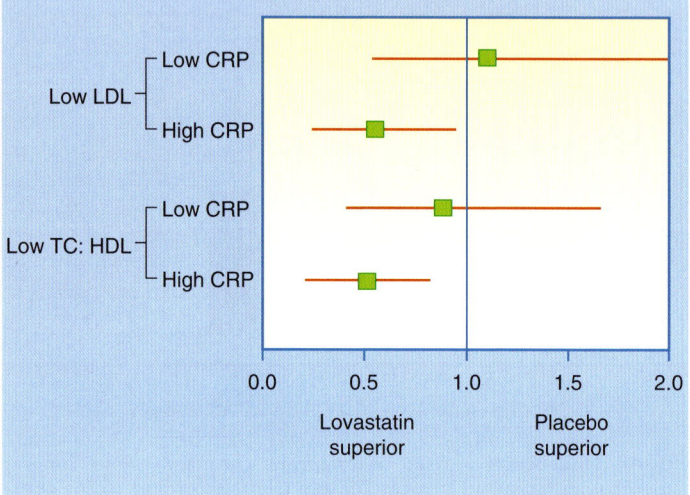

Figure 11-3. **Relative risks (and 95% confidence intervals) associated with lovastatin therapy, according to baseline lipid and CRP levels.** CRP, C-reactive protein; LDL, low-density-lipoprotein cholesterol; TC:HDL, ratio of total cholesterol to high-density-lipoprotein cholesterol. (From Ridker PM, Rifai N, Clearfield M, et al: Measurement of C-reactive protein for the targeting of statin therapy in the primary prevention of acute coronary events. N Engl J Med 344:1959-1965, 2001.

Intriguingly, baseline levels of CRP and IL-6 have also been found to predict the risk for incident type 2 diabetes.[86] Furthermore, post hoc data suggest that randomization to pravastatin in the WOSCOPS trial reduced the risk for developing type 2 diabetes.[87] These data suggest that atherosclerosis and type 2 diabetes may share a pro-inflammatory pathogenesis that statin therapy may attenuate.

The ongoing JUPITER study (Justification for the Use of Statins in Primary Prevention: An Intervention Trial Evaluating Rosuvastatin) is investigating the potential benefits of rosuvastatin compared with placebo for primary prevention among those with elevated CRP (>2 mg/L) but LDL cholesterol lower than 130 mg/dL. Exploratory analyses suggest that the potential public health gains with statin for those with high CRP could be substantial,[88] and that a strategy of CRP testing to target statin therapy for primary prevention among those without hyperlipidemia may be relatively cost-effective, especially among those at intermediate to high risk.[89]

CONCLUSION

Accumulating evidence suggests a central role for inflammatory processes in the genesis of atherosclerosis and its complications. In this regard, plasma level of C-reactive protein, a sensitive marker of vascular inflammation, is a powerful predictor of cardiovascular risk. In addition to lipid-lowering effects, statin therapy has many anti-inflammatory activities that may potentially contribute to its proven atheroprotective effects. Statin therapy has been found to lower CRP levels, and hypothesis-generating data suggest that the benefits of statin therapy may be greatest if targeted to those with elevated CRP levels, a question being directly tested in ongoing trials. Harnessing our evolving understanding of the role of inflammation in atherogenesis may provide new opportunities for the detection and prevention of cardiovascular disease, including the targeted use of statin therapy among those with evidence of vascular inflammation.

11

References

1. Scandinavian Simvastatin Survival Study Group: Randomised trial of cholesterol lowering in 4444 patients with coronary heart disease: The Scandinavian Simvastatin Survival Study (4S). Lancet 344:1383-1389, 1994.
2. The Long-term Intervention with Pravastatin in Ischaemic Disease (LIPID) Study Group: Prevention of cardiovascular events and death with pravastatin in patients with coronary heart disease and a broad range of initial cholesterol levels. N Engl J Med 339:1349-1357, 1998.
3. Downs JR, Clearfield M, Weis S, et al: Primary prevention of acute coronary events with lovastatin in men and women with average cholesterol levels: Results of AFCAPS/TexCAPS. Air Force/Texas Coronary Atherosclerosis Prevention Study. JAMA 279:1615-1622, 1998.
4. Sacks FM, Pfeffer MA, Moye LA, et al: The effect of pravastatin on coronary events after myocardial infarction in patients with average cholesterol levels. Cholesterol and Recurrent Events Trial investigators. N Engl J Med 335:1001-1009, 1996.
5. Shepherd J, Cobbe SM, Ford I, et al: Prevention of coronary heart disease with pravastatin in men with hypercholesterolemia. West of Scotland Coronary Prevention Study Group. N Engl J Med 333:1301-1307, 1995.
6. MRC/BHF Heart Protection study of cholesterol lowering with simvastatin in 20,536 high-risk individuals: A randomised placebo-controlled trial. Lancet 360:7-22, 2002.
7. Schwartz GG, Olsson AG, Ezekowitz MD, et al: Effects of atorvastatin on early recurrent ischemic events in acute coronary syndromes: The MIRACL study: A randomized controlled trial. JAMA 285:1711-1718, 2001.
8. Sever PS, Dahlof B, Poulter NR, et al: Prevention of coronary and stroke events with atorvastatin in hypertensive patients who have average or lower-than-average cholesterol concentrations, in the Anglo-Scandinavian Cardiac Outcomes Trial—Lipid-Lowering Arm

(ASCOT-LLA): A multicentre randomised controlled trial. Lancet 361:1149-1158, 2003.

9. de Groot E, Jukema JW, Montauban van Swijndregt AD, et al: B-mode ultrasound assessment of pravastatin treatment effect on carotid and femoral artery walls and its correlations with coronary arteriographic findings: A report of the Regression Growth Evaluation Statin Study (REGRESS). J Am Coll Cardiol 31:1561-1567, 1998.

10. Influence of pravastatin and plasma lipids on clinical events in the West of Scotland Coronary Prevention Study (WOSCOPS). Circulation 97:1440-1445, 1998.

11. The Lipid Research Clinics Coronary Primary Prevention Trial results: I. Reduction in incidence of coronary heart disease. JAMA 251:351-364, 1984.

12. Buchwald H, Campos CT, Boen JR, et al: Disease-free intervals after partial ileal bypass in patients with coronary heart disease and hypercholesterolemia: Report from the Program on the Surgical Control of the Hyperlipidemias (POSCH). J Am Coll Cardiol 26:351-357, 1995.

13. Cholesterol, diastolic blood pressure, and stroke: 13,000 strokes in 450,000 people in 45 prospective cohorts. Prospective studies collaboration. Lancet 346:1647-1653, 1995.

14. Libby P: Molecular bases of the acute coronary syndromes. Circulation 91:2844-2850, 1995.

15. Blake GJ, Ridker PM: Novel clinical markers of vascular wall inflammation. Circ Res 89:763-771, 2001.

16. Ross R: Atherosclerosis: An inflammatory disease. N Engl J Med 340:115-126, 1999.

17. Bellosta S, Via D, Canavesi M, et al: HMG-CoA reductase inhibitors reduce MMP-9 secretion by macrophages. Arterioscler Thromb Vasc Biol 18:1671-1678, 1998.

18. Ikeda U, Shimpo M, Ohki R, et al: Fluvastatin inhibits matrix metalloproteinase-1 expression in human vascular endothelial cells. Hypertension 36:325-329, 2000.

19. Crisby M, Nordin-Fredriksson G, Shah PK, et al: Pravastatin treatment increases collagen content and decreases lipid content, inflammation, metalloproteinases, and cell death in human carotid plaques: Implications for plaque stabilization. Circulation 103:926-933, 2001.

20. Williams JK, Sukhova GK, Herrington DM, Libby P: Pravastatin has cholesterol-lowering independent effects on the artery wall of atherosclerotic monkeys. J Am Coll Cardiol 31:684-691, 1998.

21. Sukhova GK, Williams JK, Libby P: Statins reduce inflammation in atheroma of nonhuman primates independent of effects on serum cholesterol. Arterioscler Thromb Vasc Biol 22:1452-1458, 2002.

22. Bjorkerud B, Bjorkerud S: Contrary effects of lightly and strongly oxidized LDL with potent promotion of growth versus apoptosis on arterial smooth muscle cells, macrophages, and fibroblasts. Arterioscler Thromb Vasc Biol 16:416-424, 1996.

23. Laufs U, La Fata V, Plutzky J, Liao JK: Upregulation of endothelial nitric oxide synthase by HMG CoA reductase inhibitors. Circulation 97:1129-1135, 1998.

24. Aviram M, Hussein O, Rosenblat M, et al: Interactions of platelets, macrophages, and lipoproteins in hypercholesterolemia: Antiatherogenic effects of HMG-CoA reductase inhibitor therapy. J Cardiovasc Pharmacol 31:39-45, 1998.

11

25. Giroux LM, Davignon J, Naruszewicz M: Simvastatin inhibits the oxidation of low-density lipoproteins by activated human monocyte-derived macrophages. Biochim Biophys Acta 1165:335-338, 1993.
26. Aviram M, Rosenblat M, Bisgaier CL, Newton RS: Atorvastatin and gemfibrozil metabolites, but not the parent drugs, are potent antioxidants against lipoprotein oxidation. Atherosclerosis 138:271-280, 1998.
27. Suzumura K, Yasuhara M, Tanaka K, Suzuki T: Protective effect of fluvastatin sodium (XU-62-320), a 3-hydroxy-3-methylglutaryl coenzyme A (HMG-CoA) reductase inhibitor, on oxidative modification of human low-density lipoprotein in vitro. Biochem Pharmacol 57:697-703, 1999.
28. Schonbeck U, Libby P: CD40 signaling and plaque instability. Circ Res 89:1092-1103, 2001.
29. Mach F, Schonbeck U, Sukhova GK, et al: Reduction of atherosclerosis in mice by inhibition of CD40 signaling. Nature 394:200-203, 1998.
30. Schonbeck U, Gerdes N, Varo N, et al: Oxidized low-density lipoprotein augments and 3-hydroxy-3-methylglutaryl coenzyme A reductase inhibitors limit CD40 and CD40L expression in human vascular cells. Circulation 106:2888-2893, 2002.
31. Schonbeck U, Varo N, Libby P, et al: Soluble CD40L and cardiovascular risk in women. Circulation 104:2266-2268, 2001.
32. Heeschen C, Dimmeler S, Hamm CW, et al: Soluble CD40 ligand in acute coronary syndromes. N Engl J Med 348:1104-1111, 2003.
33. Blake GJ, Ostfeld RJ, Yucel EK, et al: Soluble CD40 ligand levels indicate lipid accumulation in carotid atheroma: An in vivo study with high-resolution MRI. Arterioscler Thromb Vasc Biol 23:e11-4, 2003.
34. O'Driscoll G, Green D, Taylor RR: Simvastatin, an HMG-coenzyme A reductase inhibitor, improves endothelial function within 1 month. Circulation 95:1126-1131, 1997.
35. Pruefer D, Makowski J, Schnell M, et al: Simvastatin inhibits inflammatory properties of Staphylococcus aureus alpha-toxin. Circulation 106:2104-2110, 2002.
36. Guijarro C, Blanco-Colio LM, Ortego M, et al: 3-Hydroxy-3-methylglutaryl coenzyme a reductase and isoprenylation inhibitors induce apoptosis of vascular smooth muscle cells in culture. Circ Res 83:490-500, 1998.
37. Bustos C, Hernandez-Presa MA, Ortego M, et al: HMG-CoA reductase inhibition by atorvastatin reduces neointimal inflammation in a rabbit model of atherosclerosis. J Am Coll Cardiol 32:2057-2064, 1998.
38. Niwa S, Totsuka T, Hayashi S: Inhibitory effect of fluvastatin, an HMG-CoA reductase inhibitor, on the expression of adhesion molecules on human monocyte cell line. Int J Immunopharmacol 18:669-675, 1996.
39. Ikeda U, Shimada K: Statins and monocytes. Lancet 353:2070, 1999.
40. Rosenson RS, Tangney CC, Casey LC: Inhibition of proinflammatory cytokine production by pravastatin. Lancet 353:983-984, 1999.
41. Ferro D, Parrotto S, Basili S, et al: Simvastatin inhibits the monocyte expression of proinflammatory cytokines in patients with hypercholesterolemia. J Am Coll Cardiol 36:427-431, 2000.
42. Essig M, Nguyen G, Prie D, et al: 3-Hydroxy-3-methylglutaryl coenzyme A reductase inhibitors increase fibrinolytic activity in rat aortic endothelial cells: Role of geranylgeranylation and Rho proteins. Circ Res 83:683-690, 1998.

11

43. Weitz-Schmidt G, Welzenbach K, Brinkmann V, et al: Statins selectively inhibit leukocyte function antigen-1 by binding to a novel regulatory integrin site. Nat Med 7:687-692, 2001.
44. Ridker PM: Clinical application of C-reactive protein for cardiovascular disease detection and prevention. Circulation 107:363-369, 2003.
45. Ridker PM, Buring JE, Cook NR, Rifai N: C-reactive protein, the metabolic syndrome, and risk of incident cardiovascular events: An 8-year follow-up of 15,218 initially healthy American women. Circulation 107:391-397, 2003.
46. Ridker PM, Rifai N, Rose L, et al: Comparison of C-reactive protein and LDL cholesterol levels in the prediction of first cardiovascular events. N Engl J Med 347:1557-1565, 2002.
47. Ridker PM, Cushman M, Stampfer MJ, et al: Inflammation, aspirin, and the risk of cardiovascular disease in apparently healthy men. N Engl J Med 336:973-979, 1997.
48. Mueller C, Buettner HJ, Hodgson JM, et al: Inflammation and long-term mortality after non-ST elevation acute coronary syndrome treated with a very early invasive strategy in 1042 consecutive patients. Circulation 105:1412 1415, 2002.
49. Chew DP, Bhatt DL, Robbins MA, et al: Incremental prognostic value of elevated baseline C-reactive protein among established markers of risk in percutaneous coronary intervention. Circulation 104:992-997, 2001.
50. Walter DH, Fichtlscherer S, Sellwig M, et al: Preprocedural C-reactive protein levels and cardiovascular events after coronary stent implantation. J Am Coll Cardiol 37:839-846, 2001.
51. Buffon A, Liuzzo G, Biasucci LM, et al: Preprocedural serum levels of C-reactive protein predict early complications and late restenosis after coronary angioplasty. J Am Coll Cardiol 34:1512-1521, 1999.
52. Koenig W, Sund M, Frohlich M, et al: C-Reactive protein, a sensitive marker of inflammation, predicts future risk of coronary heart disease in initially healthy middle-aged men: Results from the MONICA (Monitoring Trends and Determinants in Cardiovascular Disease) Augsburg Cohort Study, 1984 to 1992. Circulation 99:237-242, 1999.
53. Kuller LH, Tracy RP, Shaten J, Meilahn EN: Relation of C-reactive protein and coronary heart disease in the MRFIT nested case-control study. Multiple Risk Factor Intervention Trial. Am J Epidemiol 144:537-547, 1996.
54. Danesh J, Whincup P, Walker M, et al: Low grade inflammation and coronary heart disease: Prospective study and updated meta-analyses. BMJ 321:199-204, 2000.
55. Ridker PM, Cushman M, Stampfer MJ, et al: Plasma concentration of C-reactive protein and risk of developing peripheral vascular disease. Circulation 97:425-428, 1998.
56. Ridker PM, Buring JE, Shih J, et al: Prospective study of C-reactive protein and the risk of future cardiovascular events among apparently healthy women. Circulation 98:731-733, 1998.
57. Ridker PM, Hennekens CH, Buring JE, Rifai N: C-reactive protein and other markers of inflammation in the prediction of cardiovascular disease in women. N Engl J Med 342:836-843, 2000.
58. Tracy RP, Lemaitre RN, Psaty BM, et al: Relationship of C-reactive protein to risk of cardiovascular disease in the elderly: Results from

the Cardiovascular Health Study and the Rural Health Promotion Project. Arterioscler Thromb Vasc Biol 17:1121-1127, 1997.

59. Harris TB, Ferrucci L, Tracy RP, et al: Associations of elevated interleukin-6 and C-reactive protein levels with mortality in the elderly. Am J Med 106:506-512, 1999.

60. Lowe GD, Yarnell JW, Rumley A, et al: C-reactive protein, fibrin D-dimer, and incident ischemic heart disease in the Speedwell study: Are inflammation and fibrin turnover linked in pathogenesis? Arterioscler Thromb Vasc Biol 21:603-610, 2001.

61. Albert C, Ma J, Rifai N, et al: Prospective study of C-reactive protein, homocysteine, and plasma lipid levels as predictors of sudden cardiac death. Circulation 105:2595-2599, 2002.

62. Curb JD, Abbott RD, Rodriguez BL, et al: C-reactive protein and the future risk of thromboembolic stroke in healthy men. Circulation 107:2016-2020, 2003.

63. Rost NS, Wolf PA, Kase CS, et al: Plasma concentration of C-reactive protein and risk of ischemic stroke and transient ischemic attack: The Framingham study. Stroke 32:2575-2579, 2001.

64. Ridker PM, Stampfer MJ, Rifai N: Novel risk factors for systemic atherosclerosis: A comparison of C-reactive protein, fibrinogen, homocysteine, lipoprotein(a), and standard cholesterol screening as predictors of peripheral arterial disease. JAMA 285:2481-2485, 2001.

65. Torzewski M, Rist C, Mortensen RF, et al: C-reactive protein in the arterial intima: Role of C-reactive protein receptor-dependent monocyte recruitment in atherogenesis. Arterioscler Thromb Vasc Biol 20:2094-2099, 2000.

66. Zwaka TP, Hombach V, Torzewski J: C-reactive protein-mediated low density lipoprotein uptake by macrophages: Implications for atherosclerosis. Circulation 103:1194-1197, 2001.

67. Ballou SP, Lozanski G: Induction of inflammatory cytokine release from cultured human monocytes by C-reactive protein. Cytokine 4:361-368, 1992.

68. Pasceri V, Willerson JT, Yeh ET: Direct proinflammatory effect of C-reactive protein on human endothelial cells. Circulation 102:2165-2168, 2000.

69. Pasceri V, Chang J, Willerson JT, Yeh ET: Modulation of C-reactive protein-mediated monocyte chemoattractant protein-1 induction in human endothelial cells by anti-atherosclerosis drugs. Circulation 103:2531-2534, 2001.

70. Verma S, Li SH, Badiwala MV, et al: Endothelin antagonism and interleukin-6 inhibition attenuate the proatherogenic effects of C-reactive protein. Circulation 105:1890-1896, 2002.

71. Venugopal SK, Devaraj S, Yuhanna I, et al: Demonstration that C-reactive protein decreases eNOS expression and bioactivity in human aortic endothelial cells. Circulation 106:1439-1441, 2002.

72. Verma S, Wang CH, Li SH, et al: A self-fulfilling prophecy: C-reactive protein attenuates nitric oxide production and inhibits angiogenesis. Circulation 106:913-919, 2002.

73. Devaraj S, Xu DY, Jialal I: C-reactive protein increases plasminogen activator inhibitor-1 expression and activity in human aortic endothelial cells: Implications for the metabolic syndrome and atherothrombosis. Circulation 107:398-404, 2003.

74. Ridker PM, Rifai N, Pfeffer MA, et al: Long-term effects of pravastatin

11

on plasma concentration of C-reactive protein. The Cholesterol and Recurrent Events (CARE) Investigators. Circulation 100:230-235, 1999.

75. Jialal I, Stein D, Balis D, et al: Effect of hydroxymethyl glutaryl coenzyme A reductase inhibitor therapy on high sensitive C-reactive protein levels. Circulation 103:1933-1935, 2001.

76. Ridker PM, Rifai N, Lowenthal SP: Rapid reduction in C-reactive protein with cerivastatin among 785 patients with primary hypercholesterolemia. Circulation 103:1191-1193, 2001.

77. Kinlay S, Timms T, Clark M, et al: Comparison of effect of intensive lipid lowering with atorvastatin to less intensive lowering with lovastatin on C-reactive protein in patients with stable angina pectoris and inducible myocardial ischemia. Am J Cardiol 89:1205-1207, 2002.

78. Ridker PM, Rifai N, Clearfield M, et al: Measurement of C-reactive protein for the targeting of statin therapy in the primary prevention of acute coronary events. N Engl J Med 344:1959-1965, 2001.

79. Koh KK, Schenke WH, Waclawiw MA, et al: Statin attenuates increase in C-reactive protein during estrogen replacement therapy in postmenopausal women. Circulation 105:1531-1533, 2002.

80. Albert M, Danielson E, Rifai N, Ridker PM: Effect of statin therapy on C-reactive protein levels. The Pravastatin Inflammation/CRP Evaluation (PRINCE): A Randomized Trial and Cohort Study. JAMA 286:64-70, 2001.

81. Ridker PM, Rifai N, Pfeffer MA, et al: Inflammation, pravastatin, and the risk of coronary events after myocardial infarction in patients with average cholesterol levels. Cholesterol and Recurrent Events (CARE) Investigators. Circulation 98:839-844, 1998.

82. Bickel C, Rupprecht HJ, Blankenberg S, et al: Relation of markers of inflammation (C-reactive protein, fibrinogen, von Willebrand factor, and leukocyte count) and statin therapy to long-term mortality in patients with angiographically proven coronary artery disease. Am J Cardiol 89:901-908, 2002.

83. Chan AW, Bhatt DL, Chew DP, et al: Relation of inflammation and benefit of statins after percutaneous coronary interventions. Circulation 107:1750-1756, 2003.

84. Walter DH, Fichtlscherer S, Britten MB, et al: Statin therapy, inflammation and recurrent coronary events in patients following coronary stent implantation. J Am Coll Cardiol 38:2006-2012, 2001.

85. Ridker PM: Should statin therapy be considered for patients with elevated C-reactive protein? The need for a definitive clinical trial. Eur Heart J 22:2135-2137, 2001.

86. Pradhan AD, Manson JE, Rifai N, et al: C-reactive protein, interleukin 6, and risk of developing type 2 diabetes mellitus. JAMA 286:327-334, 2001.

87. Freeman DJ, Norrie J, Sattar N, et al: Pravastatin and the development of diabetes mellitus: Evidence for a protective treatment effect in the West of Scotland Coronary Prevention Study. Circulation 103:357-362, 2001.

88. Blake GJ, Ridker PM, Kuntz KM: Projected life-expectancy gains with statin therapy for individuals with elevated C-reactive protein levels. J Am Coll Cardiol 40:49-55, 2002.

89. Blake GJ, Ridker PM, Kuntz KM: Potential cost-effectiveness of C-reactive protein screening followed by targeted statin therapy for the primary prevention of cardiovascular disease among patients without overt hyperlipidemia. Am J Med 114:485-494, 2003.

11

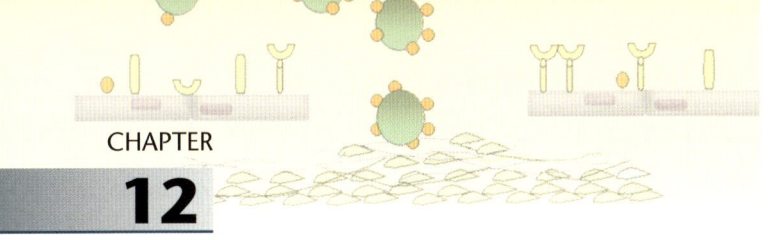

CHAPTER

12

Anticoagulant Effects of Statins

Junru Wang, Jawahar L. Mehta, Louis M. Fink,
and Martin Hauer-Jensen

Statins (3-hydroxy-3-methylglutaryl coenzyme A reductase inhibitors) have become the most frequently prescribed drug class in the Western world, with annual sales approaching $20 billion in the United States alone. Statins are potent inhibitors of cholesterol synthesis and widely used clinically for the treatment of hyperlipidemia. Several large-scale, multicenter, randomized clinical trials have demonstrated that statins are effective for primary and secondary prevention of coronary artery disease in patients with elevated cholesterol levels.[1-5] Some studies also suggest that statins have benefits beyond the coronary vascular bed and are capable of reducing ischemic stroke risk by approximately one third in patients with evidence of vascular disease.[6,7] These benefits were initially attributed to the effect of statins on blood lipids. However, several lines of evidence support the notion that the beneficial effects of statins may extend to mechanisms beyond cholesterol reduction.

The clinical benefits of statin therapy are observed much earlier than was originally predicted—in most cases within 2 years of randomization on study, and as early as 6 months.[8] Significant cholesterol reduction is associated with, at best, modest regression of atherosclerosis and luminal narrowing, as demonstrated by angiography.[9-11] Cholesterol-lowering trials suggest that the risk for myocardial infarction in individuals treated with statins is lower than in individuals treated with other cholesterol-lowering agents or modalities, despite a comparable reduction in serum cholesterol levels.[10] A retrospective study demonstrated that statin use, but not the use of other lipid-lowering drugs, was associated with a 50% risk reduction of venous thromboembolism.[12] Another retrospective cohort study showed that statins reduced the risk for deep vein thrombosis, whereas nonstatin lipid-lowering agents did not reduce that risk.[13]

The favorable clinical effects of statins have also been extended to patients with normal or average cholesterol. For

This work was supported in part by a grant from the National Institutes of Health (CA-83719).

233

example, the Long-term Intervention with Pravastatin in Ischemic Disease (LIPID) Study demonstrated a striking reduction in cardiovascular and all-cause mortality with pravastatin in patients with acute coronary syndromes, regardless of preexisting cholesterol levels.[3] The Cholesterol and Recurrent Events (CARE) study showed a significant reduction in cardiovascular deaths in patients with normal to average serum cholesterol and a history of myocardial infarction after pravastatin treatment.[14] A randomized study in more than 19,000 hypertensive patients demonstrated a marked reduction in cardiovascular and cerebrovascular events in patients with average or low cholesterol levels who received statin in addition to antihypertensive medication.[15]

Experimental and clinical evidence indicate that some of the cholesterol-independent, or pleiotropic, effects of statins involve improving or restoring endothelial function,[16-18] enhancing the stability of atherosclerotic plaques,[17,19] and decreasing oxidative stress and vascular inflammation.[20-23] Hence, statins have anticoagulant and antithrombotic effects[24-26] and ameliorate hypercoagulability.[27] Many of these effects are clearly independent of the cholesterol-lowering effects of statins.[17,25,28-30]

This chapter will review the currently available information about the anticoagulant effects of statins as well as the effects of statins on the related aspects of endothelial function, platelet aggregation, and fibrinolysis. The favorable pleiotropic effects demonstrated by statins will very likely have a profound influence on their prophylactic and therapeutic uses.

OVERVIEW OF COAGULATION, PLATELET AGGREGATION, AND FIBRINOLYSIS

Before discussing the anticoagulant effects of statins, a review of the coagulation process, platelet aggregation, and fibrinolysis is in order. A diagram of relevant parts of the coagulation system is shown in Figure 12-1.

Coagulation

Because of properties of the endothelium and the inactive form of coagulation factors and cofactors, no coagulation takes place in the bloodstream under normal conditions. The coagulation system is triggered when the blood is exposed to coagulation activators not present physiologically.[31] Mechanical injury to the endothelium exposes blood to constitutive tissue factor (TF), the primary initiator of the extrinsic coagulation pathway, and exposure to endogenous mediators, such as cytokines, induces the biosynthesis of TF.[32] TF binds to and activates factor VII. This TF-VIIa complex initiates coagulation by activating factor Xa, which catalyzes the generation of thrombin from prothrombin in the presence of activated factor Va.

The three main physiologic anticoagulant mechanisms that

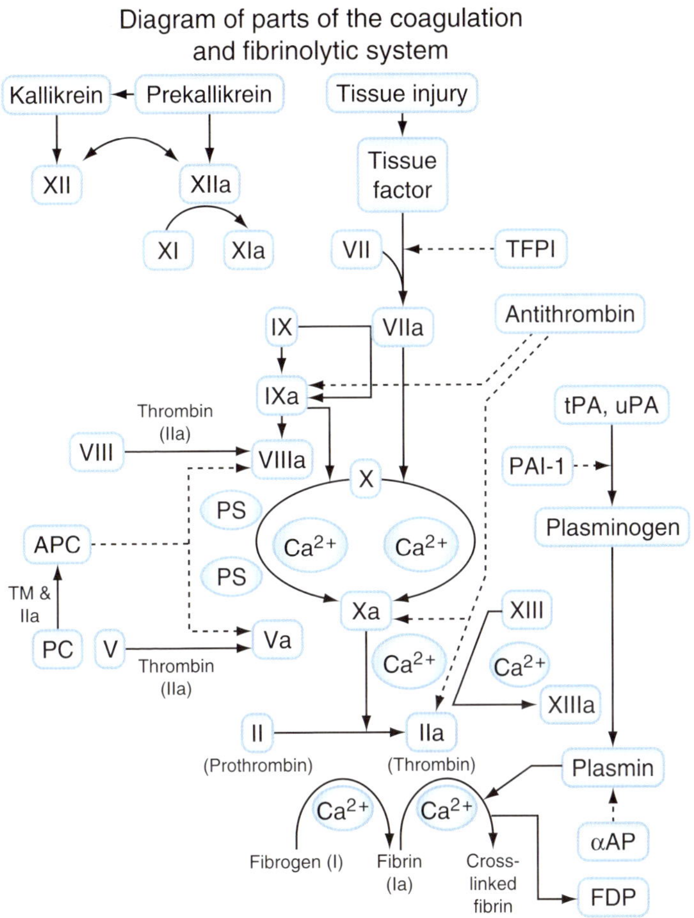

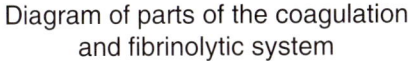

Diagram of parts of the coagulation and fibrinolytic system

Figure 12-1. Diagram depicting relevant parts of the coagulation and fibrinolytic system. αAP, α-antiplasmin; APC, activated protein C; FDP, fibrin degradation products; HK, high-molecular-weight kininogen; PAI, plasminogen activator inhibitor; PC, protein C; PS, protein S; TFPI, tissue factor pathway inhibitor; TM, thrombomodulin; tPA, tissue plasminogen activator; uPA, urokinase plasminogen activator.

counteract the accelerating coagulation pathway to maintain coagulation-anticoagulation homeostasis are (1) tissue factor pathway inhibitor (TFPI), which inhibits the TF-VIIa complex; (2) antithrombin III, which inactivates thrombin and factors Xa and IXa; and (3) the thrombomodulin–protein C system, which changes thrombin from a procoagulant to an anticoagulant and inactivates factors Va and VIIIa.

Platelet Aggregation

Platelets not only are responsible for hemostasis but also play fundamental roles in atherogenesis and in the pathophysiology of acute coronary syndromes.[33,34] Platelets are the first cellular elements at sites of vascular injury, where they initiate hemostatic and inflammatory responses and contribute to the cytokine milieu. Platelet aggregation may be triggered by shear stress, ADP, collagen, norepinephrine, and thrombin at sites of stenosis, plaque rupture, or ulceration. Integrins at the site of injury, such as von Willebrand's factor, interact with platelet receptors, resulting in platelet adherence and subsequent increase in fibrinogen receptors on the platelet surface membrane. Platelets also provide a surface for the assembly of enzyme complexes required for thrombin activation and thus serve to localize coagulation to sites of vascular injury. Platelets release a large number of mediators, notably cytokines, such as platelet-derived growth factor, transforming growth factor β, and acidic and basic fibroblast growth factors, which play important roles in tissue remodeling.

Fibrinolysis

The fibrinolytic system plays numerous physiologic roles, with the most common and well understood being the regulation of thrombus formation. Hence, fibrinolysis is the ultimate mechanism that counteracts the consequences of the coagulation process.[35] The fibrinolytic pathway converts plasminogen into the serine protease plasmin, which cleaves fibrin and dissolves clots. The generation of plasmin is mediated by plasminogen activators. Tissue plasminogen activator (tPA), released by endothelial cells upon stimulation by thrombin, is the main plasminogen activator. Plasmin cleaves fibrinogen and fibrin to produce degradation products, which inhibit thrombin action and fibrin polymerization and thus serve as natural anticoagulants. A second plasminogen activator, urokinase plasminogen activator (uPA), is synthesized by mesenchymal cells, epithelial cells, monocytes and macrophages, and stimulated endothelial cells. Plasminogen activator inhibitor-1 (PAI-1) is the major physiologic inhibitor of tPA and uPA in the regulation of fibrinolytic balance and is produced by many cell types, with the endothelial cells and adipocytes as principal sites of synthesis. Excess PAI-1 may be significant to the development and clinical course of acute and chronic cardiovascular diseases, as well as to other arterial and venous thromboembolic disease states.[36,37]

EFFECTS OF STATINS ON COAGULATION

As mentioned, an important benefit of statin therapy is the effect of these drugs on blood clotting.[20,26,29,38-42] Several potential molecular and cellular targets for the antithrombotic effects of statins have

12

been proposed, including fibrinogen, thrombin, tissue factor, thrombomodulin, and platelets, as well as other coagulation factors and cofactors.

Fibrinogen

Fibrinogen is a soluble plasma glycoprotein that is synthesized in the liver. It participates in the fluid phase of coagulation by being converted to insoluble fibrin fibers and in the cellular phase by its role in platelet aggregation.[43] High levels of fibrinogen correlate strongly with increased risk for cardiovascular disease.[44] Fibrinogen is an acute phase protein and therefore increases during many disease states, notably those associated with tissue injury and inflammation.

The effects of several statins on plasma fibrinogen have been studied, but the results are conflicting. For example, lovastatin has been shown to increase,[45,46] decrease,[47] or have no influence on plasma fibrinogen levels.[48-51] Atorvastatin has been shown to increase[50,52-54] or not change[48,55-57] plasma fibrinogen levels. Pravastatin resulted in up to a 19% reduction in some studies,[58-61] whereas other studies reported no change[62-64] or increased[65] fibrinogen levels. Simvastatin, in most studies, had little influence on fibrinogen concentrations[59,64,66-69] although increased[70] and decreased[71,72] fibrinogen levels have been reported. The results with fluvastatin are also mixed, with increased,[73] decreased,[74,75] and unchanged[76-78] fibrinogen levels being reported by different investigators.

Although differences in measurement techniques and study populations, as well as numerous other variables, may be the reason for some of these conflicting data, it is not possible to conclude if and how statins influence plasma fibrinogen.[79]

Thrombin and Antithrombin

Thrombin is a key enzyme of the blood coagulation cascade. It affects blood clotting in several ways—for example, by converting fibrinogen to fibrin, by activating platelets, and by activating other zymogens and cofactors in the coagulation cascade.[80] Hypercholesterolemic patients exhibit markedly increased thrombin generation,[72,81] and several lines of evidence point to reduced thrombin generation as an important effect of statin therapy.[81-86] Statins decrease the conversion of fibrinogen to fibrin,[24] the final aspect of the clotting cascade regulated by thrombin, and reduce circulating fibrinopeptide levels.[24,41,63,83,87] Statins also reduce the activation of factor XIII.[24,88] Factor XIIIa, formed by enzymatic cleavage of factor XIII by thrombin, transforms the loose fibrin network into a stable covalent collection of fibrin fibers.[89]

Although some studies have suggested that there is a correlation between reduced thrombin generation and lipid lowering,[81] other studies have shown that a reduction of thrombin generation in response to statin therapy occurs even in patients with only slightly elevated cholesterol.[26,41,62] The mechanisms by which statins reduce thrombin generation appear to be platelet related, but the details remain to be elucidated.[81,82,84]

The plasma proteinase inhibitor antithrombin III inactivates thrombin and enzymes involved in thrombin generation.[90] Some studies have shown that statin treatment decreases antithrombin III activity[51,61] and thrombin–antithrombin complexes.[27,61,63,72,87]

Tissue Factor

Suppression of TF expression is widely believed to be a major antithrombotic benefit of statin therapy.[20] Hence, statins have been shown to reduce monocyte TF activity independent of the reduction of cholesterol.[27,81] Analogously, animal studies have shown that statins reduce TF expression in atheromas of nonhuman primates[23] and in the vascular wall of atherosclerotic rabbits.[92,93] In vitro studies have shown that statins reduce TF expression in human aortic endothelial cells and prevent the up-regulation of TF in human aortic smooth muscle cells.[94] TF expression in cultured human monocytes and macrophages is also inhibited by statins.[95,96]

Statins may also directly affect factor VII. Several large prospective and case-control studies have shown that factor VII activity levels are elevated in hyperlipidemic patients[97,98] and predict cardiovascular events.[99-101] Many investigators have reported that statins reduce factor VII antigen levels,[61,68,72,102] the levels of activated factor VII,[104] and factor VII–dependent coagulation.[51,104-106]

Tissue factor pathway inhibitor (TFPI), synthesized primarily by vascular endothelium, binds to the TF-VIIa complex to inhibit activation of the coagulation cascade. The majority of circulating TFPI is associated with LDL, but 10% to 20% is carrier free. High plasma TFPI activity or antigen levels have been observed in patients with familial hypercholesterolemia and type II hypercholesterolemia, and statin treatment decreases TFPI levels in parallel with LDL cholesterol.[66,104,107,108] However, statins do not affect carrier-free TFPI.[104,107] Therefore, because the carrier-free TFPI is responsible for its anticoagulant actions, statin treatment may not affect the anticoagulant potency of TFPI in plasma.

Thrombomodulin and Protein C

In terms of maintaining normal endothelial cell function, a transmembrane endothelial cell glycoprotein, thrombomodulin (TM), plays a particularly prominent role (reviewed by Dittman and Nelson[109]). TM acts by forming a complex with thrombin, thereby changing its substrate specificity. Thrombin, when complexed to TM, loses its ability to cleave fibrinogen and activate cellular thrombin receptors (i.e., thrombin loses its procoagulant properties). Instead, thrombin's ability to activate protein C is enhanced 1000- to 2000-fold. Activated protein C, in concert with protein S, inactivates activated factors V and VIII and thereby limits further thrombin generation.

Clinical studies have reported decreased levels of circulating TM fragments in patients receiving statin therapy,[63,87,110,111] which suggests a decreased release of endothelial TM into the circulation and improvement of endothelial dysfunction but not necessarily altered endothelial TM expression. However, a number of clinical studies have suggested that statins enhance the thrombomodulin–protein C pathway in vivo. In a study in hypercholesterolemic patients undergoing chronic peritoneal dialysis, pravastatin treatment increased protein C levels independent of treatment response in terms of lipid lowering.[88] Furthermore, simvastatin treatment of hypercholesterolemic patients was associated with accelerated inactivation of factor Va, which was consistent with the notion that statins influence the thrombomodulin–protein C pathway.[24] A microarray study with human umbilical vein endothelial cells demonstrated that statins increased the mRNA levels of many mediators related to inflammation, vascular constriction, and coagulation, including TM.[112] Another report suggested that statin-induced increase in TM expression is a result of decreased geranyl geranylation of Rac and Cdc42.[113] However, these studies did not examine associated changes in protein functional activity or the effect of statins under conditions that normally down-regulate TM.

Studies performed in our laboratory demonstrate that atorvastatin and simvastatin potently increase TM gene expression, cellular protein, cell surface antigen, and cell surface protein C activity in four different endothelial cell types (Figs. 12-2 and 12-3). Moreover, statin treatment counteracts the down-regulatory effects of tumor necrosis factor α (TNF-α). Our preliminary observations also suggest that statins may protect against the effects of radiation on endothelial TM.[114] In contrast to the report by Masamura and co-workers,[113] our studies show rather convincingly that statins up-regulate TM, at least in part by a nitric oxide–dependent mechanism, similar to many other vasculoprotective pleiotropic statin effects.[115] Compared to the effect of statins on other mediators involved in the regulation of coagulation and fibrinolysis, the up-regulation of TM in response to statin in our study was robust, consistent with the notion that the effect on TM may be biologically relevant and clinically important. For example, whereas statin causes an approximately 50% change in TF,[92] tPA,[116] and PAI-1,[116] our study showed that statin increased TM mRNA levels at least 10-fold and resulted in strong enhancement of protein C activation. Moreover, the effects of statin on TM were equal to or exceeded those of other factors that increase TM, such as cyclic AMP, retinoids, and heat shock.[117-119]

Considering the central role of the TM–protein C system in vascular thromboresistance and for mounting an appropriate

12

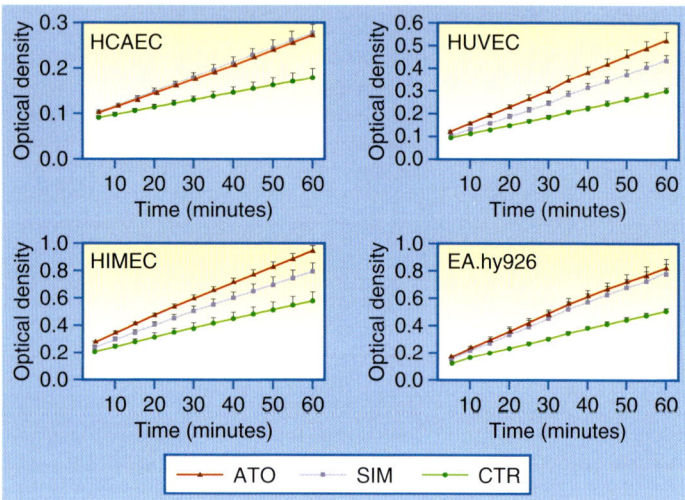

Figure 12-2. **Statins increase thrombomodulin activity (protein C activation) in four different endothelial cell lines.** Incubation for 24 hr with simvastatin (10 µM) or atorvastatin (10 µM) increases thrombomodulin activity in human coronary artery endothelial cells (HCAEC), human umbilical vein endothelial cells (HUVEC), human intestinal microvascular endothelial cells (an immortalized cell line provided by Dr. Fiocchi, Case Western Reserve University, Cleveland, OH), and EA.hy926 endothelial cells (an immortalized HUVEC line provided by Dr. Edgell, University of North Carolina, Chapel Hill, NC). ATO, atorvastatin; SIM, simvastatin; CTR, control.

response to bacterial challenge and other inflammatory stimuli, the finding that statins up-regulate TM could have major clinical implications. Acquired deficiencies of TM are thought to be pathophysiologically relevant in many disorders associated with endothelial dysfunction, including sepsis and related conditions,[120-123] adult respiratory distress syndrome (ARDS),[124] transplant rejection,[125] vein graft failure,[126] preeclampsia,[127] inflammatory bowel disease,[128] and normal tissue radiation toxicity.[129-131]

The observation that statins counteract the down-regulation effect of TNF-α on endothelial cell TM suggests a potential use of statin as an adjuvant in patients with sepsis and related disorders. During sepsis, the vascular endothelium is strongly procoagulant because of decreased expression of TM and, possibly, increased expression of TF. Despite long-standing interest in therapeutic modulation of the coagulation system in sepsis, the only approach

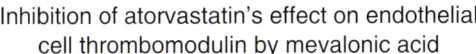

Inhibition of atorvastatin's effect on endothelial
cell thrombomodulin by mevalonic acid

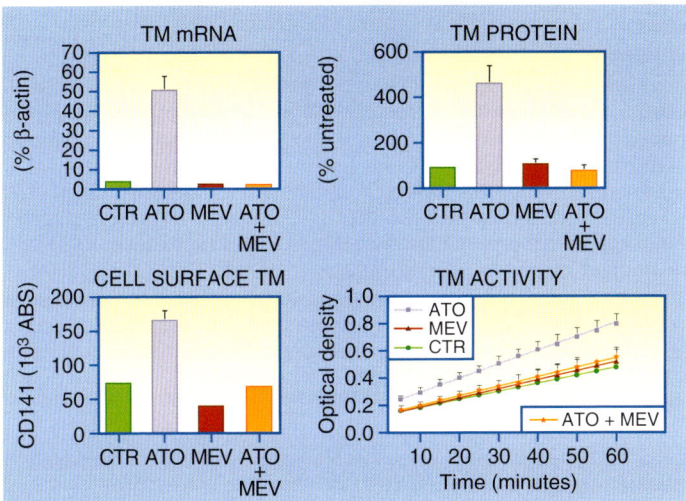

Figure 12-3. Inhibition of atorvastatin's effect on endothelial cell thrombomodulin by mevalonic acid. EA.hy926 endothelial cells were untreated (CTR) or incubated with 10 μM atorvastatin (ATO), 500 μM mevalonate (MEV), or both (ATO+MEV), for 24 hours. Thrombomodulin (TM) mRNA was measured with real-time fluorogenic probe reverse transcriptase polymerase chain reaction (TaqMan RT-PCR); thrombomodulin protein was measured with Western blot technique; cell surface thrombomodulin was measured with flow cytometry, and thrombomodulin activity was measured with the protein C activation assay. ABS, antibody binding sites.

to date that has translated into a survival benefit in the phase III clinical trial setting is the administration of recombinant activated protein C, as reported by Bernard and co-workers.[122] Importantly, these investigators showed that activated protein C infusion was equally beneficial in patients with normal and with low protein C levels, suggesting that the critical factor is not reduced availability of protein C but, rather, a defective activation mechanism. It is tempting to speculate that statins could be used to increase endothelial TM and protein C activation in patients at risk for or with established sepsis, thereby providing an inexpensive and safe prophylactic or therapeutic intervention by which to restore the anticoagulant properties of the endothelium. In support of this notion, an intriguing clinical study showed that patients who were on statin therapy when they developed sepsis were 7 times less likely to die than patients who were not on statin therapy.[132]

EFFECTS OF STATINS ON PLATELET AGGREGATION

Hyperlipidemia disorders are associated with a variety of platelet abnormalities.[133-138] Platelet-dependent thrombin generation is increased in patients with hypercholesterolemia[81,82,84] as well as in other conditions in which the cholesterol-to-phospholipids ratio in platelets is increased.[139-141] Other hyperlipidemia-associated platelet abnormalities include increases in thromboxane biosynthesis,[142,143] α-adrenergic receptor density,[144] and cytosolic calcium,[145] as well as direct activation by oxidized LDL.[146] Statins influence platelet function at several levels, notably platelet activation, platelet-dependent thrombin generation, and platelet aggregation.[147]

Platelet activation is accompanied by an altered expression of cell membrane molecules. Several studies have evaluated changes in platelet activity markers in response to statin treatment. The surface activation markers CD62 (P-selectin)[21,148-152] and CD63[149] decrease during statin therapy.

Reduction of platelet-dependent thrombin generation may be a particularly important "antiplatelet" effect of statin therapy.[81,84] It is not clear whether this effect is related to cholesterol lowering, but several studies suggest that it is cholesterol independent. For example, Puccetti and co-workers showed that cerivastatin significantly reduces platelet-dependent thrombin generation in both normal and hypercholesterolemic subjects.[82] Also, using an ex vivo thrombosis model as a surrogate for platelet reactivity, Dangas and co-workers found that statins reduced thrombus formation independent of cholesterol lowering.[25]

Numerous studies have shown that statins inhibit platelet aggregation in hypercholesterolemic patients[47,137,153,154] and in patients on chronic peritoneal dialysis.[110] Inhibition of platelet aggregation by statins is accompanied by decreased production of thromboxane,[142,148,155-157] an important platelet-generated prostaglandin that is released by activated platelets and promotes aggregation.[158] Several studies have shown that urinary 11-dehydro-thromboxane B2 excretion, which is largely a reflection of platelet TXA2 production, decreases significantly in response to statin therapy.[133,142,143,150,159] In vitro studies have shown that fluvastatin and lovastatin reduce ADP- and thrombin-induced platelet aggregation, whereas pravastatin, the hydrophilic statin, does not exhibit this effect.[155]

The precise mechanism by which statins affect platelet function is not clear. One potential mechanism may be the aforementioned reduction of thromboxane production.[160] Other suggested mechanisms include modification of the cholesterol content of platelet membranes,[145] increased endothelial cell nitric oxide synthase expression in platelets,[161,162] increased responsiveness of platelets to nitric oxide,[163] decreased cytosolic calcium,[145] decreased lipid peroxidation of platelet membranes,[164] decreased responsiveness of platelets to thrombin receptor activation,[165] and reduction in geranyl geranylation of Rap1a, a key protein in platelet aggregation.[166]

It is not clear whether the effect of statins on platelet function is dependent on or independent of cholesterol lowering. Moreover, statins exert several other effects in patients with atherosclerotic disease and hypercholesterolemia that may indirectly modify platelet function, such as favorable modification of endothelial function, stabilization of atherosclerotic plaque, and increase in the relative volume of collagen and smooth muscle cells within plaques.[16,29,38,61,167] Finally, although the majority of published studies have shown that statins decrease platelet function, a few investigators have reported that statins have no effect on platelets or even enhance platelet function.[168-172] The explanation for these contradictory findings remains elusive.

EFFECTS OF STATINS ON FIBRINOLYSIS

Clinical data related to the effects of statins on the fibrinolytic system are less conclusive than the data related to the effects of these drugs on coagulation and platelet aggregation. Several clinical studies demonstrated persuasively that statins enhance the activity of the fibrinolytic system. Statins reduced plasma PAI-1 antigen and activity in hypercholesterolemic patients, possibly by mechanisms independent of lipid lowering.[25,26,63,65,74,87] Some studies, however, suggested that statins do not alter PAI-1 antigen or activity levels significantly,[78,111,173] and others even reported increased PAI-1 activity as a result of statin therapy.[68]

Results related to the effects of statins on tPA also appear to be somewhat conflicting. Some studies have reported that statins increase plasma tPA activity or desmopressin-evoked tPA responses,[26,174,175] whereas others have demonstrated an effect on tPA antigen in the opposite direction.[65,74,151,173,174] Statin also appears to reduce plasma tPA–PAI-1 complex levels.[88] These seemingly discordant results may be explained as follows: circulating tPA forms a 1:1 complex with PAI-1,[176] which clears more slowly than free tPA. Thus, increased formation of the complex will increase tPA antigen levels but will decrease tPA activity. This is consistent with the observation that increased tPA antigen levels constitute a risk factor in cardiovascular disease.[177-179] Hence, as proposed by Emeis and Cohen, the net effect of statins is likely to enhance fibrinolysis, thereby contributing to the favorable effects of statins on cardiovascular events.[180]

Circulating D dimer, formed by plasmin digestion of cross-linked fibrin, is a frequently used test of global fibrinolytic activity. Several investigators have evaluated the effects of statins on D-dimer levels, but the results have been inconclusive. Seljeflot and co-workers reported that statins increase plasma D-dimer levels in hypercholesterolemic patients,[174] whereas other studies have found decreased[27,63,74,88] or unchanged[26,65,181,182] D-dimer levels after statin treatment.

Compared to the clinical data, in vitro data show unequivocally that statins are profibrinolytic. Several investigators have shown that statins decrease PAI-1 production and activity, while increasing tPA production and activity, in vascular endothelium[116,183-187] and smooth muscle cells.[116,183]

CONCLUSIONS

Among the many pleiotropic effects of statins, their vasculo-protective potential has been the subject of particularly intense investigation. Studies clearly show that statins profoundly influence the coagulation system, platelets, and the fibrinolytic system in a favorable direction. There is also strong preclinical and clinical evidence suggesting that, in addition to lipid lowering, these effects translate into significant benefits in patients with cardio-vascular and cerebrovascular diseases. Moreover, because of the central pathophysiologic role of the coagulation system in traumatic, infective, and degenerative disease processes, these pleiotropic effects may also be very relevant in a number of disease states not associated with hyperlipidemia and not traditionally considered vascular in origin. Although studies with statins in these disease states are still in the early stages, it is likely that they will lead to expansion of the indications for prophylactic or therapeutic use of statins. The combined uses of statins for these new indications may very well exceed their use in patients with hyperlipidemia.

References

1. Scandinavian Simvastatin Survival Study Group: Randomised trial of cholesterol lowering in 4444 patients with coronary heart disease: The Scandinavian Simvastatin Survival Study (4S). Lancet 344:1383-1389, 1994.
2. Shepherd J, Cobbe SM, Ford I, et al: Prevention of coronary heart disease with pravastatin in men with hypercholesterolemia. West of Scotland Coronary Prevention Study Group. N Engl J Med 333:1301-1307, 1995.
3. Long-term Intervention with Pravastatin in Ischaemic Disease (LIPID) Study Group: Prevention of cardiovascular events and death with pravastatin in patients with coronary heart disease and a broad range of initial cholesterol levels. The Long-term Intervention with Pravastatin in Ischaemic Disease (LIPID) Study Group. N Engl J Med 339:1349-1357, 1998.
4. Eisenberg DA: Cholesterol lowering in the management of coronary artery disease: The clinical implications of recent trials. Am J Med 104:2S-5S, 1998.
5. LaRosa JC, He J, Vupputuri S: Effect of statins on risk of coronary disease: A meta-analysis of randomized controlled trials. JAMA 282:2340-2346, 1999.

6. Vaughan CJ, Gotto AMJ, Basson CT: The evolving role of statins in the management of atherosclerosis. J Am Coll Cardiol 35:1-10, 2000.
7. Hebert PR, Gaziano JM, Chan KS, et al: Cholesterol lowering with statin drugs, risk of stroke, and total mortality. An overview of randomized trials. JAMA 278:313-321, 1997.
8. The Pravastatin Multinational Study Group for Cardiac Risk Patients: Effects of pravastatin in patients with serum total cholesterol levels from 5.2 to 7.8 mmol/liter (200 to 300 mg/dl) plus two additional atherosclerotic risk factors. Am J Cardiol 72:1031-1037, 1993.
9. Levine GN, Keaney JF, Vita JA: Cholesterol reduction in cardiovascular disease: Clinical benefits and possible mechanisms. N Engl J Med 332:512-521, 1995.
10. Brown BG, Zhao XQ, Sacco DE, et al: Lipid lowering and plaque regression: New insights into prevention of plaque disruption and clinical events in coronary disease. Circulation 87:1781-1791, 1993.
11. Brown BG, Hillger L, Zhao XQ, et al: Types of change in coronary stenosis severity and their relative importance in overall progression and regression of coronary disease: Observations from the FATS Trial. Familial Atherosclerosis Treatment Study. Ann N Y Acad Sci 748:407-417, 1995.
12. Grady D, Wenger NK, Herrington D, et al: Postmenopausal hormone therapy increases risk for venous thromboembolic disease. The Heart and Estrogen/progestin Replacement Study. Ann Intern Med 132:689-696, 2000.
13. Ray JG, Mamdani M, Tsuyuki RT, et al: Use of statins and the subsequent development of deep vein thrombosis. Arch Intern Med 161:1405-1410, 2001.
14. Sacks FM, Pfeffer MA, Moye LA, et al: The effect of pravastatin on coronary events after myocardial infarction in patients with average cholesterol levels. Cholesterol and Recurrent Events Trial investigators. N Engl J Med 335:1001-1009, 1996.
15. Sever PS, Dahlof B, Poulter NR, et al: Prevention of coronary and stroke events with atorvastatin in hypertensive patients who have average or lower-than-average cholesterol concentrations, in the Anglo Scandinavian Cardiac Outcomes Trial—Lipid-Lowering Arm (ASCOT-LLA): A multicenter randomised controlled trial. Lancet 361:1149-1158, 2003.
16. Luscher TF, Tanner FC, Noll G: Lipids and endothelial function: Effects of lipid-lowering and other therapeutic interventions. Curr Opin Lipidol 7:234-240, 1996.
17. Takemoto M, Liao JK: Pleiotropic effects of 3-hydroxy-3-methylglutaryl coenzyme a reductase inhibitors. Arterioscler Thromb Vasc Biol 21:1712-1719, 2001.
18. Dupuis J, Tardif JC, Cernacek P, et al: Cholesterol reduction rapidly improves endothelial function after acute coronary syndromes. The RECIFE (reduction of cholesterol in ischemia and function of the endothelium) trial. Circulation 99:3227-3233, 1999.
19. Wheeler DC: Are there potential non-lipid-lowering uses of statins? Drugs 56:517-522, 1998.
20. Undas A, Brozek J, Musial J: Anti-inflammatory and antithrombotic effects of statins in the management of coronary artery disease. Clin Lab 48:287-296, 2002.
21. Bickel C, Rupprecht HJ, Blankenberg S, et al: Influence of

HMG-CoA reductase inhibitors on markers of coagulation, systemic inflammation and soluble cell adhesion. Int J Cardiol 82:25-31, 2002.

22. Bickel C, Rupprecht HJ, Blankenberg S, et al: Relation of markers of inflammation (C-reactive protein, fibrinogen, von Willebrand factor, and leukocyte count) and statin therapy to long-term mortality in patients with angiographically proven coronary artery disease. Am J Cardiol 89:901-908, 2002.

23. Sukhova GK, Williams JK, Libby P: Statins reduce inflammation in atheroma of nonhuman primates independent of effects on serum cholesterol. Arterioscler Thromb Vasc Biol 22:1452-1458, 2002.

24. Undas A, Brummel KE, Musial J, et al: Simvastatin depresses blood clotting by inhibiting activation of prothrombin, factor V, and factor XIII and by enhancing factor Va inactivation. Circulation 103:2248-2253, 2001.

25. Dangas G, Smith DA, Unger AH, et al: Pravastatin: An antithrombotic effect independent of the cholesterol-lowering effect. Thromb Haemost 83:688-692, 2000.

26. Dangas G, Badimon JJ, Smith DA, et al: Pravastatin therapy in hyperlipidemia: Effects on thrombus formation and the systemic hemostatic profile. J Am Coll Cardiol 33:1294-1304, 1999.

27. Holschermann H, Hilgendorff A, Kemkes-Matthes B, et al: Simvastatin attenuates vascular hypercoagulability in cardiac transplant recipients. Transplantation 69:1830-1836, 2000.

28. Sposito AC, Chapman MJ: Statin therapy in acute coronary syndromes: Mechanistic insight into clinical benefit. Arterioscler Thromb Vasc Biol 22:1524-1534, 2001.

29. Rosenson RS: Non-lipid-lowering effects of statins on atherosclerosis. Curr Cardiol Rep 1:225-232, 1999.

30. Kearney D, Fitzgerald D: The anti-thrombotic effects of statins. J Am Coll Cardiol 33:1305-1307, 1999.

31. Roberts HR, Tabares AH: Overview of the coagulation reactions. In High KA, Roberts HR (eds): Molecular Basis of Thrombosis and Hemostasis, 1st ed. New York, Marcel Dekker, 1995, pp 35-50.

32. Morrissey JH: Tissue factor. In High KA, Roberts HR (eds): Molecular Basis of Thrombosis and Hemostasis, 1st ed. New York, Marcel Dekker, 1995, pp 101-118.

33. Fitzgerald DJ, Roy L, Catella F, et al: Platelet activation in unstable coronary disease. N Engl J Med 315:983-989, 1986.

34. Fuster V, Badimon L, Badimon JJ, et al: The pathogenesis of coronary artery disease and the acute coronary syndromes. N Engl J Med 326:310-318, 1992.

35. Bachmann F: Plasminogen-plasmin enzyme system. In Colman RW, Hirsh J, Marder VJ, et al (eds): Hemostasis and Thrombosis: Basic Principles and Clinical Practice, 4th ed. Philadelphia, Lippincott Williams & Wilkins, 2001, pp 275-320.

36. Tsikouris JP, Suarez JA, Meyerrose GE: Plasminogen activator inhibitor-1: Physiologic role, regulation, and the influence of common pharmacologic agents. J Clin Pharmacol 42:1187-1199, 2002.

37. Huber K, Christ G, Wojta J, et al: Plasminogen activator inhibitor type-1 in cardiovascular disease: Status report 2001. Thromb Res 103(Suppl 1):S7-19, 2001.

38. Bellosta S, Ferri N, Bernini F, et al: Non-lipid-related effects of statins. Ann Med 32:164-176, 2000.

12

39. Fenton JWJ, Shen GX: Statins as cellular antithrombotics. Haemostasis 29:166-169, 1999.
40. Fenton JW, Shen GX, Minnear FL, et al: Statin drugs and dietary isoprenoids as antithrombotic agents. Hematol Oncol Clin North Am 14:483-490, 2000.
41. Szczeklik A, Undas A, Musial J, et al: Antithrombotic actions of statins. Med Sci Monit 7:1381-1385, 2001.
42. Lacoste L, Lam JY, Hung J, et al: Hyperlipidemia and coronary disease: Correction of the increased thrombogenic potential with cholesterol reduction. Circulation 92:3172-3177, 1995.
43. Lord ST: Fibrinogen. In High KA, Roberts HR (eds): Molecular Basis of Thrombosis and Hemostasis, 1st ed. New York, Marcel Dekker, 1995, pp 51-74.
44. Drouet L, Bal dit Sollier C: Fibrinogen: Factor and marker of cardiovascular risk. J Mal Vasc 27:143-156, 2002.
45. Beigel Y, Fuchs J, Snir M, et al: Lovastatin therapy in hypercholesterolemia: Effect on fibrinogen, hemorrheologic parameters, platelet activity, and red blood cell morphology. J Clin Pharmacol 31:512-517, 1991.
46. Isaacsohn JL, Setaro JF, Nicholas C, et al: Effects of lovastatin therapy on plasminogen activator inhibitor-1 antigen levels. Am J Cardiol 74:735-737, 1994.
47. Mayer J, Eller T, Brauer P, et al: Effects of long-term treatment with lovastatin on the clotting system and blood platelets. Ann Hematol 64:196-201, 1992.
48. Davidson M, McKenney J, Stein E, et al: Comparison of one-year efficacy and safety of atorvastatin versus lovastatin in primary hypercholesterolemia. Atorvastatin Study Group I. Am J Cardiol 79:1475-1481, 1997.
49. Koenig W, Hehr R, Ditschuneit HH, et al: Lovastatin alters blood rheology in primary hyperlipoproteinemia: Dependence on lipoprotein(a)? J Clin Pharmacol 32:539-545, 1992.
50. Koppensteiner R, Minar E, Ehringer H: Effect of lovastatin on hemorheology in type II hyperlipoproteinemia. Atherosclerosis 83:53-58, 1990.
51. Idzior-Walu SB: Changes in the level of certain hemostatic factors during treatment with lovastatin in patients with primary hyperlipoproteinemia and phenotype IIa and IIb. Przegl Lek 49:334-339, 1992.
52. Sinzinger H, Rodrigues M, Furberg CD: Dosing of atorvastatin and increases in fibrinogen level. Atherosclerosis 147:421-422, 1999.
53. Marais AD, Firth JC, Bateman ME, et al: Atorvastatin: An effective lipid-modifying agent in familial hypercholesterolemia. Arterioscler Thromb Vasc Biol 17:1527-1531, 1997.
54. Wierzbicki AS, Lumb PJ, Semra YK, et al: Effect of atorvastatin on plasma fibrinogen. Lancet 351:569-570, 1998.
55. Bairaktari ET, Tzallas CS, Tsimihodimos VK, et al: Comparison of the efficacy of atorvastatin and micronized fenofibrate in the treatment of mixed hyperlipidemia. J Cardiovasc Risk 6:113-116, 1999.
56. Dujovne CA, Harris WS, Altman R, et al: Effect of atorvastatin on hemorheologic-hemostatic parameters and serum fibrinogen levels in hyperlipidemic patients. Am J Cardiol 85:350-353, 2000.
57. Black DM: Statins and fibrinogen. Lancet 351:1430, 1998.
58. Jay RH, Rampling MW, Betteridge DJ: Abnormalities of blood

rheology in familial hypercholesterolaemia: Effects of treatment. Atherosclerosis 85:249-256, 1990.

59. Tsuda Y, Satoh K, Kitadai M, et al: Effects of pravastatin sodium and simvastatin on plasma fibrinogen level and blood rheology in type II hyperlipoproteinemia. Atherosclerosis 122:225-233, 1996.

60. Tsuda Y, Satoh K, Takahashi T, et al: Effect of medication with pravastatin sodium on hemorheological parameters in patients with hyperlipoproteinemia. Int Angiol 12:360-364, 1993.

61. Di Garbo V, Bono M, Di Raimondo D, et al: Non lipid, dose-dependent effects of pravastatin treatment on hemostatic system and inflammatory response. Eur J Clin Pharmacol 56:277-284, 2000.

62. Salonen R, Nyyssonen K, Porkkala E, et al: Kuopio Atherosclerosis Prevention Study (KAPS): A population-based primary preventive trial of the effect of LDL lowering on atherosclerotic progression in carotid and femoral arteries. Circulation 92:1758-1764, 1995.

63. Wada H, Mori Y, Kaneko T, et al: Hypercoagulable state in patients with hypercholesterolemia: Effects of pravastatin. Clin Ther 14:829-834, 1992.

64. Branchi A, Rovellini A, Sommariva D, et al: Effect of three fibrate derivatives and of two HMG-CoA reductase inhibitors on plasma fibrinogen level in patients with primary hypercholesterolemia. Thromb Haemost 70:241-243, 1993.

65. Dangas G, Smith DA, Badimon JJ, et al: Gender differences in blood thrombogenicity in hyperlipidemic patients and response to pravastatin. Am J Cardiol 84:639-643, 1999.

66. Sandset PM, Lund H, Norseth J, et al: Treatment with hydroxymethylglutaryl-coenzyme A reductase inhibitors in hypercholesterolemia induces changes in the components of the extrinsic coagulation system. Arterioscler Thromb 11:138-145, 1991.

67. Bo M, Bonino F, Neirotti M, et al: Hemorheologic and coagulative pattern in hypercholesterolemic subjects treated with lipid-lowering drugs. Angiology 42:106-113, 1991.

68. Mitropoulos KA, Armitage JM, Collins R, et al: Randomized placebo-controlled study of the effects of simvastatin on haemostatic variables, lipoproteins and free fatty acids. The Oxford Cholesterol Study Group. Eur Heart J 18:235-241, 1997.

69. McDowell IF, Smye M, Trinick T, et al: Simvastatin in severe hypercholesterolaemia: A placebo controlled trial. Br J Clin Pharmacol 31:340-343, 1991.

70. Steinmetz A, Schwartz T, Hehnke U, et al: Multicenter comparison of micronized fenofibrate and simvastatin in patients with primary type IIA or IIB hyperlipoproteinemia. J Cardiovasc Pharmacol 27:563-570, 1996.

71. Jaeger BR, Meiser B, Nagel D, et al: Aggressive lowering of fibrinogen and cholesterol in the prevention of graft vessel disease after heart transplantation. Circulation 96(Suppl 9):II-154-158, 1997.

72. Di Garbo V, Cordova R, Avellone G: Increased thrombin generation and complement activation in patients with type IIA hyperlipoproteinemia. Curr Ther Res 58:706-723, 1997.

73. Gottsater A, Anwaar I, Lind P, et al: Increasing plasma fibrinogen, but unchanged levels of intraplatelet cyclic nucleotides, plasma endothelin-1, factor VII, and neopterin during cholesterol lowering with fluvastatin. Blood Coagul Fibrinolysis 10:133-140, 1999.

74. Lin TH, Huang CH, Voon WC, et al: The effect of fluvastatin on

fibrinolytic factors in patients with hypercholesterolemia. Kao Hsiung J Med Sci 16:600-606, 2000.

75. Rizos E, Miltiadous G, Elisaf M: The effect of fluvastatin on plasma fibrinogen levels. Curr Med Res Opin 18:154-155, 2002.

76. Rosenson RS, Tangney CC, Schaefer EJ: Comparative study of HMG-CoA reductase inhibitors on fibrinogen. Atherosclerosis 155:463-466, 2001.

77. Malyszko J, Malyszko JS, Brzosko S, et al: Effects of fluvastatin on homocysteine and serum lipids in kidney allograft recipients. Ann Transplant 7:52-54, 2002.

78. Cortellaro M, Cofrancesco E, Boschetti C, et al: Effects of fluvastatin and bezafibrate combination on plasma fibrinogen, t-plasminogen activator inhibitor and C reactive protein levels in coronary artery disease patients with mixed hyperlipidaemia (FACT study). Fluvastatin Alone and in Combination Treatment. Thromb Haemost 83:549-553, 2000.

79. Song JC, White CM: Do HMG-CoA reductase inhibitors affect fibrinogen? Ann Pharmacother 35:236-241, 2001.

80. Jenny NS, Mann KG: Thrombin. In Colman RW, Hirsh J, Marder VJ, et al (eds): Hemostasis and Thrombosis: Basic Principles and Clinical Practice, 4th ed. Philadelphia, Lippincott Williams & Wilkins, 2001, pp 171-189.

81. Aoki I, Aoki N, Kawano K, et al: Platelet-dependent thrombin generation in patients with hyperlipidemia. J Am Coll Cardiol 30:91-96, 1997.

82. Puccetti L, Bruni F, Di Renzo M, et al: Hypercoagulable state in hypercholesterolemic subjects assessed by platelet-dependent thrombin generation: In vitro effect of cerivastatin. Eur Rev Med Pharmacol Sci 3:197-204, 1999.

83. Szczeklik A, Musial J, Undas A, et al: Inhibition of thrombin generation by simvastatin and lack of additive effects of aspirin in patients with marked hypercholesterolemia. J Am Coll Cardiol 33:1286-1293, 1999.

84. Puccetti L, Bruni F, Bova G, et al: Effect of diet and treatment with statins on platelet-dependent thrombin generation in hypercholesterolemic subjects. Nutr Metab Cardiovasc Dis 11:378-387, 2001.

85. Musial J, Undas A, Undas R, et al: Treatment with simvastatin and low-dose aspirin depresses thrombin generation in patients with coronary heart disease and borderline-high cholesterol levels. Thromb Haemost 85:221-225, 2001.

86. Alessandri C, Basili S, Maurelli M, et al: Relationship between prothrombin activation fragment F1 + 2 and serum cholesterol. Haemostasis 26:214-219, 1996.

87. Wada H, Mori Y, Kaneko T, et al: Elevated plasma levels of vascular endothelial cell markers in patients with hypercholesterolemia. Am J Hematol 44:112-116, 1993.

88. Yorioka N, Masaki T, Ito T, et al: Lipid-lowering therapy and coagulation/fibrinolysis parameters in patients on peritoneal dialysis. Int J Artif Organs 23:27-32, 2000.

89. Lai T-S, Greenberg CS: Factor XIII. In High KA, Roberts HR (eds): Molecular Basis of Thrombosis and Hemostasis, 1st ed. New York, Marcel Dekker, 1995, pp 287-308.

90. Bock SC: Antithrombin III and heparin cofactor II. In Colman RW,

Hirsh J, Marder VJ, et al (eds): Hemostasis and Thrombosis: Basic Principles and Clinical Practice, 4th ed. Philadelphia, Lippincott Williams & Wilkins, 2001, pp 321-333.

91. Puccetti L, Bruni F, Bova G, et al: Role of platelets in tissue factor expression by monocytes in normal and hypercholesterolemic subjects: In vitro effect of cerivastatin. Int J Clin Lab Res 30:147-156, 2000.

92. Baetta R, Camera M, Comparato C, et al: Fluvastatin reduces tissue factor expression and macrophage accumulation in carotid lesions of cholesterol-fed rabbits in the absence of lipid lowering. Arterioscler Thromb Vasc Biol 22:692-698, 2001.

93. Camera M, Toschi V, Comparato C, et al: Cholesterol-induced thrombogenicity of the vessel wall: Inhibitory effect of fluvastatin. Thromb Haemost 87:748-755, 2002.

94. Eto M, Kozai T, Cosentino F, et al: Statin prevents tissue factor expression in human endothelial cells: Role of Rho/Rho-kinase and Akt pathways. Circulation 105:1756-1759, 2002.

95. Nagata K, Ishibashi T, Sakamoto T, et al: Rho/Rho-kinase is involved in the synthesis of tissue factor in human monocytes. Atherosclerosis 163:39-47, 2002.

96. Colli S, Eligini S, Lalli M, et al: Vastatins inhibit tissue factor in cultured human macrophages: A novel mechanism of protection against atherothrombosis. Arterioscler Thromb Vasc Biol 17:265-272, 1997.

97. Porreca E, Di Febbo C, Di Castelnuovo A, et al: Association of factor VII levels with inflammatory parameters in hypercholesterolemic patients. Atherosclerosis 165:159-166, 2002.

98. Mennen LI, Schouten EG, Grobbee DE, et al: Coagulation factor VII, dietary fat and blood lipids: A review. Thromb Haemost 76:492-499, 1996.

99. Heinrich J, Balleisen L, Schulte H, et al: Fibrinogen and factor VII in the prediction of coronary risk: Results from the PROCAM study in healthy men. Arterioscler Thromb 14:54-59, 1994.

100. Meade TW, Ruddock V, Stirling Y, et al: Fibrinolytic activity, clotting factors, and long-term incidence of ischaemic heart disease in the Northwick Park Heart Study. Lancet 342:1076-1079, 1993.

101. Ruddock V, Meade TW: Factor-VII activity and ischaemic heart disease: Fatal and non-fatal events. QJM 87:403-406, 1994.

102. Ural AU, Yilmaz MI, Avcu F, et al: Treatment with cerivastatin in primary mixed hyperlipidemia induces changes in platelet aggregation and coagulation system components. Int J Hematol 76:279-283, 2002.

103. Nordoy A, Bonaa KH, Sandset PM, et al: Effect of omega-3 fatty acids and simvastatin on hemostatic risk factors and postprandial hyperlipemia in patients with combined hyperlipemia. Arterioscler Thromb Vasc Biol 20:259-265, 2000.

104. Morishita E, Asakura H, Saito M, et al: Elevated plasma levels of free-form of TFPI antigen in hypercholesterolemic patients. Atherosclerosis 154:203-212, 2001.

105. Porreca E, Di Febbo C, Amore C, et al: Effect of lipid-lowering treatment on factor VII profile in hyperlipidemic patients. Thromb Haemost 84:789-793, 2000.

106. Sbarouni E, Melissari E, Kyriakides ZS, et al: Effects of simvastatin or hormone replacement therapy, or both, on fibrinogen, factor VII, and plasminogen activator inhibitor levels in postmenopausal women with proven coronary artery disease. Am J Cardiol 86:80-83, 2000.

12

107. Hansen JB, Huseby KR, Huseby NE, et al: Effect of cholesterol lowering on intravascular pools of TFPI and its anticoagulant potential in type II hyperlipoproteinemia. Arterioscler Thromb Vasc Biol 15:879-885, 1995.
108. Hansen JB, Huseby NE, Sandset PM, et al: Tissue-factor pathway inhibitor and lipoproteins: Evidence for association with and regulation by LDL in human plasma. Arterioscler Thromb 14:223-229, 1994.
109. Dittman WA, Nelson SC: Thrombomodulin. In High KA, Roberts HR (eds): Molecular Basis of Thrombosis and Hemostasis, 1st ed. New York, Marcel Dekker, 1995, pp 425-445.
110. Malyszko J, Malyszko JS, Hryszko T, et al: Effects of long-term treatment with simvastatin on some hemostatic parameters in continuous ambulatory peritoneal dialysis patients. Am J Nephrol 21:373-377, 2001.
111. Ambrosi P, Aillaud MF, Habib G, et al: Fluvastatin decreases soluble thrombomodulin in cardiac transplant recipients. Thromb Haemost 83:46-48, 2000.
112. Morikawa S, Takabe W, Mataki C, et al: The effect of statins on mRNA levels of genes related to inflammation, coagulation, and vascular constriction in HUVEC. Human umbilical vein endothelial cells. J Atheroscler Thromb 9:178-183, 2002.
113. Masamura K, Oida K, Kanehara H, et al: Pitavastatin-induced thrombomodulin expression by endothelial cells acts via inhibition of small G proteins of the Rho family. Arterioscler Thromb Vasc Biol 23:512-513, 2003.
114. Shi J, Wang J, Zheng H, et al: Statins increase thrombomodulin expression and function in human endothelial cells by a nitric oxide-dependent mechanism and counteract tumor necrosis factor alpha-induced thrombomodulin downregulation. Blood Coagul Fibrinolysis 14:575-585, 2003.
115. Sessa WC: Can modulation of endothelial nitric oxide synthase explain the vasculoprotective actions of statins? Trends Mol Med 7:189-191, 2002.
116. Wiesbauer F, Kaun C, Zorn G, et al: HMG CoA reductase inhibitors affect the fibrinolytic system of human vascular cells in vitro: A comparative study using different statins. Br J Pharmacol 135:284-292, 2002.
117. Archipoff G, Beretz A, Bartha K, et al: Role of cyclic AMP in promoting the thromboresistance of human endothelial cells by enhancing thrombomodulin and decreasing tissue factor activities. Br J Pharmacol 109:18-28, 1993.
118. Shibakura M, Koyama T, Saito T, et al: Anticoagulant effects of synthetic retinoids mediated via different receptors on human leukemia and umbilical vein endothelial cells. Blood 90:1545-1551, 1997.
119. Conway EM, Liu L, Nowakowski B, et al: Heat shock of vascular endothelial cells induces an up-regulatory transcriptional response of the thrombomodulin gene that is delayed in onset and does not attenuate. J Biol Chem 269:22804-22810, 1994.
120. Uchiba M, Okajima K, Murakami K, et al: Recombinant human soluble thrombomodulin reduces endotoxin-induced pulmonary vascular injury via protein C activation in rats. Thromb Haemost 74:1265-1270, 1995.
121. Mohri M, Gonda Y, Oka M, et al: The antithrombotic effects of

recombinant human soluble thrombomodulin (rhsTM) on tissue factor-induced disseminated intravascular coagulation in crab-eating monkeys *(Macaca fascicularis)*. Blood Coagul Fibrinolysis 8:274-283, 1997.

122. Bernard GR, Vincent JL, Laterre PF, et al: Efficacy and safety of recombinant human activated protein C for severe sepsis. N Engl J Med 344:699-709, 2001.

123. Faust SN, Levin M, Harrison OB, et al: Dysfunction of endothelial protein C activation in severe meningococcal sepsis. N Engl J Med 345:408-416, 2001.

124. Cone JB, Ferrer TJ, Wallace BH, et al: Alterations in endothelial thrombomodulin expression in zymosan-induced lung injury. J Trauma 54:731-736, 2003.

125. Salom RN, Maguire JA, Hancock WW: Endothelial activation and cytokine expression in human acute cardiac allograft rejection. Pathology 30:24-29, 1998.

126. Kim AY, Walinsky PL, Kolodgie FD, et al: Early loss of thrombomodulin expression impairs vein graft thromboresistance: Implications for vein graft failure. Circ Res 90:205-212, 2002.

127. Labarrere CA, Faulk WP: Microvascular perturbations in human allografts: Analogies in preeclamptic placentae. Am J Reprod Immunol 2:109-116, 1992.

128. Boehme MW, Autschbach F, Zuna I, et al: Elevated serum levels and reduced immunohistochemical expression of thrombomodulin in active ulcerative colitis. Gastroenterology 113:107-117, 1997.

129. Richter KK, Fink LM, Hughes BM, et al: Is the loss of endothelial thrombomodulin involved in the mechanism of chronicity in late radiation enteropathy? Radiother Oncol 44:65-71, 1997.

130. Hauer-Jensen M, Kong FM, Fink LM, Anscher MS: Circulating thrombomodulin during radiation therapy of lung cancer. Radiat Oncol Investig 7:238-242, 1999.

131. Wang J, Zheng H, Ou X, et al: Deficiency of microvascular thrombomodulin and up-regulation of protease-activated receptor-1 in irradiated rat intestine: Possible link between endothelial dysfunction and chronic radiation fibrosis. Am J Pathol 160:2063-2072, 2002.

132. Liappis AP, Kan VL, Rochester CG, et al: The effect of statins on mortality in patients with bacteremia. Clin Infect Dis 33:1352-1357, 2001.

133. Davi G, Ganci A, Averna M, et al: Thromboxane biosynthesis, neutrophil and coagulative activation in type IIa hypercholesterolemia. Thromb Haemost 74:1015-1019, 1995.

134. Opper C, Clement C, Schwarz H, et al: Increased number of high sensitive platelets in hypercholesterolemia, cardiovascular diseases, and after incubation with cholesterol. Atherosclerosis 113:211-217, 1995.

135. Tremoli E, Colli S, Maderna P, et al: Hypercholesterolemia and platelets. Semin Thromb Hemost 19:115-121, 1993.

136. Eynard AR, Tremoli E, Caruso D, et al: Platelet formation of 12-hydroxyeicosatetraenoic acid and thromboxane B2 is increased in type IIA hypercholesterolemic subjects. Atherosclerosis 60:61-66, 1986.

137. Fusman R, Rotstein R, Berliner S, et al: The concomitant appearance of aggregated erythrocytes, leukocytes and platelets in the peripheral blood of patients with risk factors for atherothrombosis. Clin Hemorheol Microcirc 25:165-173, 2001.

12

138. Di Minno G, Silver MJ, Cerbone AM, et al: Increased fibrinogen binding to platelets from patients with familial hypercholesterolemia. Arteriosclerosis 6:203-211, 1986.

139. Aoki I, Shimoyama K, Aoki N, et al: Platelet-dependent thrombin generation in patients with diabetes mellitus: Effects of glycemic control on coagulability in diabetes. J Am Coll Cardiol 27:560-566, 1996.

140. Hjemdahl P: Smoking, nicotine and thrombotic risk: A role for platelet dependent thrombin generation. Eur Heart J 22:16-18, 2001.

141. Kawano TA, Aoki N, Homori M, et al: Mental stress and physical exercise increase platelet-dependent thrombin generation. Heart Vessels 15:280-288, 2000.

142. Notarbartolo A, Davi G, Averna M, et al: Inhibition of thromboxane biosynthesis and platelet function by simvastatin in type IIa hypercholesterolemia. Arterioscler Thromb Vasc Biol 15:247-251, 1995.

143. Davi G, Averna M, Catalano I, et al: Increased thromboxane biosynthesis in type IIa hypercholesterolemia. Circulation 85:1792-1798, 1992.

144. Baldassarre D, Mores N, Colli S, et al: Platelet alpha 2-adrenergic receptors in hypercholesterolemia: Relationship between binding studies and epinephrine-induced platelet aggregation. Clin Pharmacol Ther 61:684-691, 1997.

145. Quan Sang KH, Levenson J, Megnien JL, et al: Platelet cytosolic Ca^{2+} and membrane dynamics in patients with primary hypercholesterolemia: Effects of pravastatin. Arterioscler Thromb Vasc Biol 15:759-764, 1995.

146. Stuart MJ, Gerrard JM, White JG: Effect of cholesterol on production of thromboxane b2 by platelets in vitro. N Engl J Med 302:6-10, 1980.

147. Puccetti L, Pasqui AL, Pastorelli M, et al: Time-dependent effect of statins on platelet function in hypercholesterolaemia. Eur J Clin Invest 32:901-908, 2002.

148. Ma LP, Nie DN, Hsu SX, et al: Inhibition of platelet aggregation and expression of alpha granule membrane protein 140 and thromboxane B2 with pravastatin therapy for hypercholesterolemia. J Assoc Acad Minor Phys 13:23-26, 2002.

149. Huhle G, Abletshauser C, Mayer N, et al: Reduction of platelet activity markers in type II hypercholesterolemic patients by a HMG-CoA-reductase inhibitor. Thromb Res 95:229-234, 1999.

150. Romano M, Mezzetti A, Marulli C, et al: Fluvastatin reduces soluble P-selectin and ICAM-1 levels in hypercholesterolemic patients: Role of nitric oxide. J Investig Med 48:183-189, 2000.

151. Seljeflot I, Tonstad S, Hjermann I, et al: Reduced expression of endothelial cell markers after 1 year treatment with simvastatin and atorvastatin in patients with coronary heart disease. Atherosclerosis 162:179-185, 2002.

152. Garlichs CD, John S, Schmeisser A, et al: Upregulation of CD40 and CD40 ligand (CD154) in patients with moderate hypercholesterolemia. Circulation 104:2395-2400, 2001.

153. Hochgraf E, Levy Y, Aviram M, et al: Lovastatin decreases plasma and platelet cholesterol levels and normalizes elevated platelet fluidity and aggregation in hypercholesterolemic patients. Metab Clin Exp 43:11-17, 1994.

154. Kaczmarek D, Hohlfeld T, Wambach G, et al: The actions of lovastatin

12

on platelet function and platelet eicosanoid receptors in type II hypercholesterolaemia. A double-blind, placebo-controlled, prospective study. Eur J Clin Pharmacol 45:451-457, 1993.

155. Osamah H, Mira R, Sorina S, et al: Reduced platelet aggregation after fluvastatin therapy is associated with altered platelet lipid composition and drug binding to the platelets. Br J Clin Pharmacol 44:77-83, 1997.

156. Aviram M, Hussein O, Rosenblat M, et al: Interactions of platelets, macrophages, and lipoproteins in hypercholesterolemia: Antiatherogenic effects of HMG-CoA reductase inhibitor therapy. J Cardiovasc Pharmacol 31:39-45, 1998.

157. Davi G, Averna M, Novo S, et al: Effects of synvinolin on platelet aggregation and thromboxane B2 synthesis in type IIa hypercholesterolemic patients. Atherosclerosis 79:79-83, 1989.

158. Funk CD: Platelet eicosanoids. In Colman RW, Hirsh J, Marder VJ, et al (eds): Hemostasis and Thrombosis: Basic Principles and Clinical Practice, 4th ed. Philadelphia, Lippincott Williams & Wilkins, 2001, pp 533-559.

159. Plana JC, Jones PH: The use of statins in acute coronary syndromes: The mechanisms behind the outcomes. Curr Atheroscler Rep 3:355-364, 2001.

160. Schror K, Lobel P, Steinhagen-Thiessen E: Simvastatin reduces platelet thromboxane formation and restores normal platelet sensitivity against prostacyclin in type IIa hypercholesterolemia. Eicosanoids 2:39-45, 1989.

161. Tannous M, Cheung R, Vignini A, et al: Atorvastatin increases ecNOS levels in human platelets of hyperlipidemic subjects. Thromb Haemost 82:1390-1394, 1999.

162. Laufs U, Gertz K, Huang P, et al: Atorvastatin upregulates type III nitric oxide synthase in thrombocytes, decreases platelet activation, and protects from cerebral ischemia in normocholesterolemic mice. Stroke 31:2442-2449, 2000.

163. Chirkov YY, Holmes AS, Willoughby SR, et al: Stable angina and acute coronary syndromes are associated with nitric oxide resistance in platelets. J Am Coll Cardiol 37:1851-1857, 2001.

164. Dmoszynska A, Kleinrok A, Dabrowski P, et al: Effect of lovastatin on platelet function in hypercholesterolemic patients. Pol Arch Med Wewn 88:287-294, 1992.

165. Hale LP, Craver KT, Berrier AM, et al: Combination of fosinopril and pravastatin decreases platelet response to thrombin receptor agonist in monkeys. Arterioscler Thromb Vasc Biol 18:1643-1646, 1998.

166. Glomset JA, Farnsworth CC: Role of protein modification reactions in programming interactions between ras-related GTPases and cell membranes. Annu Rev Cell Biol 10:181-205, 1994.

167. Rosenson RS, Tangney CC: Antiatherothrombotic properties of statins: Implications for cardiovascular event reduction. JAMA 279:1643-1650, 1998.

168. Broijersen A, Eriksson M, Leijd B, et al: No influence of simvastatin treatment on platelet function in vivo in patients with hypercholesterolemia. Arterioscler Thromb Vasc Biol 17:273-278, 1997.

169. Shalaev SV, Safiullina ZM, Zhuravleva TD, et al: Effects of lovastatin (mevacor) on platelet function in hypercholesterolemia in patients with ischemic heart disease. Kardiologiia 32:19-21, 1992.

12

170. Broijersen A, Eriksson M, Larsson PT, et al: Effects of selective LDL-apheresis and pravastatin therapy on platelet function in familial hypercholesterolaemia. Eur J Clin Invest 24:488-498, 1994.

171. Mikhailova IA, Lipovetskii BM, Konstantinov VO, et al: The thrombocyte function of subjects with atherogenic hyperlipidemias during lovastatin treatment. Kardiologiia 33:60-63, 1993.

172. Gurevich VS, Bondarenko BB, Mikhailova IA, et al: Evidence of combined therapy of dyslipoproteinemia by HMG-CoA reductase inhibitors and "essential" phospholipids. Clin Ter 142:329-334, 1993.

173. Bevilacqua M, Bettica P, Milani M, et al: Effect of fluvastatin on lipids and fibrinolysis in coronary artery disease. Am J Cardiol 79:84-87, 1997.

174. Seljeflot I, Tonstad S, Hjermann I, et al: Improved fibrinolysis after 1-year treatment with HMG CoA reductase inhibitors in patients with coronary heart disease. Thromb Res 105:285-290, 2002.

175. Nakano H, Yamada K, Nishimura M, et al: Effect of hypercholesteremia on vascular endothelial function and albumin excretion rate in patients with diabetes mellitus. Jpn J Nephrol 38:507-512, 1996.

176. Chandler WL, Levy WC, Stratton JR: The circulatory regulation of TPA and UPA secretion, clearance, and inhibition during exercise and during the infusion of isoproterenol and phenylephrine. Circulation 92:2984-2994, 1995.

177. Jansson JH, Olofsson BO, Nilsson TK: Predictive value of tissue plasminogen activator mass concentration on long-term mortality in patients with coronary artery disease: A 7-year follow-up. Circulation 88:2030-2034, 1993.

178. Ridker PM, Vaughan DE, Stampfer MJ, et al: Endogenous tissue-type plasminogen activator and risk of myocardial infarction. Lancet 341:1165-1168, 1993.

179. Thompson SG, Kienast J, Pyke SD, et al: Hemostatic factors and the risk of myocardial infarction or sudden death in patients with angina pectoris. European Concerted Action on Thrombosis and Disabilities Angina Pectoris Study Group. N Engl J Med 332:635-641, 1995.

180. Emeis JJ, Cohen LH: Another view of hydroxymethylglutaryl coenzyme A (HMG-CoA) reductase inhibitors and the fibrinolytic system. Am J Cardiol 80:977-978, 1997.

181. Chang JW, Yang WS, Min WK, et al: Effects of simvastatin on high-sensitivity C-reactive protein and serum albumin in hemodialysis patients. Am J Kidney Dis 39:1213-1217, 2002.

182. Joukhadar C, Klein N, Prinz M, et al: Similar effects of atorvastatin, simvastatin and pravastatin on thrombogenic and inflammatory parameters in patients with hypercholesterolemia. Thromb Haemost 85:47-51, 2001.

183. Bourcier T, Libby P: HMG CoA reductase inhibitors reduce plasminogen activator inhibitor-1 expression by human vascular smooth muscle and endothelial cells. Arterioscler Thromb Vasc Biol 20:556-562, 2000.

184. Lopez S, Peiretti F, Bonardo B, et al: Effect of atorvastatin and fluvastatin on the expression of plasminogen activator inhibitor type-1 in cultured human endothelial cells. Atherosclerosis 152:359-366, 2000.

185. Mussoni L, Banfi C, Sironi L, et al: Fluvastatin inhibits basal and stimulated plasminogen activator inhibitor 1, but induces tissue type

plasminogen activator in cultured human endothelial cells. Thromb Haemost 84:59-64, 2000.

186. Seeger H, Wallwiener D, Mueck AO: Lipid-independent effects of an estrogen-statin combination: Inhibition of expression of adhesion molecules and plasminogen activator inhibitor-1 in human endothelial cell cultures. Climacteric 4:209-214, 2001.

187. Essig M, Nguyen G, Prie D, et al: 3-Hydroxy-3-methylglutaryl coenzyme A reductase inhibitors increase fibrinolytic activity in rat aortic endothelial cells: Role of geranylgeranylation and Rho proteins. Circ Res 83:683-690, 1998.

12

Effects of Statins on Endothelial Progenitor Cells: Mobilization, Differentiation, and Contribution to Adult Neovascularization

Dirk H. Walter, Takayuki Asahara, and Douglas W. Losordo

Recent trials provide a wealth of data documenting the benefit of cholesterol-lowering therapy with HMG-CoA reductase inhibitors, or statins, in both primary and secondary prevention of coronary heart disease and stroke.[1-3] A growing body of evidence indicates that statins possess favorable effects independent of, or at least in addition to, their lipid-lowering capacity. These effects include inhibition of smooth muscle cell proliferation, reduction of platelet aggregation, and attenuation of vascular inflammation.[4] Statins have also been shown to decrease neointimal thickening and clinical events and angiographic restenosis after coronary stent implantation.[5,6] In vivo studies have established that statins may also promote angiogenesis in ischemic limbs in a manner analogous to that seen with endothelial cell mitogens such as vascular endothelial growth factors (VEGFs), beta-fibroblast growth factor (β-FGF), or estrogens,[7-12] suggesting a direct influence on endothelial biology.

Intriguing experimental data and clinical studies suggest that the beneficial effect of statins on cardiovascular disease[13] and bone fractures[14] may be based on a common mechanism—that is, neovascularization. In this respect, the vascular endothelium represents the key regulatory component of the vessel wall. Evidence has accumulated that statins might specifically exert their beneficial effects by modulating endothelial cell function.[15-17] Statins have been shown to alter endothelium-derived nitric oxide (NO) bioavailability, thereby attenuating endothelial dysfunction and atherosclerotic disease progression.[18]

In this regard, it is important to recognize that withdrawal or discontinuation of statins can abrogate their clinical effect and immediately reverse the beneficial effect based on NO bioavailability.[19,20]

ROLE OF ENDOTHELIAL PROGENITOR CELLS IN ANGIOGENESIS

In recent years, the understanding of the processes responsible for the formation of new blood vessels after tissue ischemia has dramatically changed. In the past, the vascularization of ischemic tissues was believed to be caused by the migration and proliferation of mature endothelial cells—a process termed angiogenesis. Experimental evidence suggests that circulating endothelial progenitor cells (EPCs) derived from the bone marrow exhibit features of endothelial cells, go to (or *home* to) sites of ischemia, and contribute to the formation of new blood vessels, a process referred to as vasculogenesis.[21,22] Further, it appears that mature endothelial cells and immature EPCs together contribute to neovascularization after critical ischemia.

Importantly, mobilization of bone marrow–derived EPCs augments neovascularization of ischemic tissue and represents a potentially useful strategy for clinical therapy.[23] The isolation of bone marrow–derived circulating progenitor cells from peripheral blood, their differentiation into an endothelial phenotype under culture conditions, and their contribution to adult neovascularization was first described in 1997.[23] Since then, other groups have shown that bone marrow–derived or peripheral blood CD34+ cells, or mononuclear cells, give rise to endothelial cells under appropriate culture conditions.[23-30] These cells are characterized by their uptake of diacetylated low-density lipoprotein (LDL) and positive staining for CD31, typical features of endothelial cells and monocytic cell lineages.[23] Expression of the endothelial NO-synthase and the receptor for VEGF (i.e., VEGF receptor 2, Flk-1/KDR), as well as von Willebrand factor, vascular endothelial (VE) cadherin, CD146, or endoglin (CD105), was detected in the outgrowing cells (Fig. 13-1).[27,31,32]

Characterization of these "endothelial" progenitor cells, determination of their contribution to adult neovascularization, and identification of potential means of mobilization are currently being investigated. The pharmacologic modulation of functional properties and the determination of the fate of these cells in different microenvironments are also under intense investigation.[33]

Novel insights into the molecular and cellular processes contributing to the formation of new blood vessels may lead to new therapeutic applications. By using this approach, several groups have demonstrated that ex vivo expanded EPCs or bone marrow transplanted cells home to sites of ischemia and contribute to the formation of new blood vessels.[31,32,34] Transplantation of ex vivo

Important markers for hematopoietic and endothelial progenitor cells

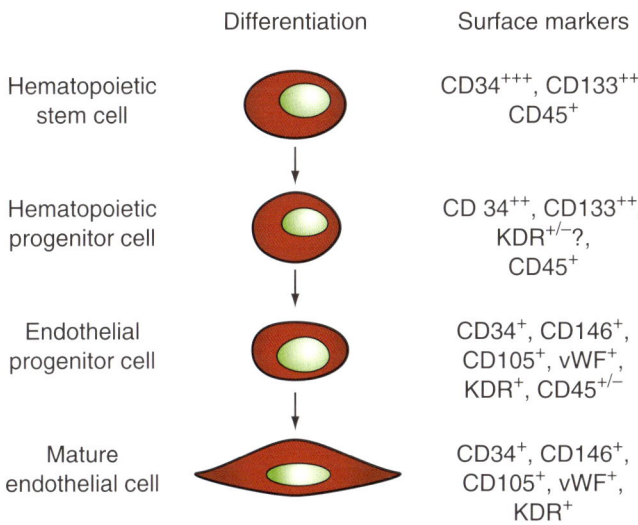

	Differentiation	Surface markers
Hematopoietic stem cell		$CD34^{+++}$, $CD133^{++}$, $CD45^+$
Hematopoietic progenitor cell		$CD\ 34^{++}$, $CD133^{++}$, $KDR^{+/-}$?, $CD45^+$
Endothelial progenitor cell		$CD34^+$, $CD146^+$, $CD105^+$, vWF^+, KDR^+, $CD45^{+/-}$
Mature endothelial cell		$CD34^+$, $CD146^+$, $CD105^+$, vWF^+, KDR^+

Figure 13-1 Important markers for hematopoietic and endothelial progenitor cells. During differentiation from hematopoietic stem cells, surface marker expression varies or changes.

13

expanded EPCs or isolated hematopoietic progenitor cells has been shown to improve blood flow recovery and capillary density after peripheral limb ischemia[28,29,32] and after myocardial infarction.[35-37] Importantly, transplantation of EPCs after myocardial infarction has been shown to increase cardiac function and reduce left ventricular fibrosis.

Soon after evaluation of the concept of progenitor cell transplantation for regeneration of ischemic tissues (Fig. 13-2), clinical studies were begun and demonstrated safety and feasibility of autologous progenitor cell or bone marrow cell transplantation in patients with ischemic heart disease.[38-41] These studies were highly suggestive of a beneficial effect on the postinfarction remodeling processes. These effects were seen despite the fact that relatively low numbers of progenitor cells, somewhere between 3% and 25%, have been shown in animal models to incorporate into ischemic tissues.[34,42-44] Of note, chemokines and cytokines that are released during tissue ischemia or vascular trauma are capable of activating the endogenous regeneration mechanisms that attract circulating EPCs to the site of injury.

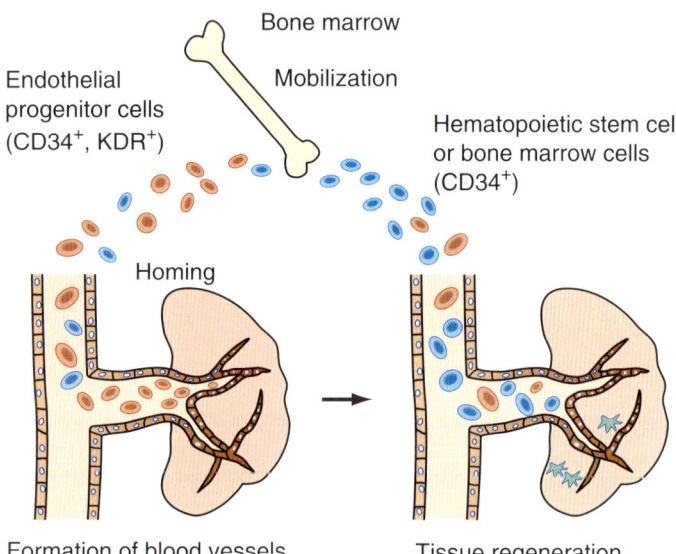

Figure 13-2 Potential of current cell therapy using CD34[+] hematopoietic progenitor cells, bone marrow cells, or ex vivo expanded circulating endothelial progenitor cells: contribution to neovascularization and tissue regeneration.

13

MOBILIZATION OF PROGENITOR CELLS BY CYTOKINES

Several cytokines and chemokines have been shown to promote mobilization of hematopoietic stem cells and EPCs (Fig. 13-3). Granulocyte colony-stimulating factor (G-CSF) is a widely used and the best characterized cytokine in clinical stem cell transplantation. G-CSF mobilizes stem cells by disrupting the surface receptors that are required for homing of stem cells in the bone marrow. This is accomplished by proteolytic cleavage of adhesion receptors or the chemokine receptor CXCR4,[45,46] a common mechanism in stem cell mobilization. In animal models, cytokine-induced stem cell mobilization with G-CSF resulted in improved cardiac function after myocardial ischemia.[47] In addition, reinjection of isolated, G-CSF–mobilized adult human CD34[+] cells with properties of embryonic hemangioblasts stimulated neo-angiogenesis in the infarcted tissue.[35] However, recent data indicate that G-CSF results in an impairment of the activity of EPCs from patients with ischemic heart disease (S. Dimmeler, personal communication, 2003), suggesting the need for other pharmacologic

Mechanisms of stem cell mobilization from the bone marrow niche

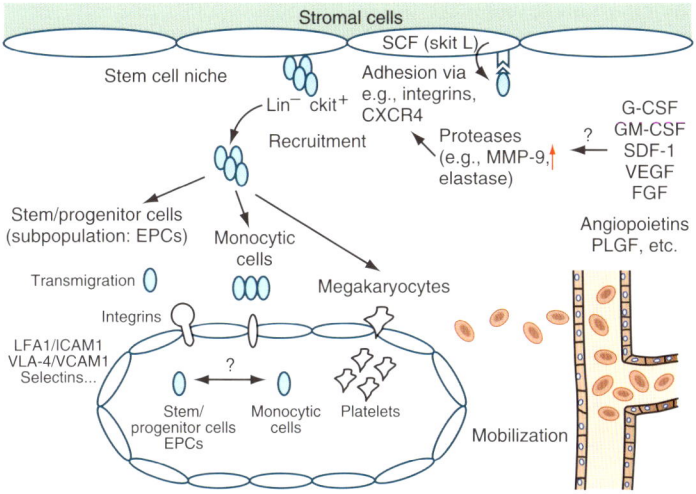

Figure 13-3 Mechanisms of stem cell mobilization from the bone marrow niche. Mobilizing agents recruit stem cells by disruption of cell-cell or cell-stroma contact. Transmigrating cells enter the bloodstream via endothelial sinusoids. Progenitor cells circulate and home to sites of ischemia. EPCs, endothelial progenitor cells; FGF, fibroblast growth factor; G-CSF, granulocyte colony-stimulating factor; GM-CSF, granulocyte-macrophage colony-stimulating factor; MMP, matrix metalloproteinase; PLGF, placental growth factor; SCF, stem cell factor; SDF-1, stromal cell–derived factor-1; VEGF, vascular endothelial growth factor.

strategies to amplify therapeutic cell transplantation by altering functional parameters.

Another cytokine, granulocyte-macrophage colony-stimulating factor (GM-CSF), was also shown to promote mobilization of EPCs with a corresponding improvement in hind-limb neovascularization.[48] Interestingly, clinical studies indicate that collateral flow to the myocardial vascular bed is increased after GM-CSF application.[49]

Angiogenic growth factors, including VEGF, angiopoietins, and FGFs, also act as EPC-mobilizing agents and promote incorporation of these cells into sites of postnatal neovascularization.[50,51] Furthermore, placental growth factor (PLGF), previously known to have a synergistic effect with VEGF,[52] was also shown to stimulate angiogenesis and collateral growth in ischemic hearts and limbs with an efficiency at least comparable to that of VEGF,[53] and to induce recruitment of bone marrow–derived EPCs.[54] Synergistic effects have been shown for angiopoietins such as Ang-1, the ligand for Tie-2, which is also expressed on EPCs. Stromal cell–derived factor-1, the ligand for the chemokine receptor CXCR4, represents an important stimulus for the recruitment of EPCs and influences their homing to sites of ischemic neovascularization.[55-58] Endogenous mobilization of stem or progenitor cells by exogenous colony-stimulating factors or angiogenic growth factors might thus be one way to modulate recruitment of bone marrow–derived EPCs and thereby induce therapeutic neovascularization.

Naturally, elucidating and understanding the mechanisms involved in stem cell mobilization will be crucial for therapeutic applications.[59]

STATINS AND PROGENITOR CELL DIFFERENTIATION AND MOBILIZATION

In vitro experiments have demonstrated that statins potently augment the differentiation of EPCs out of mononuclear cells and CD34-positive hematopoietic stem cells isolated from peripheral blood.[27,60] Treatment of mice with statins was shown to augment c-kit+/Sca-1+–positive hematopoietic stem cells in the bone marrow and to further increase the number of differentiated EPCs.

Indeed, in patients with stable coronary artery disease,[61] treatment with statins was shown to enhance the number of circulating EPCs, and the results were comparable to those in patients undergoing VEGF gene transfer for ischemia.[62] The functional consequence of EPC mobilization by statins was illustrated in recent studies showing endothelial repair at the site of arterial injury.[63,64] It was long believed that the endothelial regeneration process involved proliferation and migration from mature endothelial cells adjacent to the site of injury. However, circulating bone marrow–derived EPCs home to the sites of endothelial disruption and incorporate into nascent endothelium.

Bone marrow–derived cells of endothelial lineage mobilized in response to statins exhibit enhanced adhesion as well as integrin expression involving integrin receptors $\alpha_5\beta_1$ and $\alpha_v\beta_5$, receptors for two classic integrins known to play a crucial role in angiogenesis signaling.[65,66] These findings suggest that statins modulate adhesiveness of EPCs to support homing to the sites of vascular injury (Fig. 13-4).

Thus, in addition to the number (or differentiation) of circulating cells, the functions of cells involving migratory activity, adhesiveness, and homing capacity appear to be critical parameters for therapeutic cell transplantation.

It is noteworthy that EPCs from patients with coronary artery disease[30] or diabetes[67] are functionally impaired, resulting in reduced migratory activity and homing capacity. The functional capacity of EPCs has been shown to tightly correlate with risk factors for coronary artery disease. Given the important role of

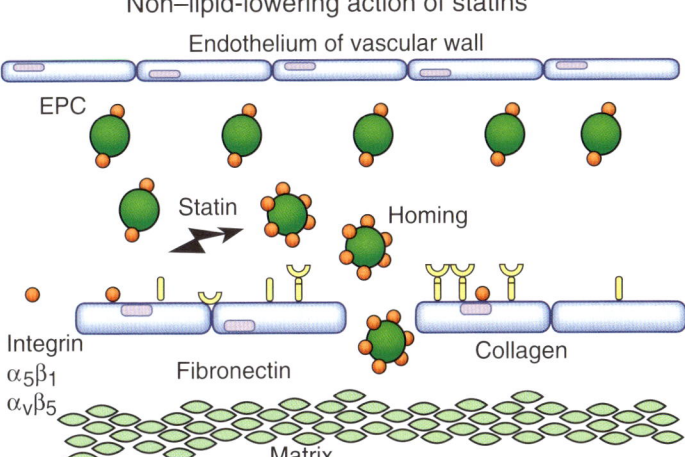

Figure 13-4 Non–lipid-lowering action of statins. Statins up-regulate integrin receptor expression to promote adhesion and modulate homing of bone marrow–derived endothelial progenitor cells to sites of endothelial disruption following balloon denudation of carotid arteries. EPC, endothelial progenitor cell.

EPCs in the neovascularization of ischemic tissue, the decrease in EPC numbers and the impairment of their activity may contribute to impaired neovascularization in these patients, perhaps partly explaining the impaired angiogenesis reported in previous studies.[68,69] Hill and colleagues have shown that the number of EPCs may be a surrogate biologic marker for vascular function and cumulative cardiovascular risk in apparently healthy men.[70]

These findings suggest that endothelial injury in the absence of sufficient circulating progenitor cells may affect the progression of cardiovascular disease. Therefore, interfering with the mechanisms underlying the functional impairment of EPCs from patients with coronary artery disease, and investigating the signal transduction pathways responsible for this phenomenon, will be crucial to improve therapy.

In addition to influencing the number and differentiation of endothelial progenitor cells, statin treatment offers a useful tool to increase functional activity of EPCs from patients with coronary artery disease.[27,61,63] Nevertheless, controversy exists regarding the potential pro- and antiangiogenic effects of statins.[71,72] Pro-angiogenic effects, in line with EPC mobilization and differentiation, occur at low doses corresponding to physiologic levels achieved in clinical practice, whereas antiangiogenic effects are seen at high or toxic doses that are never reached by oral administration of statins in clinical settings. Importantly, in addition to the dose dependency, there appears to be a class effect among different types of statins.

The mechanism by which statins affect EPC differentiation and function is not completely understood, but it appears to be unrelated to a reduction in serum cholesterol. Statins and growth factors such as VEGF seem to share a common signaling pathway involving activation of the phosphatidylinositol 3-kinase (PI3K)/Akt cascade, but it is still not known how statins activate PI3K/Akt. Recent studies indicated that statin-mediated activation of Akt is the result of the inhibition of mevalonate formation, but further studies are required to fully elucidate the underlying mechanisms.[7,27, 60] Alternatively, statins might play a central role for the survival of EPCs in ischemic tissues. Activation of the PI3K/Akt pathway might also have further downstream targets involving inhibition of apoptosis, modulation of migratory activity, and expression of cell cycle regulatory proteins.

Statins also inhibit senescence of EPCs. This effect appears to be mediated by the regulation of various cell cycle proteins.[73] Thus, inhibition of senescence of EPCs and induction of their proliferation by statins in vitro may result in improvement of their functional activity. Other studies demonstrate that EPCs from healthy volunteers and from patients with coronary artery disease can also transdifferentiate in vitro into functionally active cardiomyocytes when co-cultivated with cardiomyocytes. This requires either cell-to-cell contact or cellular fusion to mediate the EPC transdifferentiation. However, this issue has not been fully resolved.[74-76] Overall, the therapeutic use of autologous EPCs may aid in cardiomyocyte regeneration, at least to some extent, in patients with ischemic heart disease, thereby potentially contributing to organ-specific regeneration.

In summary, statins are potent drugs with effects on mobilization, differentiation, and survival of EPCs. These agents may also reverse impaired functional capacity of EPCs in patients with risk factors for coronary artery disease or documented active coronary artery disease. Augmentation of functionally active EPCs with improved homing capacity will be a critical step in advancing therapeutic neovascularization.

References

1. Scandinavian Simvastatin Survival Study Group: Randomised trial of cholesterol lowering in 4444 patients with coronary heart disease: The Scandinavian Simvastatin Survival Study (4S). Lancet 344:1383-1389, 1994.
2. The Long-Term Intervention with Pravastatin in Ischaemic Disease (LIPID) Study Group: Prevention of cardiovascular events and death with pravastatin in patients with coronary heart disease and a broad range of initial cholesterol levels. N Engl J Med 339:1349-1357, 1998.

3. Sacks FM, Pfeffer MA, Moye LA, et al: The effect of pravastatin on coronary events after myocardial infarction in patients with average cholesterol levels. Cholesterol and Recurrent Events Trial investigators. N Engl J Med 335:1001-1009, 1996.

4. Rosenson RS, Tangney CC: Antiatherothrombotic properties of statins: Implications for cardiovascular event reduction. JAMA 279:1643-1650, 1998.

5. Indolfi C, Cioppa A, Stabile E, et al: Effects of hydroxymethylglutaryl coenzyme A reductase inhibitor simvastatin on smooth muscle cell proliferation in vitro and neointimal formation in vivo after vascular injury. J Am Coll Cardiol 35:214-221, 2000.

6. Walter DH, Schachinger V, Elsner M, et al: Effect of statin therapy on restenosis after coronary stent implantation. Am J Cardiol 85:962-968, 2000.

7. Kureishi Y, Luo Z, Shiojima I, et al: The HMG-CoA reductase inhibitor simvastatin activates the protein kinase Akt and promotes angiogenesis in normocholesterolemic animals. Nat Med 6:1004-1010, 2000.

8. Takeshita S, Zheng LP, Brogi E, et al: Therapeutic angiogenesis: A single intraarterial bolus of vascular endothelial growth factor augments revascularization in a rabbit ischemic hind limb model. J Clin Invest 93:662-670, 1994.

9. Meurice T, Bauters C, Auffray JL, et al: Basic fibroblast growth factor restores endothelium-dependent responses after balloon injury of rabbit arteries. Circulation 93:18-22, 1996.

10. Pare G, Krust A, Karas RH, et al: Estrogen receptor-alpha mediates the protective effects of estrogen against vascular injury. Circ Res 90:1087-1092, 2002.

11. Krasinski K, Spyridopoulos I, Asahara T, et al: Estradiol accelerates functional endothelial recovery after arterial injury. Circulation 95:1768-1772, 1997.

12. Mendelsohn ME, Karas RH: The protective effects of estrogen on the cardiovascular system. N Engl J Med 340:1801-1811, 1999.

13. Laufs U, Liao JK: Rapid effects of statins: From prophylaxis to therapy for ischemic stroke. Arterioscler Thromb Vasc Biol 23:156-157, 2003.

14. Wierzbicki AS, Reynolds TM: Statins and fractures. Lancet 357:1887-1889, 2001.

15. Wolfrum S, Jensen KS, Liao JK: Endothelium-dependent effects of statins. Arterioscler Thromb Vasc Biol 23:729-736, 2003.

16. Treasure CB, Klein JL, Weintraub WS, et al: Beneficial effects of cholesterol-lowering therapy on the coronary endothelium in patients with coronary artery disease. N Engl J Med 332:481-487, 1995.

17. Dupuis J, Tardif JC, Cernacek P, Theroux P: Cholesterol reduction rapidly improves endothelial function after acute coronary syndromes. The RECIFE (Reduction of Cholesterol in Ischemia and Function of the Endothelium) trial. Circulation 99:3227-3233, 1999.

18. Laufs U, La Fata V, Plutzky J, Liao JK: Upregulation of endothelial nitric oxide synthase by HMG CoA reductase inhibitors. Circulation 97:1129-1135, 1998.

19. Heeschen C, Hamm CW, Laufs U, et al: Withdrawal of statins in patients with acute coronary syndromes. Circulation 107:e27, 2003.

20. Laufs U, Endres M, Custodis F, et al: Suppression of endothelial nitric oxide production after withdrawal of statin treatment is mediated by

13

negative feedback regulation of rho GTPase gene transcription. Circulation 102:3104-3110, 2000.

21. Isner JM, Asahara T: Angiogenesis and vasculogenesis as therapeutic strategies for postnatal neovascularization. J Clin Invest 103:1231-1236, 1999.

22. Carmeliet P: Mechanisms of angiogenesis and arteriogenesis. Nat Med 6:389-395, 2000.

23. Asahara T, Murohara T, Sullivan A, et al: Isolation of putative progenitor endothelial cells for angiogenesis. Science 275:964-967, 1997.

24. Shi Q, Rafii S, Wu MH, et al: Evidence for circulating bone marrow-derived endothelial cells. Blood 92:362-367, 1998.

25. Bhattacharya V, McSweeney PA, Shi Q, et al: Enhanced endothelialization and microvessel formation in polyester grafts seeded with CD34(+) bone marrow cells. Blood 95:581-585, 2000.

26. Peichev M, Naiyer AJ, Pereira D, et al: Expression of VEGFR-2 and AC133 by circulating human CD34(+) cells identifies a population of functional endothelial precursors. Blood 95:952-958, 2000.

27. Dimmeler S, Aicher A, Vasa M, et al: HMG-CoA reductase inhibitors (statins) increase endothelial progenitor cells via the PI 3-kinase/Akt pathway. J Clin Invest 108:391-397, 2001.

28. Murohara T, Ikeda H, Duan J, et al: Transplanted cord blood-derived endothelial precursor cells augment postnatal neovascularization. J Clin Invest 105:1527-1536, 2000.

29. Schatteman GC, Hanlon HD, Jiao C, et al: Blood-derived angioblasts accelerate blood-flow restoration in diabetic mice. J Clin Invest 106:571-578, 2000.

30. Vasa M, Fichtlscherer S, Aicher A, et al: Number and migratory activity of circulating endothelial progenitor cells inversely correlate with risk factors for coronary artery disease. Circ Res 89:E1-7, 2001.

31. Asahara T, Masuda H, Takahashi T, et al: Bone marrow origin of endothelial progenitor cells responsible for postnatal vasculogenesis in physiological and pathological neovascularization. Circ Res 85:221-228, 1999.

32. Kalka C, Masuda H, Takahashi T, et al: Transplantation of ex vivo expanded endothelial progenitor cells for therapeutic neovascularization. Proc Natl Acad Sci USA 97:3422-3427, 2000.

33. Blau HM, Brazelton TR, Weimann JM: The evolving concept of a stem cell: Entity or function? Cell 105:829-841, 2001.

34. Crosby JR, Kaminski WE, Schatteman G, et al: Endothelial cells of hematopoietic origin make a significant contribution to adult blood vessel formation. Circ Res 87:728-730, 2000.

35. Kocher AA, Schuster MD, Szabolcs MJ, et al: Neovascularization of ischemic myocardium by human bone-marrow-derived angioblasts prevents cardiomyocyte apoptosis, reduces remodeling and improves cardiac function. Nat Med 7:430-436, 2001.

36. Kawamoto A, Gwon HC, Iwaguro H, et al: Therapeutic potential of ex vivo expanded endothelial progenitor cells for myocardial ischemia. Circulation 103:634-637, 2001.

37. Orlic D, Kajstura J, Chimenti S, et al: Bone marrow cells regenerate infarcted myocardium. Nature 410:701-705, 2001.

38. Strauer BE, Brehm M, Zeus T, et al: Repair of infarcted myocardium by autologous intracoronary mononuclear bone marrow cell transplantation in humans. Circulation 106:1913-1918, 2002.

13

39. Assmus B, Schachinger V, Teupe C, et al: Transplantation of Progenitor Cells and Regeneration Enhancement in Acute Myocardial Infarction (TOPCARE-AMI). Circulation 106:3009-3017, 2002.

40. Stamm C, Westphal B, Kleine HD, et al: Autologous bone-marrow stem-cell transplantation for myocardial regeneration. Lancet 361:45-46, 2003.

41. Tse HF, Kwong YL, Chan JK, et al: Angiogenesis in ischaemic myocardium by intramyocardial autologous bone marrow mononuclear cell implantation. Lancet 361:47-49, 2003.

42. Jackson KA, Majka SM, Wang H, et al: Regeneration of ischemic cardiac muscle and vascular endothelium by adult stem cells. J Clin Invest 107:1395-1402, 2001.

43. Murayama T, Tepper OM, Silver M, et al: Determination of bone marrow-derived endothelial progenitor cell significance in angiogenic growth factor-induced neovascularization in vivo. Exp Hematol 30:967-972, 2002.

44. Aicher A, Brenner W, Zuhayra M, et al: Assessment of the tissue distribution of transplanted human endothelial progenitor cells by radioactive labeling. Circulation 107:2134-2139, 2003.

45. Levesque JP, Hendy J, Takamatsu Y, et al: Disruption of the CXCR4/CXCL12 chemotactic interaction during hematopoietic stem cell mobilization induced by GCSF or cyclophosphamide. J Clin Invest 111:187-196, 2003.

46. Petit I, Szyper-Kravitz M, Nagler A, et al: G-CSF induces stem cell mobilization by decreasing bone marrow SDF-1 and up-regulating CXCR4. Nat Immunol 3:687-694, 2002.

47. Orlic D, Kajstura J, Chimenti S, et al: Mobilized bone marrow cells repair the infarcted heart, improving function and survival. Proc Natl Acad Sci USA 98:10344-10349, 2001.

48. Takahashi T, Kalka C, Masuda H, et al: Ischemia- and cytokine-induced mobilization of bone marrow-derived endothelial progenitor cells for neovascularization. Nat Med 5:434-438, 1999.

49. Seiler C, Pohl T, Wustmann K, et al: Promotion of collateral growth by granulocyte-macrophage colony-stimulating factor in patients with coronary artery disease: A randomized, double-blind, placebo-controlled study. Circulation 104:2012-2017, 2001.

50. Asahara T, Takahashi T, Masuda H, et al: VEGF contributes to postnatal neovascularization by mobilizing bone marrow-derived endothelial progenitor cells. EMBO J 18:3964-3972, 1999.

51. Rafii S, Heissig B, Hattori K: Efficient mobilization and recruitment of marrow-derived endothelial and hematopoietic stem cells by adenoviral vectors expressing angiogenic factors. Gene Ther 9:631-641, 2002.

52. Carmeliet P, Moons L, Luttun A, et al: Synergism between vascular endothelial growth factor and placental growth factor contributes to angiogenesis and plasma extravasation in pathological conditions. Nat Med 7:575-583, 2001.

53. Luttun A, Tjwa M, Moons L, et al: Revascularization of ischemic tissues by PlGF treatment, and inhibition of tumor angiogenesis, arthritis and atherosclerosis by anti-Flt1. Nat Med 8:831-840, 2002.

54. Hattori K, Heissig B, Wu Y, et al: Placental growth factor reconstitutes hematopoiesis by recruiting VEGFR1(+) stem cells from bone-marrow microenvironment. Nat Med 8:841-849, 2002.

55. Yamaguchi J, Kusano KF, Masuo O, et al: Stromal cell-derived factor-1

effects on ex vivo expanded endothelial progenitor cell recruitment for ischemic neovascularization. Circulation 107:1322-1328, 2003.

56. Mohle R, Bautz F, Rafii S, et al: The chemokine receptor CXCR-4 is expressed on CD34+ hematopoietic progenitors and leukemic cells and mediates transendothelial migration induced by stromal cell-derived factor-1. Blood 91:4523-4530, 1998.

57. Wright DE, Bowman EP, Wagers AJ, et al: Hematopoietic stem cells are uniquely selective in their migratory response to chemokines. J Exp Med 195:1145-1154, 2002.

58. Peled A, Petit I, Kollet O, et al: Dependence of human stem cell engraftment and repopulation of NOD/SCID mice on CXCR4. Science 283:845-848, 1999.

59. Rafii S, Lyden D: Therapeutic stem and progenitor cell transplantation for organ vascularization and regeneration. Nat Med 9:702-712, 2003.

60. Llevadot J, Murasawa S, Kureishi Y, et al: HMG-CoA reductase inhibitor mobilizes bone marrow–derived endothelial progenitor cells. J Clin Invest 108:399-405, 2001.

61. Vasa M, Fichtlscherer S, Adler K, et al: Increase in circulating endothelial progenitor cells by statin therapy in patients with stable coronary artery disease. Circulation 103:2885-2890, 2001.

62. Kalka C, Masuda H, Takahashi T, et al: Vascular endothelial growth factor(165) gene transfer augments circulating endothelial progenitor cells in human subjects. Circ Res 86:1198-1202, 2000.

63. Walter DH, Rittig K, Bahlmann FH, et al: Statin therapy accelerates reendothelialization: A novel effect involving mobilization and incorporation of bone marrow-derived endothelial progenitor cells. Circulation 105:3017-3024, 2002.

64. Werner N, Priller J, Laufs U, et al: Bone marrow-derived progenitor cells modulate vascular reendothelialization and neointimal formation: Effect of 3-hydroxy-3-methylglutaryl coenzyme a reductase inhibition. Arterioscler Thromb Vasc Biol 22:1567-1572, 2002.

65. Friedlander M, Brooks PC, Shaffer RW, et al: Definition of two angiogenic pathways by distinct alpha v integrins. Science 270:1500-1502, 1995.

66. Eliceiri BP, Cheresh DA: The role of alpha v integrins during angiogenesis: Insights into potential mechanisms of action and clinical development. J Clin Invest 103:1227-1230, 1999.

67. Tepper OM, Galiano RD, Capla JM, et al: Human endothelial progenitor cells from type II diabetics exhibit impaired proliferation, adhesion, and incorporation into vascular structures. Circulation 106:2781-2786, 2002.

68. Rivard A, Silver M, Chen D, et al: Rescue of diabetes-related impairment of angiogenesis by intramuscular gene therapy with adeno-VEGF. Am J Pathol 154:355-363, 1999.

69. Rivard A, Fabre JE, Silver M, et al: Age-dependent impairment of angiogenesis. Circulation 99:111-120, 1999.

70. Hill JM, Zalos G, Halcox JP, et al: Circulating endothelial progenitor cells, vascular function, and cardiovascular risk. N Engl J Med 348:593-600, 2003.

71. Urbich C, Dernbach E, Zeiher AM, Dimmeler S: Double-edged role of statins in angiogenesis signaling. Circ Res 90:737-744, 2002.

72. Weis M, Heeschen C, Glassford AJ, Cooke JP: Statins have biphasic effects on angiogenesis. Circulation 105:739-745, 2002.

73. Assmus B, Urbich C, Aicher A, et al: HMG-CoA reductase inhibitors

13

reduce senescence and increase proliferation of endothelial progenitor cells via regulation of cell cycle regulatory genes. Circ Res 92:1049-1055, 2003.

74. Badorff C, Brandes RP, Popp R, et al: Transdifferentiation of blood-derived human adult endothelial progenitor cells into functionally active cardiomyocytes. Circulation 107:1024-1032, 2003.

75. Anversa P, Nadal-Ginard B: Myocyte renewal and ventricular remodelling. Nature 415:240-243, 2002.

76. Vassilopoulos G, Wang PR, Russell DW: Transplanted bone marrow regenerates liver by cell fusion. Nature 422:901-904, 2003.

13

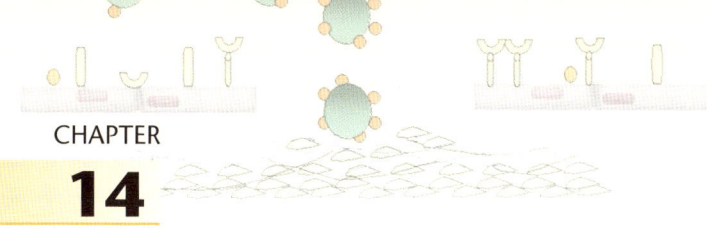

Statins and Angiogenesis

Michael Weis and John P. Cooke

Angiogenesis is the sprouting of new capillaries from preexisting blood vessels. This is a multistep process that involves proliferation, migration, and differentiation of endothelial cells, remodeling of the extracellular matrix, and functional maturation of the newly assembled vessels. Therapeutic modulation of angiogenesis is a promising new therapeutic avenue under investigation. In patients with coronary and peripheral arterial disease, angiogenic growth factors are being used to induce "biologic bypasses" to relieve ischemia-induced symptoms and to preserve end-organ function. It is therefore incumbent upon workers in this area to understand how common coexisting medical conditions (such as hyper-cholesterolemia) and medications (such as statins) may influence the response to native and exogenous angiogenic agents. In this chapter, we review the somewhat discordant literature regarding the effects of statins on angiogenesis, and we arrive at a synthesis that unites the disparate observations. In brief, statins have a biphasic effect on angiogenesis that is dose dependent. At low doses, statins enhance angiogenesis, in large part as a result of their activation of the nitric oxide (NO) synthase pathway. At high doses, antiangiogenic effects of statins predominate, because of their inhibition of isoprenoid synthesis (Fig. 14-1). These effects of statins on angiogenesis may be of therapeutic utility and are deserving of further study and possibly targeted application to diseases characterized by inadequate or pathologic angiogenesis.

EFFECT OF HYPERCHOLESTEROLEMIA ON ANGIOGENESIS

Hypercholesterolemia is a major risk factor for cardiovascular morbidity and mortality. Accordingly, modification of cardio-

This work was supported by grants from the National Heart, Lung and Blood Institute (R01 HL-63685, R01 AT/HL00204, P01 AG18784, and PO1AI50153), the Tobacco Related Disease Research Program (7RT-0128), Philip Morris External Research Program, and a grant from Sanofi-Synthelabo. Dr. Cooke is an Established Investigator of the American Heart Association.

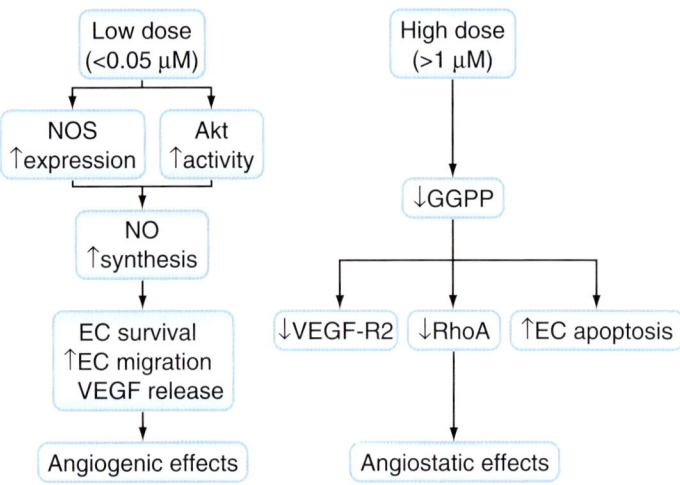

Biphasic effects of statins on angiogenesis

Figure 14-1 Biphasic effects of statins on angiogenesis. Low-dose statins mediate angiogenic effects by increasing nitric oxide synthase (NOS) expression, activating the protein kinase Akt, and thereby increasing NO synthesis. Endothelium-derived NO has several angiogenic effects, including increased survival, proliferation, and migration of endothelial cells (EC), as well as increased EC release of vascular endothelial growth factor (VEGF). High-dose statins impair angiogenesis by reducing geranylgeranyl pyrophosphate (GGPP) with resultant decrease in VEGF-receptor-2 (VEGF-R2), diminished RhoA activity, and enhanced apoptosis.

vascular risk includes treatment of hypercholesterolemia. For healthy subjects without cardiovascular disease, mild elevations of cholesterol should be first treated with lifestyle changes (i.e., diet and exercise) and then the lipid profile reevaluated. In these individuals, a low-density-lipoprotein (LDL) cholesterol under 130 mg/dL is acceptable. For patients with clinical evidence of atherosclerosis, or for diabetics, even mild elevations of cholesterol are life threatening, and LDL cholesterol should be reduced to under 100 mg/dL. For many people, the lipid profile remains unfavorable even after dietary and exercise regimens have been implemented. These individuals require drug therapy to reduce their cholesterol. Of the available agents, the most commonly used are the 3-hydroxy-3-methylglutaryl coenzyme A (HMG-CoA) reductase inhibitors, or statins. These agents are popular because they are very effective antilipid agents, they are well tolerated, and they have been shown in large randomized clinical trials to reduce cardiovascular morbidity and overall mortality. These agents reduce cholesterol by inhibiting the biosynthesis of L-mevalonate. L-mevalonate is a precursor for cholesterol, as well as isoprenoid intermediates such as farnesyl pyrophosphate (FPP) and geranyl-geranyl pyrophosphate (GGP). Because hypercholesterolemia impairs angiogenesis, as will be discussed, any antilipid agent, including statins, could be anticipated to have a favorable effect on native or therapeutic angiogenesis in a hypercholesterolemic individual.

INTERACTION OF HYPERCHOLESTEROLEMIA AND NITRIC OXIDE SYNTHASE

The impairment of angiogenesis by hypercholesterolemia appears to be the result, at least in part, of its impairment of the NO synthase (NOS) pathway. Endothelium-derived NO plays an important role in the actions of angiogenic factors. A number of angiogenic factors up-regulate the expression of endothelial NOS and stimulate the release of endothelium-derived NO. Vascular endothelial growth factor (VEGF) stimulates the release of NO from cultured human umbilical venous endothelial cells and up-regulates the expression of NOS.[1,2] Vascular segments of rabbit thoracic aorta release NO in response to VEGF; preincubation with L-arginine increases basal and VEGF-stimulated NO release twofold.[2] Similar observations have been made when the angiogenic stimulus was transforming growth factor β (TGF-β) or basic fibroblast growth factor (bFGF).[3-5]

The release of NO by these factors appears to play a critical role in their angiogenic actions. In a three-dimensional fibrin gel, human umbilical venous endothelial cells elaborate NO and form capillary-like structures when stimulated by bFGF or VEGF, effects that are blocked by the NOS antagonist Nω-nitro-L-arginine methylester (L-NAME).[6,7] Similar effects have been observed in vitro using substance P or TGF-β.[8,9] In the rabbit cornea model of angiogenesis, VEGF-induced angiogenesis is blocked by L-NAME.[10]

The mechanisms by which NO promotes angiogenesis are not fully elucidated. NO may exert its effect as an endothelial survival factor, inhibiting apoptosis[11,12] and/or enhancing endothelial cell proliferation.[13,14] Alternatively, NO may enhance endothelial migration[9,15] by stimulating endothelial cell podokinesis,[16] by enhancing the expression of $\alpha_v\beta_3$ integrin,[15] and/or by increasing dissolution of the extracellular matrix via the bFGF–induced up-regulation of urokinase-type plasminogen activator.[14] Finally, the hemodynamic effects of this potent vasodilator may play a role in its angiogenic effects. It is known that increased flow (induced by prazosin) in the skeletal microcirculation is associated with increased endothelial cell proliferation (as indicated by uptake of bromodeoxyuridine by capillary endothelial cells).[17]

Hypercholesterolemia is known to impair the synthesis and bioactivity of endothelium-derived NO.[18] When NO bioactivity is reduced, angiogenesis is attenuated. Vascular explants from rabbit thoracic aorta or human coronary artery manifest capillary-like outgrowth when placed into a collagen matrix, a phenomenon that is inhibited by oxidized LDL cholesterol,[21,22] an agent also known to reduce NO bioactivity.[21] In hypercholesterolemic rabbits, endo-thelium-dependent, NO-mediated vasodilation is blunted, as is the angiogenic response to hind-limb ischemia.[22] These data indicate that hypercholesterolemia impairs angiogenesis in part by impairing NO synthase activity. They are also consistent with observations that the angiogenic response to hind-limb ischemia is impaired in eNOS-deficient mice, an effect that cannot be reversed by VEGF.[23]

HOW DOES HYPERCHOLESTEROLEMIA IMPAIR NITRIC OXIDE-DEPENDENT ANGIOGENESIS?

Hypercholesterolemia is known to impair NO bioactivity by increasing endothelial oxidative stress. Impaired endothelium-dependent, NO-mediated vasodilation is associated with an increased vascular elaboration of superoxide anion. Superoxide anion reacts extremely rapidly with nitric oxide to form the cytotoxic free radical peroxynitrite anion.

Recently, a new mechanism for hypercholesterolemia-induced impairment of the NO synthase pathway has been elucidated. An endogenous antagonist of NOS has been described, N(G)-dimethylarginine, or asymmetric dimethylarginine (ADMA). This is an arginine analogue that competes with L-arginine for NOS.[24] The competitive inhibition of NOS by ADMA is reversed by supplemental L-arginine.[25,26]

Because NO appears to play a role in angiogenesis, and because in certain disorders (such as hypercholesterolemia) plasma ADMA is sufficiently elevated to interfere with NO synthesis, we hypothesized that ADMA may be an endogenous antiangiogenic factor that contributes to lipid-induced impairment of angiogenesis. We used the apoE-deficient mouse to investigate the effects of hypercholesterolemia on angiogenesis and to determine if any impairment may be mediated by ADMA.

Normal (C57Bl/6J) and apoE-deficient mice underwent sub-cutaneous placement of a disc angiogenesis system (DAS), which involves a disc (11 mm in diameter and 1 mm thick) made of a polyvinyl alcohol sponge (Fig. 14-2). Nitrocellulose cell-impermeable filters were affixed to each side of the sponge, so cells (and thus vessels) penetrated or exited only through the rim of the disc.[27,28] To study the direct effect of an angiogenic or an antagonist substance, these agents were added directly to a pellet inserted in the center of the disc (see Fig. 14-2). To determine the local effects of ADMA (40 or 400 µg) or FGF (20 µg), these agents were dissolved in 20 µL of phosphate-buffered saline (PBS) and added to the pellet. The pellet was coated with ethylene-vinyl acetate

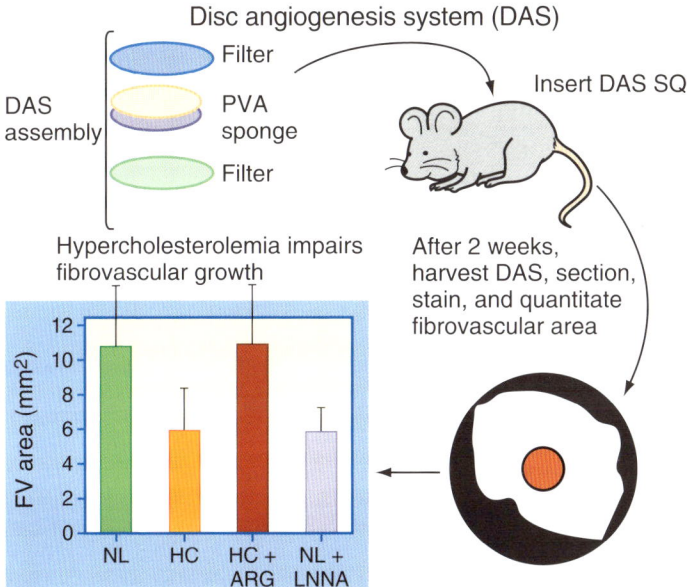

Figure 14-2 The disc angiogenesis system (DAS) is a useful in vivo assay for angiogenesis that can be used to quantitate the angiogenic effects of agents added locally to the disc or administered exogenously. (See text for description of the assay.) The results observed in the DAS correlate very well with other in vivo assays for angiogenesis. In the study shown, hypercholesterolemia reduced fibrovascular growth, an effect that was reversed by L-arginine (Arg), and that was mimicked in normocholesterolemic mice (HC) by the systemic administration of the NO synthase antagonist L-nitroarginine (LNNA). FV, fibrovascular; NL, normal; PVA, polyvinyl alcohol; SQ, subcutaneously.

copolymer to provide a slow release of the solution from the pellet into the disc. The pellet was inserted into the disc before sealing the disc with the Millipore filters. In this study, some animals also received oral L-arginine (LA, 6 g/100 mL, Sigma) or L-nitro-arginine (LNA, 6 mg/100 mL, Sigma) in their drinking water, a dose that we have found effectively inhibits NO synthesis in vivo.[29]

Two weeks after disc implantation, the mice were sacrificed with an overdose of 4% chloral hydrate and cervical dislocation. The disc was removed through an incision in the skin at the implantation site. The discs were then fixed in 10% formalin and embedded in paraffin. Subsequently, 5-μm sections were made in a plane through the center of the disc and parallel to the disc surface.

Implantation of the disc caused ingrowth of fibrovascular tissue. The area occupied by this fibrovascular growth was directly proportional to the total area of the disc occupied by blood vessels at a given stage of growth.[27,28] Therefore, the measurement of this total area was used as an index of angiogenesis.

The plasma concentrations of ADMA, measured by high-performance liquid chromatography, were elevated in apoE-deficient mice (1.9 ± 0.6 versus 1.2 ± 0.2 μmol/L in the normal controls, $P = .04$).[30] The elevation of plasma ADMA was associated with an impairment of angiogenesis. Specifically, the fibrovascular growth area in the discs implanted in hypercholesterolemic E⁻ mice was about half of that in the discs from the E⁺ animals (5.9 ± 2.1 versus 10.8 ± 2.2 mm², $P < .01$) (see Fig. 14-2). Furthermore, fibrovascular growth in response to bFGF was reduced by half in the hypercholesterolemic mice (10.1 ± 2.0 versus 23.3 ± 4.0 mm², $P < .01$).[30]

When we administered L-arginine in the drinking water (6 g/100 mL) to the apoE-deficient mice (E⁻ + LA), fibrovascular growth in the E⁻ mice was restored to levels observed in normocholesterolemic mice. Oral administration of the NOS antagonist L-nitro-arginine mimicked the effect of (lipid-induced) systemic elevation of ADMA, reducing the fibrovascular growth area to approximately half the usual response in normocholesterolemic animals (see Fig. 14-2).[30] These studies are consistent with the idea that endogenous or exogenous inhibition of NO synthesis impairs angiogenesis. They further indicate that a portion of the impaired angiogenic response in hypercholesterolemic animals is mediated by the endogenous NOS inhibitor ADMA.

Plasma levels of ADMA are elevated in humans with hyper-cholesterolemia, diabetes mellitus, insulin resistance, hypertension, or homocysteinemia.[26,31-36] A recent study from our group in humans revealed a positive correlation between the plasma L-arginine-to-ADMA ratio and NO-dependent vasodilation, as well as between this ratio and urinary nitrate excretion.[26]

ADMA is metabolized to citrulline by the enzyme dimethyl-arginine dimethylaminohydrolase (DDAH).[37] Inhibition of ADMA degradation leads to its accumulation and adverse effects on the vasculature. Pharmacologic inhibition of DDAH causes a gradual vasoconstriction of vascular segments, which is reversed by L-arginine.[38] We found that DDAH activity in vascular cells is impaired by hypercholesterolemia.[39] Oxidized LDL cholesterol, but not native LDL cholesterol, caused ADMA to accumulate in the conditioned medium of endothelial cells. This effect was associated with a decline in the activity (but not the expression) of DDAH. Similarly, DDAH activity was impaired in segments of thoracic aorta from hypercholesterolemic rabbits.[39] Studies from our group have revealed that DDAH is exquisitely sensitive to oxidative stress induced by elevated levels of cholesterol, glucose, or homocysteine.[39-41] A lipid-induced impairment of DDAH activity causes an increase in cellular and systemic ADMA levels, which reduce NO synthesis and thereby impair angiogenesis. Therefore, by reducing hypercholesterolemia, and in particular levels of LDL

14

cholesterol, statins can improve NO bioactivity and synthesis. In addition, statins are known to increase the endothelial expression of NO synthase.[42] By these actions, at lower doses, statins enhance angiogenesis.

ANTIANGIOGENIC EFFECTS OF STATINS

Statins block the synthesis of L-mevalonate, the precursor of cholesterol. However, L-mevalonate is also the precursor for the isoprenoids geranyl and farnesyl phosphate. The isoprenoids are important lipid moieties added during posttranslational modification of a variety of proteins, including G protein and G-protein subunits, Ras, and Ras-like proteins, such as Rho, Rab, Rae, Ral, and Ra.[43] At higher doses, statins inhibit angiogenesis by interfering with isoprenylation of these proteins.

Prior to recognition of this dose dependency of the modulation of angiogenesis by statins, the literature regarding the effects of statins on angiogenesis was discordant. Some reported that statins reduced endothelial cell proliferation and migration[44-49] and enhanced the antitumor effect of tumor necrosis factor α.[50] These observations tend to favor an antiangiogenic role for statins. In contrast, statins have been shown to promote angiogenesis by decreasing the small transmembrane protein caveolin and by activating the endothelial protein kinase Akt/PKB.[38,51,52] The discrepant data are largely explained by the dose dependency of these effects.

DOSE-DEPENDENT EFFECTS OF STATINS ON ANGIOGENESIS: IN VITRO OBSERVATIONS

We and others have reported dose-dependent effects of statins on angiogenesis.[47,48] Statins in low concentrations ($<1 \mu M$) enhance angiogenesis via eNOS activation.[48,52] As mentioned, NO promotes angiogenesis by enhancing endothelial cell proliferation, migration, and podokinesis.[53] By contrast, statins in high concentrations ($>1 \mu M$) decrease angiogenesis, at least in part by reducing GGP.[47] The angiostatic effects of statins at high therapeutic concentrations are lipid independent and are reversible by supplementation with mevalonate and GGP.[47] As mentioned, GGP is required for the membrane localization of small GTP-binding proteins such as Rho family members.[43] In fact, statins inhibit membrane localization of RhoA with concentration dependence similar to that for the inhibition of tube formation, whereas geranylgeranyl pyrophosphate, the substrate for the geranylation of Rho, reverses the statin-induced antiangiogenic effects.[39]

We found that endothelial cell proliferation, migration, and differentiation were each enhanced at low statin concentrations ($0.005\text{-}0.01 \mu M$) but significantly inhibited at high statin concentrations (0.05-1 μM) of cerivastatin.[47] At higher concentrations, we observed a negative effect on these endothelial processes that was associated with decreased endothelial release of VEGF and with increased endothelial apoptosis. These antiangiogenic effects were reversed by GGP. A similar biphasic dose-dependent effect on endothelial angiogenic processes was observed with atorvastatin.[47]

Other antiangiogenic effects of statins may include inhibition of the expression or activity of monocyte chemoattractant protein-1,[54] metalloproteinase and angiotensin-II,[55,56] pre-proendothelin gene,[57] and actin filament and focal adhesion formation.[58]

Endothelial cell survival factors are involved in angiogenesis.[59] Dysfunction of Rho and Ras induces apoptosis.[60] High-dose statins increase endothelial cell apoptosis,[47,48,61] most probably by reducing geranyl geranylation of Rho proteins known to modulate the activity of vascular endothelial growth factor receptor-2.[62] In contrast, low-dose statin therapy inhibits endothelial cell apoptosis.[47]

Another mechanism by which statins might interfere with angiogenic signaling is immunomodulation. It is well established that the immune system plays an important role in the regulation of angiogenesis via leukocyte-cytokine activation.[2] Statins reduce T-lymphocyte activation[63] and cytokine activity[64] and thereby may interfere with the pro-angiogenic actions mediated by inflammatory cells.

STATINS AND ANGIOGENESIS IN VIVO

To determine if the biphasic dose-dependent effects of statins on angiogenesis could be observed in vivo, we used the disc angiogenesis system described earlier. In normocholesterolemic mice, inflammation-induced angiogenesis was enhanced with low-dose statin therapy (0.5 mg/kg/day) but significantly inhibited by high concentrations of cerivastatin or atorvastatin (2.5 mg/kg/day) (Fig. 14-3). Despite the fact that high-dose statin treatment was effective at reducing lipid levels in hyperlipidemic apoE$^{-/-}$ mice, it impaired (rather than enhanced) angiogenesis at high doses.[47]

In a model of pathologic angiogenesis, we injected Lewis lung cancer cells into the flanks of C57BL/6 mice. The mice were treated with cerivastatin (0.5 or 2.5 mg/kg/day) in drinking water. After 14 or 24 days, just prior to sacrifice, 2-mL fluorescent microspheres were injected into the left ventricle over 4 minutes. Tumor tissue was explanted, measured, weighed, and prepared for histomorphometry. Tumor vascularization was quantitated by analyzing the vessel density using fluorescent microscopy and Scion Image software. High-dose (but not low-dose) cerivastatin decreased tumor growth and tumor vascularization in this murine Lewis lung cancer model.[47]

Others have shown that statins impair angiogenesis in a mouse corneal pocket assay and in a chick chorioallantoic membrane

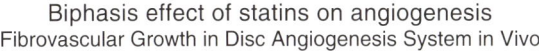

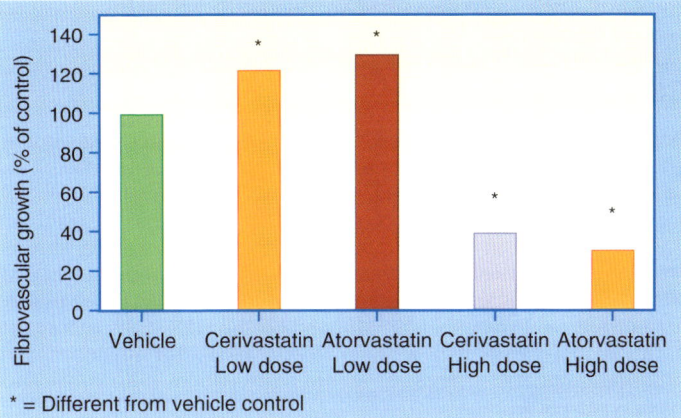

Biphasis effect of statins on angiogenesis
Fibrovascular Growth in Disc Angiogenesis System in Vivo

* = Different from vehicle control

Figure 14-3 Histogram showing the biphasic, lipid-independent effects of statins on the fibrovascular growth observed in the disc angiogenesis system (DAS) in normocholesterolemic animals. Low-dose (0.5 mg/kg/day, subcutaneously) atorvastatin or cerivastatin enhanced fibrovascular growth, whereas a high dose (2.5 mg/kg) suppressed fibrovascular growth. Of note, mice metabolize statins more effectively than humans. The dose range used in our study is based on published biotransformation studies with statins in mice, and on our own studies of the lipid-lowering effects of statins in hypercholesterolemic apoE$^{-/-}$ mice. We observed a reduction in cholesterol levels of approximately 35% and 15% after 7 days of treatment with 2.5 or 0.5 mg/kg/day cerivastatin, respectively. (See reference 47 for more details.)

assay.[46,49] In contrast, simvastatin promoted angiogenesis in ischemic limbs of normocholesterolemic rabbits.[42] We propose that these seemingly discordant observations may be explained by the biphasic, dose-dependent, and lipid-independent effects of HMG-CoA reductase inhibition on angiogenesis.[47]

Blais and co-workers recently explored the association between statins and cancer incidence in humans.[65] Patients treated with statins were found to be 28% less likely than users of bile acid–binding resins to be diagnosed as having any cancer (odds ratio, 0.72; 95% confidence interval, 0.57-0.92). In the 4S trial, fewer cancer-related deaths were observed in patients receiving long-term simvastatin therapy.[66] It is possible that some of the antiangiogenic effects that we observed are responsible for these intriguing findings.

Plaque growth is also dependent on angiogenesis.[67] Pro-angiogenic agents such as VEGF and nicotine increase plaque neovascularization and progression.[68,69] By contrast, inhibition of plaque angiogenesis reduces plaque growth.[67] Accordingly, it is possible that the known benefit of statins on the progression of coronary atherosclerosis is in part related to inhibition of plaque neovascularization.

CONCLUSION

HMG-CoA reductase inhibition has a biphasic and dose-dependent effect on angiogenesis that is mainly independent of its effects on blood cholesterol. High-dose statins decrease angiogenesis by inducing endothelial cell apoptosis, an effect related to the reduced formation of geranylated proteins. In contrast, low-dose statins enhance angiogenesis by increasing the expression and activity of NOS and by reducing the oxidative degradation of NO. The observation that angiogenesis is modulated by the HMG-CoA reductase pathway may establish a mechanistic basis for some of the lipid-independent effects of statins on cancer mortality and cardiovascular events.

References

1. Hood JD, Meininger CJ, Ziche M, Granger HJ: VEGF upregulates ecNOS message, protein, and NO production in human endothelial cells. Am J Physiol 274:H1054-1058, 1998.
2. van der Zee R, Murohara T, Luo Z, et al: Vascular endothelial growth factor/vascular permeability factor augments nitric oxide release from quiescent rabbit and human vascular endothelium. Circulation 95:1030-1037, 1997.
3. Inoue N, Venema RC, Sayegh HS, et al: Molecular regulation of the bovine endothelial cell nitric oxide synthase by transforming growth factor-beta 1. Arterioscler Thromb Vasc Biol 15:1255-1261, 1995.
4. Wu HM, Yuan Y, McCarthy M, Granger HJ: Acidic and basic FGFs dilate arterioles of skeletal muscle through a NO-dependent mechanism. Am J Physiol 271:H1087-1093, 1996.
5. Tiefenbacher CP, Chilian WM: Basic fibroblast growth factor and heparin influence coronary arteriolar tone by causing endothelium-dependent dilation. Cardiovasc Res 34:411-417, 1997.
6. Babaei S, Teichert-Kuliszewska K, Monge JC, et al: Role of nitric oxide in the angiogenic response in vitro to basic fibroblast growth factor. Circ Res 82:1007-1015, 1998.
7. Papapetropoulos A, Garcia-Cardena G, Madri JA, Sessa WC: Nitric oxide production contributes to the angiogenic properties of vascular endothelial growth factor in human endothelial cells. J Clin Invest 100:3131-3139, 1997.
8. Papapetropoulos A, Desai KM, Rudic RD, et al: Nitric oxide synthase inhibitors attenuate transforming-growth-factor-beta 1-stimulated capillary organization in vitro. Am J Pathol 150:1835-1844, 1997.
9. Ziche M, Morbidelli L, Masini E, et al: Nitric oxide mediates angiogenesis in vivo and endothelial cell growth and migration in vitro promoted by substance P. J Clin Invest 94:2036-2044, 1994.
10. Ziche M, Morbidelli L, Choudhuri R, et al: Nitric oxide synthase lies downstream from vascular endothelial growth factor-induced but not

basic fibroblast growth factor-induced angiogenesis. J Clin Invest 99:2625-2634, 1997.

11. Dimmeler S, Hermann C, Galle J, Zeiher AM: Upregulation of superoxide dismutase and nitric oxide synthase mediates the apoptosis-suppressive effects of shear stress on endothelial cells. Arterioscler Thromb Vasc Biol 19:656-664, 1999.

12. Rossig L, Fichtlscherer B, Breitschopf K, et al: Nitric oxide inhibits caspase-3 by S-nitrosation in vivo. J Biol Chem 274:6823-6826, 1999.

13. Morbidelli L, Chang CH, Douglas JG, et al: Nitric oxide mediates mitogenic effect of VEGF on coronary venular endothelium. Am J Physiol 270:H411-415, 1996.

14. Ziche M, Parenti A, Ledda F, et al: Nitric oxide promotes proliferation and plasminogen activator production by coronary venular endothelium through endogenous bFGF. Circ Res 80:845-852, 1997.

15. Murohara T, Asahara T, Takahashi T: Role of endothelial nitric oxide synthase in endothelial cell migration: Endogenous nitric oxide maintains integrin $\alpha_v\beta_3$ expression in endothelial cells. Circulation 98(Suppl):I730, 1998.

16. Noiri E, Lee E, Testa J, et al: Podokinesis in endothelial cell migration: Role of nitric oxide. Am J Physiol 274:C236-244, 1998.

17. Hudlicka O: Is physiological angiogenesis in skeletal muscle regulated by changes in microcirculation? Microcirculation 5:7-23, 1998.

18. Chen CH, Cartwright J Jr, Li Z, et al: Inhibitory effects of hypercholesterolemia and ox-LDL on angiogenesis-like endothelial growth in rabbit aortic explants: Essential role of fibroblast growth factor. Arterioscler Thromb Vasc Biol 17:1303-1312, 1997.

19. Chen CH, Henry PD: Atherosclerosis as a microvascular disease: Impaired angiogenesis mediated by suppressed basic fibroblast growth factor expression. Proc Assoc Am Phys 109:351-361, 1997.

20. Cooke JP, Dzau VJ: Nitric oxide synthase: Role in the genesis of vascular disease. Annu Rev Med 48:489-509, 1997.

21. Simon BC, Cunningham LD, Cohen RA: Oxidized low-density lipoproteins cause contraction and inhibit endothelium-dependent relaxation in the pig coronary artery. J Clin Invest 86:75-79, 1990.

22. Van Belle E, Rivard A, Chen D, et al: Hypercholesterolemia attenuates angiogenesis but does not preclude augmentation by angiogenic cytokines. Circulation 96:2667-2674, 1997.

23. Murohara T, Asahara T, Silver M, et al: Nitric oxide synthase modulates angiogenesis in response to tissue ischemia. J Clin Invest 101:2567-2578, 1998.

24. Vallance P, Leone A, Calver A, et al: Endogenous dimethylarginine as an inhibitor of nitric oxide synthesis. J Cardiovasc Pharmacol 20(Suppl 12):S60-S62, 1992.

25. Bode-Boger SM, Boger RH, Kienke S, et al: Elevated L-arginine/dimethylarginine ratio contributes to enhanced systemic NO production by dietary L-arginine in hypercholesterolemic rabbits. Biochem Biophys Res Commun 219:598-603, 1996.

26. Boger RH, Bode-Boger SM, Szuba A, et al: Asymmetric dimethylarginine (ADMA): A novel risk factor for endothelial dysfunction: Its role in hypercholesterolemia. Circulation 98:1842-1847, 1998.

27. Fajardo LF, Kowalski J, Kwan HH, et al: Methods in laboratory investigation: The disc angiogenesis system. Lab Invest 58:718-724, 1988.

14

28. Kowalski J, Kwan HH, Prionas SD, et al: Characterization and applications of the disc angiogenesis system. Exp Mol Pathol 56:1-19, 1992.

29. Maxwell AJ, Schauble E, Bernstein D, Cooke JP: Limb blood flow during exercise is dependent on nitric oxide. Circulation 98:369-374, 1998.

30. Jang JJ, Ho HK, Kwan HH, et al: Angiogenesis is impaired by hypercholesterolemia: Role of asymmetric dimethylarginine. Circulation 102:1414-1419, 2000.

31. Chan JR, Boger RH, Bode-Boger SM, et al: Asymmetric dimethylarginine increases mononuclear cell adhesiveness in hypercholesterolemic humans. Arterioscler Thromb Vasc Biol 20:1040-1046, 2000.

32. Lundman P, Eriksson MJ, Stuhlinger M, et al: Mild to moderate hypertriglyceridemia in young men is associated with endothelial dysfunction and increased plasma concentrations of asymmetric dimethylarginine. J Am Coll Cardiol 38:111-116, 2001.

33. Abbasi F, Asagmi T, Cooke JP, et al: Plasma concentrations of asymmetric dimethylarginine are increased in patients with type 2 diabetes mellitus. Am J Cardiol 88:1201-1203, 2001.

34. Stuhlinger MC, Abbasi F, Chu JW, et al: Relationship between insulin resistance and an endogenous nitric oxide synthase inhibitor. JAMA 287:1420-1426, 2002.

35. Asagmi T, Abbasi F, Stuehlinger M, et al: Metformin treatment lowers asymmetric dimethylarginine concentrations in patients with type 2 diabetes. Metabolism 51:843-846, 2002.

36. Stuhlinger MC, Oka RK, Graf EE, et al: Endothelial dysfunction induced by hyperhomocysteinemia: Role of ADMA. Circulation 108:933-938, 2003.

37. MacAllister RJ, Fickling SA, Whitley GSJ, Vallance P: Metabolism of methylarginines by human vasculature: Implications for the regulation of nitric oxide synthesis. Br J Pharmacol 112:43-48, 1994.

38. MacAllister RJ, Parry H, Kimoto M, et al: Regulation of nitric oxide synthesis by dimethylarginine dimethyl-aminohydrolase. Br J Pharmacol 119:1533-1540, 1996.

39. Ito A, Tsao PS, Adimoolam S, et al: A novel mechanism for endothelial dysfunction: Dysregulation of dimethylarginine dimethylaminohydrolase. Circulation 99:3092-3095, 1999.

40. Lin KY, Ito A, Asagami T, et al: Dysregulation of dimethylarginine dimethylaminohydrolase: A mechanism for endothelial dysfunction in diabetes mellitus. Circulation 106:987-992, 2002.

41. Stuhlinger MC, Tsao PS, Her J-H, et al: Homocysteine impairs the NO synthase pathway: Role of asymmetric dimethylarginine. Circulation 104:2569-2575, 2001.

42. Wolfrum S, Jensen KS, Liao JK: Endothelium-dependent effects of statins. Arterioscler Thromb Vasc Biol 23:729-736, 2003.

43. Edwards PA, Ericsson J: Sterols and isoprenoids: Signaling molecules derived from the cholesterol biosynthetic pathway. Annu Rev Biochem 68:157-185, 1999.

44. Negre-Aminou P, van Vliet AK, van Erck M, et al: Inhibition of proliferation of human smooth muscle cells by various HMG-CoA reductase inhibitors: Comparison with other human cell types. Biochim Biophys Acta 1345:259-268, 1997.

14

45. Vincent L, Chen W, Hong L, et al: Inhibition of endothelial cell migration by cerivastatin, an HMG-CoA reductase inhibitor: Contribution to its anti-angiogenic effect. FEBS Lett 495:159-166, 2001.

46. Vincent L, Soria C, Mirshahi F, et al: Cerivastatin, an inhibitor of 3-hydroxy-3-methylglutaryl coenzyme a reductase, inhibits endothelial cell proliferation induced by angiogenic factors in vitro and angiogenesis in in vivo models. Arterioscler Thromb Vasc Biol 22:623-629, 2002.

47. Weis M, Heeschen C, Glassford AJ, Cooke JP: Statins have biphasic effects on angiogenesis. Circulation 105:739-745, 2002.

48. Urbich C, Dernbach E, Zeiher AM, Dimmeler S: Double-edged role of statins in angiogenesis signaling. Circ Res 90:737-744, 2002.

49. Park HJ, Kong D, Iruela-Arispe L, et al: 3-Hydroxy-3-methylglutaryl coenzyme A reductase inhibitors interfere with angiogenesis by inhibiting the geranylgeranylation of RhoA. Circ Res 91:143-150, 2002.

50. Feleszko W, Balkowiec EZ, Sieberth E, et al: Lovastatin and tumor necrosis factor-alpha exhibit potentiated antitumor effects against Ha-ras-transformed murine tumor via inhibition of tumor-induced angiogenesis. Int J Cancer 81:560-567, 1999.

51. Brouet A, Sonveaux P, Dessy C, et al: Hsp90 and caveolin are key targets for the proangiogenic nitric oxide-mediated effects of statins. Circ Res 89:866-873, 2001.

52. Kureishi Y, Luo Z, Shiojima I, et al: The HMG-CoA reductase inhibitor simvastatin activates the protein kinase akt and promotes angiogenesis in normocholesterolemic animals. Nat Med 6:1004-1010, 2000.

53. Goligorsky MS, Budzikowski AS, Tsukahara H, Noiri E: Co-operation between endothelin and nitric oxide in promoting endothelial cell migration and angiogenesis. Clin Exp Pharmacol Physiol 26:269-271, 1999.

54. Romano M, Diomede L, Sironi M, et al: Inhibition of monocyte chemotactic protein-1 synthesis by statins. Lab Invest 80:1095-1100, 2000.

55. Ikeda U, Shimpo M, Ohki R, et al: Fluvastatin inhibits matrix metalloproteinase-1 expression in human vascular endothelial cells. Hypertension 36:325-329, 2000.

56. Nickenig G, Baumer AT, Temur Y, et al: Statin-sensitive dysregulated AT1 receptor function and density in hypercholesterolemic men. Circulation 100:2131-2134, 1999.

57. Hernandez-Perera O, Perez-Sala D, Navarro-Antolin J, et al: Effects of the 3-hydroxy-3-methylglutaryl-CoA reductase inhibitors, atorvastatin and simvastatin, on the expression of endothelin-1 and endothelial nitric oxide synthase in vascular endothelial cells. J Clin Invest 101:2711-2719, 1998.

58. Aepfelbacher M, Essler M, Huber E, et al: Bacterial toxins block endothelial wound repair: Evidence that Rho GTPases control cytoskeletal rearrangements in migrating endothelial cells. Arterioscler Thromb Vasc Biol 17:1623-1629, 1997.

59. Dimmeler S, Zeiher AM: Endothelial cell apoptosis in angiogenesis and vessel regression. Circ Res 87:434-439, 2000.

60. Rowinsky EK, Windle JJ, Von Hoff DD: Ras protein farnesyltransferase: A strategic target for anticancer therapeutic development. J Clin Oncol 17:3631-3652, 1999.

61. Knapp AC, Huang J, Starling G, Kiener PA: Inhibitors of HMG-CoA

reductase sensitize human smooth muscle cells to fas-ligand and cytokine-induced cell death. Atherosclerosis 152:217-227, 2000.

62. Gingras D, Lamy S, Beliveau R: Tyrosine phosphorylation of the vascular endothelial-growth-factor receptor-2 (VEGFR-2) is modulated by Rho proteins. Biochem J 348:273-280, 2000.

63. Kwak B, Mulhaupt F, Myit S, Mach F: Statins as a newly recognized type of immunomodulator. Nat Med 6:1399-1402, 2000.

64. Weis M, Pehlivanli S, Meiser BM, von Scheidt W: Simvastatin treatment is associated with improvement in coronary endothelial function and decreased cytokine activation after heart transplantation. J Am Coll Cardiol 38:814-818, 2001.

65. Blais L, Desgagne A, LeLorier J: 3-Hydroxy-3-methylglutaryl coenzyme A reductase inhibitors and the risk of cancer: A nested case-control study. Arch Intern Med 160:2363-2368, 2000.

66. Pedersen TR, Wilhelmsen L, Faergeman O, et al: Follow-up study of patients randomized in the Scandinavian simvastatin survival study (4S) of cholesterol lowering. Am J Cardiol 86:257-262, 2000.

67. Moulton KS, Heller E, Konerding MA, et al: Angiogenesis inhibitors endostatin or TNP-470 reduce intimal neovascularization and plaque growth in apolipoprotein E-deficient mice. Circulation 99:1726-1732, 1999.

68. Heeschen C, Jang JJ, Weis M, et al: Nicotine stimulates angiogenesis and promotes tumor growth and atherosclerosis. Nat Med 7:833-839, 2001.

69. Celletti F, Waugh J, Amabile P, et al: Vascular endothelial growth factor enhances atherosclerotic plaque progression. Nat Med 7:425-429, 2001.

14

Effects of Statins on Lymphocyte Function–Associated Antigen-1

Gabriele Weitz-Schmidt

3-Hydroxy-3-methylglutaryl coenzyme A (HMG-CoA) reductase inhibitors, or statins, can be divided into two groups: natural or fungi-derived statins (e.g., lovastatin, simvastatin, pravastatin) and synthetically derived statins (e.g., atorvastatin, fluvastatin, rosuvastatin).[1,2] Some of the statins are administered in their active form (e.g., pravastatin, fluvastatin), whereas others are given as lactone prodrugs that are enzymatically hydrolyzed in vivo to their respective active β-hydroxy acid forms (e.g., lovastatin, simvastatin).[1]

Statins competitively block the enzyme HMG-CoA reductase, which catalyzes the conversion of HMG-CoA to mevalonate. The inhibition of this rate-limiting step of the mevalonate pathway results in decreased levels of mevalonate and its downstream products—that is, cholesterol and isoprenoids such as farnesyl pyrophosphate and geranylgeranyl pyrophosphate. The decrease of intracellular cholesterol in hepatocytes leads to an increased uptake of low-density-lipoprotein (LDL) cholesterol and ultimately to decreased plasma cholesterol levels.[1,2] The reduced synthesis of isoprenoids may impair the posttranslational modification of proteins (prenylation), known to be important for many different cellular functions. Target proteins include small GTP-binding proteins such as Rho, Ras, and Rac.[3]

Statins are mainly prescribed to lower plasma cholesterol levels and thereby reduce the risk for cardiovascular disease.[4] Clinical trials have further demonstrated that their use is associated with the long-term reduction in cerebrovascular events.[5] Other proposed benefits of statins include immunomodulatory effects in recipients of heart transplants.[6,7] More recent investigations suggest a link between statin use and a decreased risk for Alzheimer's disease[8,9] or bone fractures in older adults.[10,11]

These diverse clinical effects indicate that statins may have effects beyond the effects on cholesterol synthesis. Indeed, there is compelling evidence, in particular from preclinical studies, that statins exert a variety of effects involving non–lipid-related mechanisms. Statins have been shown to be efficacious in animal models of acute inflammation in the absence of cholesterol-lowering effects.[12,13] More recent studies suggest that statins can reduce symptoms in murine experimental autoimmune encephalomyelitis, an experimentally induced rodent autoimmune disease,[14,15] and in an animal model of arthritis.[16] Furthermore, statins were found to enhance new bone formation in rodents.[17] These findings in animals are supported by in vitro studies that show direct, non–lipid-related effects of statins on bone cell, endothelial cell, and leukocyte functions.[17-23] At the level of individual cellular pathways, statins have been demonstrated to increase endothelial nitric oxide synthase (eNOS) activity in endothelial cells and as a consequence may improve endothelial function through enhanced release of NO.[18] Moreover, statins have been shown to inhibit inducible major histocompatibility complex (MHC) class II expression in endothelial cells and monocytes/macrophages.[19] There are also reports showing that statins reduce the secretion of proinflammatory cytokines (e.g., interleukin [IL] 6, IL-1β),[20] chemokine expression (e.g., monocyte chemotactic protein [MCP]-1),[21] and adhesion molecule expression (e.g., intercellular adhesion molecule [ICAM]-1, Mac-1).[22,23] The latter effects in particular may impair leukocyte migration to sites of inflammation and may thereby contribute to antiatherosclerotic and immunomodulatory activity in patients.

Most of these non–lipid-related, or pleiotropic, effects of statins are considered to depend on HMG-CoA reductase inhibition.[12,14,15,17-19,21-23] They are thought to be related to the reduced prenylation of proteins important for diverse cellular functions. Only recently, a novel mechanism of statin action has been described that, in contrast to these previously described effects, has proved to be unrelated to the mevalonate pathway (Fig. 15-1).[24] This statin effect, the inhibition of the integrin lymphocyte function-associated antigen-1 (LFA-1, $\alpha_L\beta_2$, CD11a/CD18) is the main subject of this chapter.

LYMPHOCYTE FUNCTION–ASSOCIATED ANTIGEN-1 AS THERAPEUTIC TARGET

LFA-1 is an α/β heterodimeric glycoprotein belonging to the β_2 integrin family.[25] The integrin is constitutively expressed in an inactive state on all leukocytes. In response to different stimuli, including T-cell activation via the T-cell receptor (TCR), LFA-1 is converted from a non–ligand-binding (inactive) state to a ligand-binding (active) state.[25,26] The ligands of LFA-1 include ICAM-1 and -2, which are expressed on endothelial cells, and ICAM-3, which is expressed on leukocytes.[25,26] As do all the members of the β_2 integrin family, LFA-1 contains an inserted (I) domain. Within the I domain, a divalent cation coordination site (named metal

Statins inhibit the LFA-1/ICAM-1 interaction independent of the mevalonate pathway

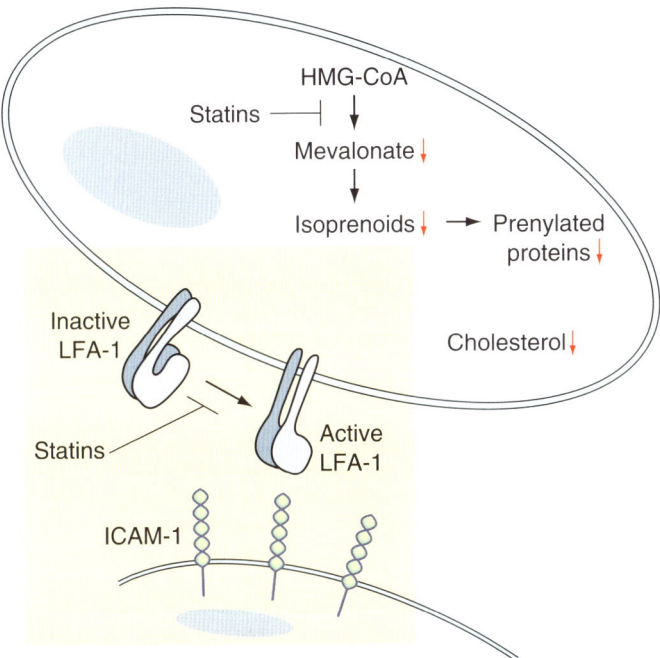

Figure 15-1 Inhibition of the LFA-1–ICAM-1 interaction by statins, independent of the mevalonate pathway. The leukocyte integrin LFA-1 needs to be converted by intracellular signals from an inactive to an active state to bind to its major ligand, ICAM-1. Certain statins bind to an extracellular allosteric site of LFA-1, thereby locking LFA-1 in an inactive (non–ligand-binding) state *(yellow box)*. This activity of statins is unrelated to their intracellular effect on HMG-CoA reductase and the mevalonate pathway. HMG-CoA, 3-hydroxy-3-methylglutaryl coenzyme A; ICAM-1, intercellular adhesion molecule-1; LFA-1, lymphocyte function–associated antigen-1.

ion–dependent adhesion site or MIDAS) interacts directly with the ICAM ligands.[25,26]

LFA-1 plays an important role in lymphocyte recirculation and also participates in the migration of leukocytes through the endothelium to sites of inflammation and antigen presentation.[25] In addition, during T-cell activation, the β_2 integrin participates in the formation of the immunologic synapse and provides a co-stimulatory activation signal.[27,28] These multiple functions make LFA-1 an attractive therapeutic target in inflammatory and immunologic diseases. Indeed, anti–LFA-1 monoclonal antibodies (mAbs) have been shown to be efficacious in animal models of dermatitis,[29] arthritis,[30] transplant rejection,[31] and ischemia/reperfusion injury.[32] Moreover, clinical studies suggest that anti–LFA-1 therapy may be beneficial in bone marrow and solid organ transplantation.[33,34] The most convincing clinical data reported so far have been in studies of chronic plaque psoriasis, where a humanized anti–LFA-1 mAb is in stage III development.[35] However, the use of biologicals poses significant limitations in clinical practice—e.g., the need for parenteral application. Thus the availability of orally active low-molecular-weight inhibitors of LFA-1 would be highly desirable.

INHIBITION OF LFA-1 BY STATINS INDEPENDENT OF THE MEVALONATE PATHWAY

Many low-molecular-weight compounds have been recognized as inhibiting the LFA-1–ICAM-1 interaction. They are of different chemical classes and have different modes of action.[36-38] The statin lovastatin was among the first molecules found to extracellularly block LFA-1 function.[39] This unexpected activity of the HMG-CoA reductase inhibitor was identified by random screening of more than 100,000 agents in an LFA-1–dependent cell adhesion assay. Further investigations revealed that the compound also blocked the LFA-1–ICAM-1 interaction in a cell-free, enzyme-linked immunosorbent (ELISA)-type binding assay utilizing immobilized purified LFA-1 and recombinant ICAM-1 (Fig. 15-2).[39] Moreover, the proliferative response of T cells induced by the engagement of both LFA-1 and the T-cell receptor was inhibited by lovastatin.[24] However, mevalonate partially reversed this T-cell proliferative response, indicating that mechanisms contributing to the effect were both HMG-CoA reductase dependent and independent. In contrast, an analogue of lovastatin, des-oxo-lovastatin, was able to completely block T-cell co-stimulation in the presence of mevalonate.[24] Des-oxo-lovastatin cannot be hydrolyzed to the HMG-CoA reductase active β-hydroxy acid form but inhibits LFA-1 with the same potency as lovastatin (see Fig. 15-2).[24] These findings indicated that lovastatin is able to inhibit both LFA-1-mediated leukocyte adhesion and T-cell co-stimulation unrelated to HMG-CoA reductase inhibition and the mevalonate pathway. Inhibition by lovastatin was found to be highly selective for LFA-1 over other integrins. Thus, the binding of ICAM-1 to the β_2 integrin Mac-1 (α_M/β_2, CD11b/CD18), which also contains an I domain, was not affected.[24] Moreover, lovastatin was inactive in assays assessing adhesion or T-cell co-stimulation mediated by the integrin VLA-4 ($\alpha_4\beta_1$, CD49d/CD29), which lacks an I domain.[24]

Utilizing x-ray crystallography, lovastatin was found to bind to the I domain of the α_L chain of LFA-1.[39] Surprisingly, the statin

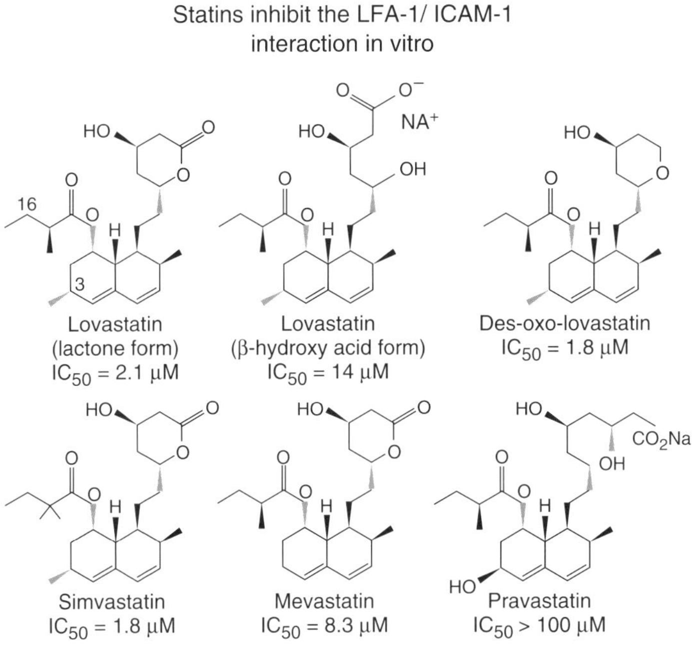

Statins inhibit the LFA-1/ ICAM-1
interaction in vitro

| Lovastatin (lactone form) $IC_{50} = 2.1\ \mu M$ | Lovastatin (β-hydroxy acid form) $IC_{50} = 14\ \mu M$ | Des-oxo-lovastatin $IC_{50} = 1.8\ \mu M$ |
| Simvastatin $IC_{50} = 1.8\ \mu M$ | Mevastatin $IC_{50} = 8.3\ \mu M$ | Pravastatin $IC_{50} > 100\ \mu M$ |

Figure 15-2 **Mechanism of inhibition of the LFA-1–ICAM-1 interaction by statins in vitro.** The IC_{50} values shown were determined in the enzyme-linked immunosorbent (ELISA)-type LFA-1–ICAM-1 binding assay.

bound to a previously unidentified hydrophobic pocket underneath the C-terminal α-helix of the I domain distant from the MIDAS (Fig. 15-3).[39] An overlay of the structure of the LFA-1 I domain in solution[40] and co-crystallized with lovastatin[39] suggests a displacement of the C-terminal helix and thus provides the structural basis for an allosteric inhibition of LFA-1 by lovastatin (see Fig. 15-3). A mutant LFA-1 "locked" in a high-affinity (ligand-binding) state has recently been found to be resistant to lovastatin inhibition.[41] This finding is in agreement with the assumption that lovastatin blocks LFA-1 indirectly via an allosteric mechanism. Because the HMG-CoA reductase inhibitor lovastatin was the first molecule shown to interact with this novel allosteric site on the I domain, the site was termed lovastatin site, or L-site.[24]

Besides lovastatin and des-oxo-lovastatin, the β-hydroxy acid form of lovastatin and the natural statins simvastatin, mevastatin, and pravastatin have been investigated in LFA-1 binding assays in

15

C-terminal helix α_7 of the LFA-1 I domain

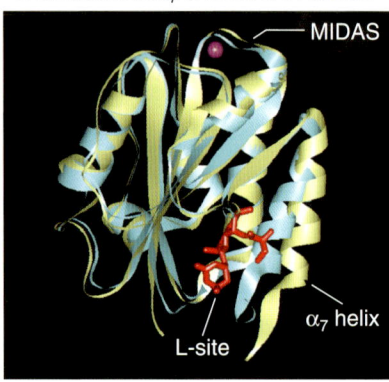

Figure 15-3 **The C-terminal helix α_7 of the LFA-1 I domain** is flexible and may be displaced upon lovastatin binding. An overlay of the structure of the LFA-1 I domain in solution *(blue color)* and co-crystallized with the small-molecular-weight inhibitor lovastatin *(yellow color)* suggests a displacement of the C-terminal helix α_7 of the I domain as the structural basis for the allosteric inhibition of LFA-1 by lovastatin. L-site, lovastatin binding site; MIDAS, metal ion–dependent adhesion site.

vitro.[24] The β-hydroxy acid form of lovastatin was found to be less potent than lovastatin, the lactone form (see Fig. 15-2) prodrug.[24] Simvastatin inhibited the LFA–1/ICAM-1 interaction at concentrations comparable to those used for lovastatin, whereas mevastatin and pravastatin (see Fig. 15-2) were less active or inactive.[24] These findings correlated with the affinity of the compounds for the L-site as assessed by nuclear magnetic resonance analysis.[24] The observed structure-activity relationship is well explained by the x-ray structure of the I-domain–lovastatin complex. The weaker activity of mevastatin compared with lovastatin could be the result of the missing methyl group at C3, which reduces the number of van der Waals interactions formed between the statin and the L-site. The lack of activity of pravastatin is likely to be because its C3 hydroxyl group would reside in the unfavorable hydrophobic environment of the L-site.[24]

Further investigations showed that the L-site is also utilized by other small-molecule LFA-1 inhibitors chemically different from statins, and thus it constitutes a major principle for selective LFA-1 inhibition.[42,43]

Taken together, these results indicate that statins are able to modulate leukocyte adhesion and T-cell activation via their binding to the L-site of LFA-1, independent of the mevalonate pathway. The evidence suggesting that this effect of statins on LFA-1 contributes to the overall biologic effects of statins is reviewed next.

LFA-1 INHIBITION BY STATINS: RELEVANCE TO THEIR BENEFIT

The first evidence that some anti-inflammatory or immunomodulatory effects of statins are unrelated to their cholesterol-lowering activity emerged from clinical trials assessing the effect of statins in recipients of heart transplants. In these patients, treatment with simvastatin or pravastatin not only decreased the incidence of acute rejection episodes but also lowered the incidence or progression of transplant coronary vasculopathy and improved patient survival rates.[6,7] On the basis of current knowledge, two major mechanisms are proposed by which statins can potentially modulate the immune response in these patients. First, statins inhibit interferon (IFN)-γ–inducible MHC class II expression on macrophages and endothelial cells, and second, statins directly interfere with LFA-1 binding to ICAM-1.[19,24] Both events would impair the activation of the host T cells and thus promote graft survival. The relevance of LFA-1 inhibition for the immunosuppressive effects is supported by the finding that LFA-1 blockade alone (by mAbs) prolongs cardiac allograft survival in primates[31] and exhibits beneficial effects in kidney transplant recipients.[34] However, it needs to be noted that pravastatin, which does not block LFA-1 in vitro, exhibits immunomodulatory effects in transplant recipients as well.[6,24] This seeming discrepancy between clinical observations and in vitro results may be explained by active metabolites or could indicate that the statin effect on LFA-1 is not essential for the overall biologic effects of these drugs in transplant recipients.

Recently, an increasing number of reports have suggested that statins may be efficacious in autoimmune diseases such as multiple sclerosis (MS) and rheumatoid arthritis (RA).[44,45] Preliminary data reported by Vollmer and colleagues suggest that patients with MS who receive simvastatin for 6 months have fewer relapses and fewer intracerebral lesions.[44] However, randomized controlled studies need to be conducted to definitively ascertain the effect of statin treatment in MS. Moreover, anti-inflammatory effects of simvastatin have been reported in patients with RA.[45] These clinical observations are supported by findings in rodent models of experimental autoimmune encephalomyelitis (EAE) and RA.[14,15,46] In both models, statins were shown to suppress disease activity either when given prophylactically or after clinical onset of the disease. It was demonstrated in these studies that statins are able to modify Th1/Th2 responses in vitro and in vivo. Specifically, in the collagen-induced arthritis model, simvastatin significantly suppressed the development and expansion of Th1 cells in the absence of cholesterol-lowering effects.[46] In the EAE model, atorvastatin was shown to promote the differentiation of Th0 cells into Th2 cells.[14,15] The finding that inhibition of the LFA-1–ICAM-1 interaction by monoclonal antibodies evokes Th2 cytokine predominance in a murine heart allograft model supports the hypothesis that LFA-1 blockade contributes to the immuno-modulatory effects in the arthritis and EAE models.[47]

It is unknown to what extent LFA-1 inhibition by statins may contribute to the well-established antiatherosclerotic effects of this drug class. Atherosclerosis has many features of a chronic inflammatory process.[48,49] Adhesion molecules, including LFA-1 and ICAM-1, are known to mediate the recruitment of monocytes and T lymphocytes to the developing atherosclerotic plaques.[48,49] Thus, an interruption of the LFA-1–ICAM-1 interaction by statins may be one mechanism by which statin therapy achieves a faster and more efficient reduction of coronary events when compared with other cholesterol-lowering therapies, including ileal bypass surgery.[4,50] The finding that simvastatin, which inhibits LFA-1 in vitro, exhibits antiatherosclerotic activity in a well-established rodent model of atherosclerosis supports this hypothesis.[51]

In summary, it is not entirely clear at this point to what extent LFA-1 inhibition contributes to the immunomodulatory and antiatherosclerotic effects of statins. It certainly needs to be noted that micromolar concentrations of statins are necessary to achieve LFA-1 inhibition in vitro. These concentrations may or may not be reached at sites of inflammation or antigen presentation with standard doses of statins. Also, it is difficult to differentiate between the statin effects that result from their powerful cholesterol-lowering activity and those that result from their non–lipid-lowering effects, such as LFA-1 inhibition. In conclusion, further investigations are needed to assess the contribution of LFA-1 inhibition by statins and to provide the data required for clinicians to consider prescribing statins as immunomodulators.

FUTURE DIRECTIONS

Statins currently used to lower cholesterol and the risk for cardio-vascular disease preferentially affect HMG-CoA reductase and not LFA-1 activity. One approach to improve their effect on LFA-1 on the one hand and to elucidate the biologic relevance of LFA-1 inhibition by statins on the other is to design statin-like compounds optimized for LFA-1 blockade. The synthesis of the lovastatin analogue des-oxo-lovastatin and the statin-based LFA-1 inhibitors LFA703 and LFA451 may serve as the first successful examples of this approach.[24,38] Differentially optimizing statins for their various biologic effects may result in new drugs of different therapeutic indications, including transplant rejection and autoimmune diseases.

References

1. Corsini A, Maggi FM, Catapano AL: Pharmacology of competitive inhibitors of HMG-CoA reductase. Pharmacol Res 31:9, 1995.

15

2. Chong PH: Lack of therapeutic interchangeability of HMG-CoA reductase inhibitors. Ann Pharmacother 36:1907, 2002.
3. Liao JK: Isoprenoids as mediators of the biological effects of statins. J Clin Invest 110:285, 2002.
4. Maron DJ, Fazio S, Linton MF: Current perspectives of statins. Circulation 101:207, 2000.
5. Byington RP, Davis BR, Plehn JF, et al: Reduction of stroke events with pravastatin: The Prospective Pravastatin Pooling (PPP) Project. Circulation 103:387, 2001.
6. Kobashigawa JA, Katznelson S, Laks H, et al: Effect of pravastatin on outcomes after cardiac transplantation. N Engl J Med 333:621, 1995.
7. Wenke K, Meiser B, Thiery J, et al: Simvastatin reduces graft vessel disease and mortality after heart transplantation. Circulation 96:1398, 1997.
8. Wolozin B, Kellman W, Ruosseau P, et al: Decreased prevalence of Alzheimer disease associated with 3-hydroxy-3-methylglutaryl coenzyme A reductase inhibitors. Arch Neurol 57:1439, 2000.
9. Bonetta L: Potential neurological value of statins increases. Nat Med 8:541, 2002.
10. Meier CR, Schlienger RG, Kraenzlin ME, et al: HMG-CoA reductase inhibitors and the risk of fractures. JAMA 283:3205, 2000.
11. Wang PS, Solomon DH, Mogun H, et al: HMG-CoA reductase inhibitors and the risk of hip fractures in elderly patients. JAMA 283:3211, 2000.
12. Diomede L, Albani D, Sottocorno M, et al: In vivo anti-inflammatory effect of statins is mediated by nonsterol mevalonate products. Arterioscler Thromb Vasc Biol 21:1327, 2001.
13. Kimura M, Kurose I, Russell J, et al: Effects of fluvastatin on leukocyte-endothelial cell adhesion in hypercholesterolemic rats. Arterioscler Thromb Vasc Biol 17:1521, 1997.
14. Youssef S, Stueve O, Patarroyo JC, et al: The HMG-CoA reductase inhibitor, atorvastatin, promotes a Th2 bias and reverses paralysis in central nervous system autoimmune disease. Nature 420:78, 2002.
15. Aktas O, Waiczies S, Smorodchenko A, et al: Treatment of relapsing paralysis in experimental encephalomyelitis by targeting Th1 cells through atorvastatin. J Exp Med 197:725, 2003.
16. Leung BP, Sattar N, Crilly A, et al: A novel anti-inflammatory role for simvastatin in inflammatory arthritis. J Immunol 170:1524, 2003.
17. Mundy G, Garrett R, Harris S, et al: Stimulation of bone formation in vitro and in rodents by statins. Science 286:1946, 1999.
18. Laufs U, La Fata V, Plutzky J, et al: Upregulation of endothelial nitric oxide synthase by HMG CoA reductase inhibitors. Circulation 97:1129, 1998.
19. Kwak B, Mulhaupt F, Myit S, et al: Statins as a newly recognized type of immunomodulator. Nat Med 6:1399, 2000.
20. Inoue I, Goto S, Mizotani K, et al: Lipophilic HMG-CoA reductase inhibitor has an anti-inflammatory effect: Reduction of mRNA levels for interleukin-1beta, interleukin-6, cyclooxygenase-2, and p22phox by regulation of peroxisome proliferator-activated receptor alpha (PPARalpha) in primary endothelial cells. Life Sci 67:863, 2000.
21. Romano M, Diomede L, Sironi M, et al: Inhibition of monocyte chemotactic protein-1 synthesis by statins. Lab Invest 80:1095, 2000.
22. Takeuchi S, Kawashima S, Rikitake Y, et al: Cerivastatin suppresses lipopolysaccharide-induced ICAM-1 expression through inhibition of Rho GTPase in BAEC. Biochem Biophys Res Commun 269:102, 2000.

23. Weber C, Erl W, Weber KS, et al: HMG-CoA reductase inhibitors decrease CD11b expression and CD11b-dependent adhesion of monocytes to endothelium and reduce increased adhesiveness of monocytes isolated from patients with hypercholesterolemia. J Am Coll Cardiol 30:1212, 1997.
24. Weitz-Schmidt G, Welzenbach K, Brinkmann V, et al.: Statins selectively inhibit leukocyte function antigen-1 by binding to a novel regulatory integrin site. Nat Med 7:687, 2001.
25. Springer TA: Traffic signals for lymphocyte recirculation and leukocyte emigration: The multistep paradigm. Cell 76:301, 1994.
26. Hogg N, Leitinger B: Shape and shift changes related to the function of leukocyte integrins LFA-1 and Mac-1. J Leukoc Biol 69:893, 2001.
27. Grakoui A, Bromley SK, Sumen C, et al: The immunological synapse: A molecular machine function controlling T cell activation. Science 285:221, 1999.
28. Van Seventer GA, Shimizu Y, Horgan KJ, et al: The LFA-1 ligand ICAM-1 provides an important costimulatory signal for T cell receptor-mediated activation of resting T cells. J Immunol 144:4579, 1990.
29. Scheynius A, Camp RL, Pure E: Unresponsiveness to 2,4-dinitro-1-fluoro-benzene after treatment with monoclonal antibodies to leukocyte function-associated molecule-1 and intercellular adhesion molecule-1 during sensitization. J Immunol 156:1804, 1996.
30. Issekutz AC: Adhesion molecules mediating neutrophil migration to arthritis in vivo and across endothelium and connective tissue barriers in vitro. Inflamm Res 47(Suppl. 3):S123, 1998.
31. Poston RS, Robbins RC, Chan B, et al: Effects of humanized monoclonal antibody to rhesus CD11a in rhesus monkey cardiac allograft recipients. Transplantation 69:2005, 2000.
32. Martin X, Da Silva M, Virieux SR, et al: Protective effect of an anti-LFA 1 monoclonal antibody (odulimomab) on renal damage due to ischemia and kidney autotransplantation. Transplant Proc 32:481, 2000.
33. Cavazzana-Calvo M, Jabado N, Bordigoni P, et al: In vivo infusion of anti-LFA-1 and anti-CD2 antibodies prevents graft failure after HLA partially incompatible bone marrow transplantation in children with high risk acute lymphoblastic leukaemia. Leuk Lymphoma 28:103, 1997.
34. Hourmant M, Bedrossian J, Durand D, et al: A randomized multicenter trial comparing leukocyte function-associated antigen-1 monoclonal antibody with rabbit antithymocyte globulin as induction treatment in first kidney transplantations. Transplantation 62:1565, 1996.
35. Gottlieb AB, Krueger JG, Wittkowski K, et al: Psoriasis as a model for T-cell-mediated disease: Immunobiologic and clinical effects of treatment with multiple doses of efalizumab, an anti-CD11a antibody. Arch Dermatol 138:591, 2002.
36. Liu G: Inhibitors of LFA-1/ICAM-1 interaction: From monoclonal antibodies to small molecules. Drugs Future 26:767, 2001.
37. Wattanasin S, Albert R, Ehrhardt C, et al: 1,4-Diazepane-2-ones as novel inhibitors of LFA-1. Bioorg Med Chem Lett 13:499, 2003.
38. Welzenbach K, Hommel U, Weitz-Schmidt G: Small molecule inhibitors induce conformational changes in the I domain and the I-like domain of lymphocyte function-associated antigen-1: Molecular insights into integrin inhibition. J Biol Chem 277:10590, 2002.
39. Kallen J, Welzenbach K, Ramage P, et al: Structural basis for LFA-1 inhibition upon lovastatin binding to the CD11a I domain. J Mol Biol 292:1, 1999.

15

40. Legge GB, Kriwacki RW, Chung J, et al: NMR solution structure of the inserted domain of human leukocyte function associated antigen-1. J Mol Biol 295:1251, 2000.
41. Lu C, Shimaoka M, Ferzly M, et al: An isolated, surface-expressed I domain of the integrin alphaLbeta2 is sufficient for strong adhesive function when locked in the open conformation with a disulfide bond. Proc Natl Acad Sci U S A 98:2387, 2001.
42. Liu G, Link JT, Pei Z, et al: Discovery of novel p-arylthio cinnamides as antagonists of leukocyte function-associated antigen-1/intracellular adhesion molecule-1 interaction: 1. Identification of an additional binding pocket based on an anilino diaryl sulfide lead. J Med Chem 43:4025, 2000.
43. Last-Barney K, Davidson W, Cardozo M, et al: Binding site elucidation of hydantoin-based antagonists of LFA-1 using multidisciplinary technologies: Evidence for the allosteric inhibition of a protein-protein interaction. J Am Chem Soc 123:5643, 2001.
44. Vollmer T, Durkalski V, Corboy J, et al: An open-label, single arm study of simvastatin as a therapy for multiple sclerosis. Neurology 60(Suppl 1):A84, 2003.
45. Kanda H, Hamasaki K, Kubo K, et al: Antiinflammatory effect of simvastatin in patients with rheumatoid arthritis. J Rheumatol 29:2024, 2002.
46. Leung BP, Sattar N, Crilly A, et al: A novel anti-inflammatory role for simvastatin in inflammatory arthritis. J Immunol 170:1524, 2003.
47. Suzuki J, Isobe M, Izawa A, et al: Differential Th1 and Th2 cell regulation of murine cardiac allograft acceptance by blocking cell adhesion of ICAM-1/LFA-1 and VCAM-1/VLA-4. Transplant Immunol 7:65, 1999.
48. Ross R: Atherosclerosis: An inflammatory disease. N Engl J Med 340:115, 1999.
49. Watanabe T, Fan J: Atherosclerosis and inflammation: Mononuclear cell recruitment and adhesion molecules with reference to the implication of ICAM-1/LFA-1 pathway in atherogenesis. Int J Cardiol 66(Suppl 1):S45, 1998.
50. Vaughan CJ, Murphy MB, Buckley BM: Statins do more than just lower cholesterol. Lancet 348:1079, 1996.
51. Sparrow CP, Burton CA, Hernandez M, et al: Simvastatin has anti-inflammatory and antiatherosclerotic activities independent of plasma cholesterol lowering. Arterioscler Thromb Vasc Biol 21,115, 2001.

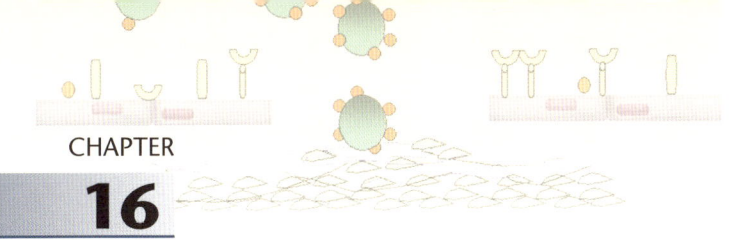

Statins and Bone

I. Ross Garrett and Gregory R. Mundy

CHEMICAL NATURE OF STATINS

Specific competitive inhibitors of the 3-hydroxy-3-methylglutaryl coenzyme A (HMG-CoA) reductase, such as lovastatin, simvastatin, pravastatin, atorvastatin, fluvastatin, and cerivastatin, widely used agents for lowering cholesterol and reducing heart attack rates, provide an important and effective approach to the treatment of hyperlipidemia and arteriosclerosis.[1,2] These orally prescribed statin drugs, some prescribed for over 10 years for lowering cholesterol, appear to have relatively good safety profiles. Newer, recently synthesized statin compounds are in clinical trials and should be on the market in the near future.[3-5] These appear to have reduced side effects while still being efficacious for the treatment of patients with hypercholesterolemia.

The chemical structures of the first three HMG-CoA reductase inhibitors in Table 16-1 are closely related, but the physicochemical properties of lovastatin and simvastatin (Zocor) differ from those of pravastatin (Pravachol). Fluvastatin (Lescol) represents the first synthetic HMG-CoA reductase inhibitor and shares physicochemical characteristics with pravastatin as well as with lovastatin and simvastatin. Atorvastatin (Lipitor), which is also a synthetic HMG-CoA reductase inhibitor, lowers plasma cholesterol levels by inhibiting endogenous cholesterol synthesis. In large trials involving patients with hypercholesterolemia, atorvastatin produced greater reductions in total cholesterol, low-density-lipoprotein (LDL) cholesterol, apolipoprotein B, and triglyceride levels than lovastatin, pravastatin, or simvastatin.[6]

Atorvastatin shares physicochemical characteristics with pravastatin as well as with lovastatin and simvastatin (see Table 16-1). Simvastatin and pravastatin contain chemical modifications of lovastatin originally derived from a fungal source.[7-9] Both lovastatin and simvastatin, administered as prodrug or lactone forms, differ from the other statins administered as the active or β-hydroxy acid. The conversion of prodrug to the β-hydroxy acid form occurs primarily in the gut and liver by the action of local enzymes. The β-hydroxy acid form is responsible for inhibition of

16

Table 16–1

Physiochemical and Pharmacokinetic Properties of the Current Statins

	Lovastatin	Simvastatin	Pravastatin	Fluvastatin	Atorvastatin	Cerivastatin
Prodrug	Yes	Yes	No	No	No	No
Bioavailability (%)	<5	<5	17	24	14	60
Relative lipid-lowering potency	3	6	2	1	12	200
Lipophilicity	Yes	Yes	No	Yes	Yes	Yes
Protein binding (%)	>95	95	50	96	>96	99
Renal excretion (%)	30	13	60	<6	<2	24
Hepatic first-pass extraction (%)	40-70	50-80	50-70	40-70	20-30	50-60
Metabolic enzymes	CPY3A4	CPY3A4	Hydroxylase	CPY2C9	CPY3A4	CPY3A4 and CPY2C8
Number of active metabolites	3	3	2	No	2	2
Plasma elimination ($t_{1/2}$) (hr)	2	3	2	3	15	3

16

the HMG-CoA reductase enzyme. The lactone prodrugs of lovastatin and simvastatin are almost three orders of magnitude more lipophilic than their corresponding β-hydroxy acid forms, which are in turn approximately 100 times more lipophilic than pravastatin.[10] The differences in lipophilicity reflect the potential of these various substances to cross cellular membranes nonselectively by passive diffusion, and they help explain why pravastatin does not easily cross cellular membranes, whereas both lovastatin and simvastatin do. A pyridine derivative, cerivastatin (Baycol), is a newer, synthetic, and enantiomerically pure inhibitor of HMG-CoA reductase. As a sodium salt, cerivastatin is present in the active or β-hydroxy acid form. It is 100 times more potent at inhibiting HMG-CoA reductase in liver microsomal fractions than simvastatin, and it is more potent in vivo at lowering liver cholesterol. Because the primary site of cholesterol synthesis is the liver, the pharmaceutical industry designed these agents to be hepatoselective. The enzyme HMG-CoA reductase catalyzes the rate-limiting step in cholesterol biosynthesis, and although cholesterol is the main product of the pathway controlled by this enzyme, its direct product mevalonate is a precursor to a number of nonsterol compounds vital to a variety of cellular functions.

BONE METABOLISM

Bone is a metabolically active organ in which the organizational pattern of the mineral and organic components determines the successful mechanical function of the skeleton. This is achieved by a combination of dense, compact bone and cancellous (trabecular) bone, reinforced at points of stress.[11,12] Distinct agents and mechanisms regulate bone formation and bone resorption, the two major processes of bone remodeling.

The formation of new bone occurs by the production of a new bone matrix by the osteoblast and its subsequent mineralization by mechanisms that are as yet poorly understood. Because the formation of new bone is primarily a function of the osteoblast, agents regulating bone formation can act by either increasing or decreasing the replication of cells of osteoblastic lineage or by modifying the differentiated function of the osteoblast.

Both systemic hormones and local factors control bone formation. The local regulators of bone formation are growth factors that act directly on cells of osteoblastic lineage. Growth factors are polypeptides with important effects on cell function. Some polypeptide growth factors are also present in the circulation and may function as systemic agents, but for the most part they work locally in specific tissues as regulators of cell metabolism. Production of new bone during embryogenesis occurs through a complex series of cellular interactions that communicate the information needed for correct pattern formation and the signals required for differentiation of cells into cartilage and bone. Most bones in the body start as cartilage models and then are ultimately replaced by bone through the process of endochondral bone formation. In contrast, bones of the craniofacial skeleton form directly by the conversion of mesenchymal progenitors into osteoblasts through intramembranous bone formation. The result of either developmental path is bone surrounded by a periosteal layer rich in progenitor cells and containing a mature marrow cavity and vascular supply.

In young healthy adults, remodeling of the existing skeleton is a continuous process resulting in no net bone formation. This highly regulated process is sensitive to both hormonal fluctuations and aging. Imbalances in this process between bone resorption and bone formation often result in either osteopenia or osteosclerosis. Although intense periods of new bone formation take place in adults during fracture healing, the matrix degradation occurring during these repair phases causes the release of many growth factors known to be stored in bone.[13] These growth factors play a critical role in the bone repair process by controlling the rate and extent of new bone growth.

A wide variety of growth factors are stored in and released from bone. These include insulin-like growth factors (IGFs), fibroblast growth factors (FGFs), transforming growth factor β (TGF-β), and bone morphogenetic proteins (BMPs), which are unique osteoinductive growth factors. The BMPs have bone-forming activity and account for the major proportion of the osteo-inductive potential of bone extracts.[14] The BMP family of proteins has been characterized, and at least six related proteins, termed BMP-2 through BMP-7, exist.[15] There appear to be two subgroups of these proteins, one composed of the closely related proteins BMP-2 and BMP-4, and a second composed of BMP-5, BMP-6, and BMP-7. All these BMPs are members of the TGF-β superfamily.

One promising use of this family of proteins is local application to repair bone or stimulate new bone formation where loss has occurred. However, it appears that BMPs are not effective as systemic treatments, probably because of their pharmacokinetics. It would therefore be beneficial to stimulate the production of these potent active agents at local sites in bone, resulting in bone formation where needed.

To date, there is one anabolic agent on the market, teriparatide, which will be sold under the name of Fortéo. Fortéo is a portion of human parathyroid hormone (PTH). Another bone anabolic agent currently under investigation is fluoride. Although both these agents cause substantial increases in bone formation, fluoride is associated with impaired bone integrity and a lack of concomitant improvement in fracture rates. In addition, although Fortéo appears to be effective as a bone anabolic agent, it is a peptide that is expensive to manufacture and can only be given by injection, which limits its use for the treatment of osteoporosis.

DISCOVERY OF THE EFFECTS OF STATINS ON BONE

In attempts to identify small-molecular-weight bone anabolic compounds, attention has focused on the growth regulatory factors responsible for the control of normal bone remodeling. Growth factors incorporated into the bone matrix and released in active form during resorption are themselves available locally to control all of the subsequent events involved in the formation of bone and to complete the normal remodeling cascade.[13] These growth factors are responsible for enhancing osteoclast apoptosis, causing chemotaxis of osteoblast precursors to sites of resorption defects, and stimulating the proliferation of osteoblast precursors to lead to a sufficient number of osteoblasts to ensure that normal bone formation can take place. The bone morphogenetic proteins, in contrast, are responsible for enhancing osteoblast differentiation, including stimulation of the expression of the structural proteins of bone such as type 1 collagen and the mineralization of the bone matrix. BMP-2 injected over bone surfaces in vivo causes a powerful enhancement of new bone formation. It has been hypothesized that BMP-2 is very likely an autocrine factor involved in osteoblastic differentiation, and that it is expressed by osteoblasts as they differentiate to further enhance mineralization.[16] The BMP-2 promoter has been characterized, and on the basis of the properties of BMP-2, it has been utilized as a target to identify new compounds that stimulate its transcription and subsequent osteoblast differentiation.

A cell-based screening assay was used to identify the small molecules that enhance BMP-2 transcription. This assay employed an osteoblast cell line from transgenic mice; the transgene was targeted to the osteoblast lineage and comprised the SV40 large T antigen.[17] These immortalized cells derived from the transgenic mice were then transfected with the BMP-2 promoter operatively linked to the firefly luciferase reporter. Screening of a natural products collection led to the identification of an extract that specifically stimulated the BMP-2 promoter in these cells. By purification of this extract, the HMG-CoA reductase inhibitor lovastatin was identified as the active constituent. Further investigations found that inhibitors of the HMG-CoA reductase stimulate bone formation both in vitro and in vivo in animal models of osteoporosis.[18] This was associated with increased expression of the BMP-2 gene in bone cells.[18]

IN VITRO EFFECTS

Effect of Statins on Bone Formation

Commercially available lovastatin increases BMP-2 transcription in a manner similar to that seen with simvastatin, mevastatin, and atorvastatin. Cerivastatin, however, is 10- to 100-fold more potent in stimulating the BMP-2 promoter than these other statins. On the other hand, pravastatin does not stimulate BMP-2 promoter activity at all. Investigations of the effects of statins on endogenous BMP-2 mRNA expression by human MG63 osteoblastic cells treated with simvastatin showed a twofold increase in BMP-2 mRNA with no obvious effect on BMP-4 mRNA. In parallel, statins also increased BMP-2 protein expression by cultured human MG63 osteoblasts. Sugiyama and co-workers confirmed these findings, where they showed that compactin and simvastatin, but not pravastatin, induced BMP-2 in human osteosarcoma cells.[19] These results were further supported by Maeda and colleagues, who showed that not only does simvastatin increase alkaline phosphatase activity and mineralization of osteoblastic cells in vitro at doses as low as 0.01 μM, but it also increases BMP-2 and collagen type-1 mRNA expression in these cells.[20] Furthermore, lovastatin has been shown to increase BMP-2 expression in human vascular smooth muscle cells, suggesting a role for the statins in plaque stabilization.[21]

Local stimulation of BMP-2 protein production, a major growth regulatory factor for the morphogenesis of bone and for postnatal bone formation, leads to new bone formation. Because statins have the capacity to stimulate BMP-2 transcription and increase protein expression, it was important to determine if an accompanying parallel biologic effect existed—namely, the stimulation of bone formation. An in vitro model of bone formation was employed that utilizes cultures of neonatal murine calvaria to determine the potential of agents to stimulate bone formation. These calvarial bone cultures respond to known bone growth factors by increasing new bone formation over a 4- to 7-day period. Simvastatin caused marked increases in osteoblast accumulation and new bone formation over 4 to 7 days of culture.

Other statins, such as lovastatin, atorvastatin, and fluvastatin, also stimulated bone formation in this assay. This effect was striking when bones were exposed to 0.06 μM cerivastatin for only 24 hours. The studies showed marked increases in new bone formation and osteoblast numbers compared with controls. This suggests that transient exposure of bone cultures to statins is enough to initiate a cascade of bone formation, which is probably induced by the local production of the osteogenic protein BMP-2. Pravastatin was unable to stimulate BMP-2 promoter activity[19,20] and it was also unable to stimulate new bone formation. Pravastatin cannot enter cells other than hepatocytes,[22-24] resulting in the reduced pleiotropic effects of this drug. These effects also correlate with its inability to stimulate new bone formation.

Simvastatin and lovastatin given as prodrugs, or lactones, are unable to inhibit HMG-CoA reductase in this form. Conversion of these compounds to the active, or β-hydroxy acid form, occurs in the intestine and liver of patients receiving this therapy. Studies to determine if either the lactone or the β-hydroxy acid form were active on bone were carried out by preparing these forms of simvastatin[25] and checking for their ability to inhibit HMG-CoA reductase. Only the β-hydroxy acid form of the drug was successful in inhibiting HMG-CoA reductase activity, whereas the prodrug or lactone form did not. In contrast, both the lactone and the β-hydroxy acid forms of simvastatin stimulated bone formation in neonatal murine calvaria. These findings indicate that the local bone environment probably activates the lactone prodrug to the β-hydroxy acid form by bone cellular enzymes such as esterases.

Effect of Statins on Osteoclasts

HMG-CoA reductase inhibitors induce apoptosis of many animal cells by inhibiting the synthesis of mevalonate and its downstream products farnesyl pyrophosphate and geranylgeranyl pyrophosphate, which are substrates of prenyltransferases, and subsequently prevent prenylation of target proteins. It has been reported that compactin (mevastatin) at concentrations of 1 to 100 μM suppresses osteoclastic bone resorption in vitro by inducing apoptosis of osteoclasts.[26] The apoptosis induced by this compound results from the inhibition of mevalonate farnesyl pyrophosphate and geranylgeranyl pyrophosphate, preventing the prenylation of target proteins. A more recent study confirms these findings and indicates that this inhibition results from the inhibition of the fusion of preosteoclastic cells and the disruption of the actin ring in osteoclasts.[27] These authors indicated that these effects are a consequence of the inhibition of prenylation of target proteins by prenyl protein transferases through decreases in their substrates.

These in vitro findings suggest that statins, although able to stimulate osteoblasts to increase their bone-forming activity, are also capable of inhibiting resorbing osteoclasts. However, these in vitro effects occur at markedly different concentrations: the inhibition of osteoclastic activity occurs between 1 and 100 μM, whereas the bone anabolic effects of these agents occur at concentrations as low as 0.06 μM. Given the hepatoselective nature of these statin drugs and the high concentrations required for the effect, it is unlikely that statins are able to inhibit bone resorption in vivo as suggested previously.[26] Alternatively, it is clear that statins have anabolic effects in vitro, and there is increasing evidence that they also have these effects in vivo.

IN VIVO EFFECTS

Local Bone Formation

The stimulation of local bone formation by either local or systemic application of bone anabolic agents would vastly improve the clinical treatment and repair of bone fractures, help the integration and stabilization of orthopedic implants, and markedly improve the repair of isolated bony defects, such as those found in periodontitis. Growth factors, including recombinant BMP-2 and FGF, have the ability to stimulate bone formation and increase repair rates in animal models. Because of the lack of systemic availability, the use of these factors is restricted to their local application. Furthermore, the use these recombinant human growth factors for local application to stimulate bone formation in humans has unfortunately been variable, and concerns have been raised about the expense and drug stability in such therapies.[28]

An alternative may be to use locally active bone-modulating drugs normally used to treat systemic bone diseases. For instance, local application of bisphosphonates in animal studies has been shown to increase bone area next to dental implants[29] and to reduce bone resorption following surgical trauma.[30,31] Unfortunately, these drugs (bisphosphonates, calcitonin, estrogen, vitamin D analogues) inhibit bone resorption (i.e., they stabilize current bone levels) instead of primarily stimulating new bone formation and are therefore of limited benefit.

The local administration of low-molecular-weight bone anabolic agents would be of great benefit for the treatment of bone disorders requiring new bone growth. Injections of bone anabolic agents over the calvaria of normal mice have provided a simple assessment model to determine local anabolic effects. A 1999 study using this model indicated that statins stimulate local bone formation in mice[18] and result in a 30% to 50% increase in bone thickness after 21 days, a result similar to that seen with the growth factor acidic FGF (aFGF). This approach might have a practical corollary in periodontal therapy, which would require single doses capable of causing a stimulatory effect. In addition, short-term bone formation needs to create lasting increases in bone volume. However, lovastatin incorporated into polymer discs (manufactured to release lovastatin at a constant rate) resulted in a 50% to 70% increase in cranial bone thickness over a 21-day period in mice. This bone anabolic effect with controlled-release lovastatin was much better than lovastatin alone injected directly over the same cranial surface in mice.[32] Others have shown that a single high dose of simvastatin formulated in a gel can stimulate cranial bone apposition, and the bone thus formed remained for up to 22 days after dosing.[33]

These findings are of great interest, because they indicate that statins directly stimulate bone formation when applied locally, in a manner similar to that of local application of BMP-2 to bone surfaces. This poses the possibility of statins being used for local generation of new bone, at sites of repair, for periodontal disease or for nonunion fracture. To date, no known low-molecular-weight compounds exist to stimulate the formation of new bone locally. Because of the physicochemical nature of statins, they can be incorporated into matrixes for local controlled release, which improves their local bone anabolic activity. Statins have numerous advantages for local stimulation of bone formation. These include their low manufacturing cost compared with recombinant proteins such as BMPs or FGFs, their known safe toxicity profiles, the relative ease of incorporating them into controlled-release matrices, and their marked increase in effectiveness when they are applied in this fashion. The possible uses of locally administered statins include orthopedic indications such as device stabilization, surgical repair of bone defects, and other bone loss conditions such as periodontal bone disease.

Systemic Bone Formation

What is needed now is an orally available bone anabolic agent that stimulates systemic new bone formation for the treatment of bone loss diseases such as osteoporosis. Because statins stimulate new bone formation both in vitro and by local administration in mice, they may be good candidates. Assessment of candidate drugs to treat osteoporosis involves the use of animal models such as the ovariectomized rat, which serves as a model of postmenopausal bone loss. Lovastatin given to ovariectomized rats daily for 35 days resulted in a marked increase in bone density when compared to the vehicle-treated ovariectomized rats. Evidence of the anabolic nature of statins on bone in vivo was derived in a series of experiments that compared the effects of treating intact rats with simvastatin, cerivastatin, or acidic FGF, a bone anabolic agent known to increase bone formation in rats.[34]

Long bones of rats treated orally with cerivastatin or simvastatin showed increases of 43% and 38% in tibial trabecular volumes, respectively.[35] Both cerivastatin and simvastatin increase trabecular bone in rats in a manner similar to that previously seen with acidic FGF.[34] The anabolic nature of any treatment can be determined by measuring bone formation indices using fluorescent markers to pre-label areas of active bone growth. These indices, bone formation rate (BFR) and mineral apposition rate (MAR), indicate the presence of new bone formation, and a significant increase in these dynamic measurements indicates that the therapy has had an anabolic effect on bone. There was a 46% increase in BFR and a 32% increase in MAR in the tibia of rats treated with cerivastatin at 0.1 mg/kg per day.[35] This indicates that statins have an anabolic effect by increasing the rate at which bone is forming, and it shows that statins have the potential to stimulate bone formation both in vitro and in vivo in rats. Presumably, this systemic increase in bone formation in rats is the result of an increase in the local production of BMP-2, a known bone growth factor. Cerivastatin has also been shown to improve cortical bone strength in ovariectomized rats when used in doses as low as 0.1 mg/kg per day, and in addition it significantly increased bone mineral density (BMD), BFR, osteocalcin mRNA levels, and resistance to fracture.[36] Other studies showed that simvastatin given orally to rats significantly increases cancellous bone compressive strength in the vertebral bodies.[37] Other studies showed an increase in cortical bone in young male rats given a single local administration of statins.[38] A recent paper showed that in mice given a diet prepared with simvastatin, there was a marked improvement in fracture healing. At 14 days, the callus of the simvastatin-treated mice had a 53% larger transverse area than controls (P = .001), the force required to break the bone was 63% greater (P = .001), and the energy uptake was increased by 150% (P = .0008). The authors indicated that the results point to a new possibility in the treatment of bone fractures.[39]

These antihypercholesterolemic drugs target the liver, the site of synthesis of a major proportion of the circulating cholesterol. This first-pass effect limits the systemic distribution of the drugs, especially to the bone (see Table 16-1). To circumvent this, lovastatin was made into a dermally absorbable gel. When used for only 5 days, this preparation was more potent and effective on bone formation than long-term oral dosing (35 days) because of its ability to avoid the first-pass effect. In 5 days, this preparation of lovastatin increased bone volume up to 33%; 30 days after the last dose, the BFR was still increased by 166%.[40]

MECHANISM OF ACTION

Role of the Mevalonate Pathway

The reduction in mevalonate pathway intermediates with a subsequent inhibition of prenylation by statins is responsible for a large proportion of the pleiotropic effects of these drugs. To determine if this was the case for bone, cultures of neonatal murine calvaria were treated with simvastatin to stimulate bone formation in the presence or absence of downstream metabolites. Mevalonate, farnesyl pyrophosphate, or geranylgeranyl pyrophosphate inhibited statin-stimulated bone formation, indicating that the effect of statins on bone is the result of the inhibition of the formation of one or more of these downstream metabolites by inhibitors of the HMG-CoA reductase enzyme. Furthermore, because geranylgeranyl pyrophosphate can reverse these effects, inhibition of prenylation caused by geranyl geranylation may play a major role in the stimulation of bone formation by this drug. Many proteins are known to require this form of prenylation for their activity, including GTPases such as Rho, Rac, and Rap. These proteins play important roles in cellular proliferation and differentiation, and therefore any perturbation of their activity influences cellular activity. A number of the pleiotropic effects of statins result from their effects on prenylation, as discussed previously. One role prenylation plays in cellular activity is to control endothelial nitric oxide synthase (eNOS), because prenylated Rho GTPase appears to controls the activity of this enzyme.[41]

Role of Nitric Oxide Synthase

Studies of statins in endothelial cells have shown that inhibition of Rho GTPase prenylation is important in up-regulating eNOS activity, thus providing beneficial effects in the endothelium.[42] This results from the posttranslational regulation of endothelial NOS stability by Rho GTPase. Both eNOS activity and NO[43] have been shown to be needed for bone formation in mice and in cultured mouse calvaria.[44,45]

Further analysis of the effects of these drugs on statin-stimulated bone formation revealed that they also up-regulated eNOS mRNA in murine osteoblasts. In parallel with this increased expression of eNOS mRNA, probably resulting from enhanced mRNA stability,[46] there was increased expression of mRNA for BMP-2. Interestingly, the expression of both eNOS and BMP-2 mRNAs occurred 6 hours after exposure to the drug and disappeared by 24 hours. Furthermore, both eNOS protein levels and NO production increased by 24 hours in human osteoblastic MG63 cells, and at the same time BMP-2 protein levels were found to be increased in cells treated with statins.[45,47] These findings link the expression of eNOS protein and BMP-2 mRNA in time, although the mechanism whereby activation of eNOS activity and presumably NO activity might lead to BMP-2 protein increases is still under investigation.

Role of BMP-2

Because BMP-2 is an important regulator of bone formation in skeletal development as well as postnatal bone formation, the enhancement of BMP-2 expression in bone cells following statin treatment illustrates the potential for treatment of osteoporosis. To determine if BMP-2 was involved in statin-stimulated bone formation, noggin, a naturally occurring antagonist of BMP activity, was found to inhibit bone formation stimulated both by BMP-2 and by simvastatin.[47] Noggin, however, did not affect bone formation stimulated by aFGF. These results indicate that BMP, presumably BMP-2, is important for bone formation stimulated by statins. Further evidence using truncated BMP receptor-type 1B, the receptor used by BMP-2, clearly shows that BMP is important for statin-stimulated bone formation.[47]

CLINICAL DATA

Statins have been orally administered as bone anabolic agents in rats, and their relative toxicity is low in humans. These agents could provide an important treatment for osteoporosis, particularly when significant amounts of trabecular bone have been lost. Current therapies for the treatment of osteoporosis, including estrogen replacement therapy, selective estrogen receptor modulators, and bisphosphonates, are primarily based on blunting the resorption component of bone remodeling.

Bone morphogenetic protein-2 is a central growth factor in osteoblast differentiation.[13] BMP-2 belongs to a large family of bone-derived growth factors, which include homologues in the TGF family as well as other unrelated growth factors such as IGF, the FGF family, and the platelet-derived growth factors. These growth factors are incorporated into the bone matrix during bone formation and are subsequently released, in an active form, during bone resorption. The TGFs are responsible for osteoblast chemotaxis to sites of resorption defects, which is required to initiate the process of formation and to stimulate proliferation of those osteoblast precursors. TGFs are probably also responsible for apoptosis of osteoclasts and cessation of the resorption phase of the remodeling cycle. BMPs, in contrast, are responsible for enhancing osteoblast differentiation, including stimulation of expression of the structural proteins of bone, such as type I collagen, and the mineralization of bone matrix.[17] BMP-2 applied to bone surfaces in vivo causes a powerful stimulation of new bone formation. BMP-2 is probably an autocrine factor involved in osteoblast differentiation, it is expressed by osteoblasts as they differentiate, and it further enhances mineralization.[17] Thus, statins, which stimulate transcription of BMP-2, may further enhance this process of osteoblast differentiation and new bone formation.

Of course, the question is whether statins will have similar effects on human bone. It has been shown that statins increase BMP-2 expression in human osteoblastic (MG-63) cells,[47] and perhaps these agents exert the same effects in human cells in vivo. On the basis of previous findings,[16] Bauer and Cummings examined their large databases to determine if there was any previously unrecognized association between statin usage and skeletal status. They found that there was indeed a possible relationship between statin use, bone mineral density, and subsequent fracture.[48] Since then, numerous published studies have indicated a significant increase of BMD associated with taking statins in postmenopausal women.[49] A recent study showed that statins seemed to be protective against nonpathologic fracture among older women.[50] One study supported an association between statin use by older adults and reduction in the risk of hip fracture,[51] and another study suggested current exposure to statins is associated with a decreased risk of bone fractures in individuals aged 50 years and older.[52,53] One study found the odds ratio for fracture associated with statin use to be 0.40 (95% confidence interval [CI], 0.23-0.71). Adjusting for BMD at the femoral neck, spine, and whole body increased the odds ratios to 0.45 (95% CI, 0.25-0.80), 0.42 (95% CI, 0.24-0.75), and 0.43 (95% CI, 0.24-0.78), respectively. Adjusting for age, weight, concurrent medications, and lifestyle factors had no substantial effect on the odds ratio for fracture. The conclusion was that there was a 60% reduction in fracture risk associated with statin use, a percentage that is greater than would be expected from increases in BMD alone.[54] Another study showed similar findings in men.[55] Finally, a study suggested that HMG-CoA reductase inhibitors may increase BMD of the femur in male patients with type 2 diabetes mellitus.[56]

A recent prospective 1-year study looked at the effects of a 40 mg/day dose of simvastatin on BMD and bone turnover.[57] Thirty consecutive postmenopausal hypercholesterolemic women (61.2 ± 4.9 years) were treated for 12 months with 40 mg/day simvastatin, and 30 normocholesterolemic age-matched postmenopausal women provided control data. Simvastatin treatment resulted in a significant increase in bone alkaline phosphatase, indicating increased osteoblastic activity, whereas there was no significant decrease in the bone resorption marker, carboxy-terminal fragment of type I collagen, over the study period. Simvastatin increased BMD at 6 and 12 months in these women, and the authors concluded that simvastatin had a positive effect on bone formation and BMD. Another recent study indicated that simvastatin was able to increase serum osteocalcin concentrations in patients.[58]

Other preliminary reports (one from the same database as a positive published report) suggested no effect.[59-62] Major drawbacks of these studies include that these are retrospective; the compliance of patients taking statins is unknown; in some cases, statins that are ineffective on bone metabolism, such as pravastatin, are included; and the dosages of the statins used vary considerably.

CONCLUSION

These results in toto suggest statins have the capacity to increase BMP-2 expression and stimulate osteoblast differentiation, leading to new bone formation. All statins currently on the market have been selected for their capacity to target the liver and decrease cholesterol biosynthesis there, and therefore they are poorly delivered to bone. Moreover, many of them are highly subject to first-pass metabolism by cytochrome P-450 enzymes in the liver and intestinal wall. Consequently, the biodistribution of active statin or metabolites to bone and other peripheral tissues is small. This makes it uncertain whether current statins will have beneficial effects on bone in humans when given orally. There are several possible ways to improve biodistribution to bone. The more potent statins such as atorvastatin may get past the liver in sufficient amounts to cause beneficial effects on bone, and animal studies suggest that this may well be the case. Alternative modes of administration of the statins, such as topical application through a skin patch, may also solve the problem of poor biodistribution to bone. Finally, other drugs of this class that were not selected for development as cholesterol-lowering agents because of their greater biodistribution to peripheral tissues may be ideal drugs for use as bone-active agents.

Perhaps the most important consequence of these findings is not that the statins themselves may be effective drugs for diseases of bone loss, but rather that these results focus attention on the cholesterol biosynthetic pathway and its relationship to BMP-2 expression and bone formation. This is further emphasized by recent observations that the nitrogen-containing bisphosphonates, drugs that reduce bone resorption and have a large market for the treatment of osteoporosis, target enzymes in this pathway. This knowledge may lead to the identification of new drugs and other therapeutic approaches to enhance bone formation and produce an ideal anabolic agent for osteoporosis.

References

1. Hunninghake DB: Therapeutic efficacy of the lipid-lowering armamentarium: The clinical benefits of aggressive lipid-lowering therapy. Am J Med 104:9S-13S, 1998.
2. Spin JM, Vagelos RH: Early use of statins in acute coronary syndromes. Curr Atheroscler Rep 5:44-51, 2003.
3. Igel M, Sudhop T, von Bergmann K: Pharmacology of 3-hydroxy-3-methylglutaryl-coenzyme A reductase inhibitors (statins), including rosuvastatin and pitavastatin. J Clin Pharmacol 42:835-845, 2002.
4. Cheng-Lai A: Rosuvastatin: A new HMG-CoA reductase inhibitor for the treatment of hypercholesterolemia. Heart Dis 5:72-78, 2003.
5. Noji Y, Higashikata T, Inazu A, et al: Long-term treatment with pitavastatin (NK-104), a new HMG-CoA reductase inhibitor, of patients with heterozygous familial hypercholesterolemia. Atherosclerosis 163:157-164, 2002.
6. Lea AP, McTavish D: Atorvastatin: A review of its pharmacology and therapeutic potential in the management of hyperlipidaemias. Drugs 53:828-847, 1997.
7. Todd PA, Goa KL: Simvastatin: A review of its pharmacological properties and therapeutic potential in hypercholesterolaemia. Drugs 40:583-607, 1990.
8. Kishida Y, Naito A, Iwado S, et al: [Research and development of pravastatin]. Yakugaku Zasshi 111:469-487, 1991.
9. Henwood JM, Heel RC: Lovastatin: A preliminary review of its pharmacodynamic properties and therapeutic use in hyperlipidaemia. Drugs 36:429-454, 1988.
10. Serajuddin AT, Ranadive SA, Mahoney EM: Relative lipophilicities, solubilities, and structure-pharmacological considerations of 3-hydroxy-3-methylglutaryl-coenzyme A (HMG-CoA) reductase inhibitors pravastatin, lovastatin, mevastatin, and simvastatin. J Pharm Sci 80:830-834, 1991.
11. Glimcher MJ: Comparison, structure and organization of bone and other mineralized tissues and the mechanism of calcification. In Aubarch GD (ed): Handbook of Physiology, Endocrinology, Parathyroid Gland. Washington, DC, American Physiological Society, 1976, pp 25-48.
12. Glimcher MJ, Krane SM: The organizational and structure of bone and the mechanism of calcification. In Ramachandran GN, Goudl BS (eds): A Treatise on Collagen: Biology of Collagens. New York, Academic Press, 1968, pp 68-91.

13. Mundy GR, Boyce B, Hughes D, et al: The effects of cytokines and growth factors on osteoblastic cells. Bone 17:71S-75S, 1995.
14. Hoffmann A, Gross G: BMP signaling pathways in cartilage and bone formation. Crit Rev Eukaryot Gene Expr 11:23-45, 2001.
15. Wozney JM, Rosen V: Bone morphogenetic proteins. In Mundy GR, Martin TJ (eds): Physiology and Pharmacology of Bone. New York, Springer-Verlag, 1998, pp 725-748.
16. Harris SE, Bonewald LF, Harris MA, et al: Effects of transforming growth factor beta on bone nodule formation and expression of bone morphogenetic protein 2, osteocalcin, osteopontin, alkaline phosphatase, and type I collagen mRNA in long-term cultures of fetal rat calvarial osteoblasts. J Bone Miner Res 9:855-863, 1994.
17. Ghosh-Choudhury N, Windle JJ, Koop BA, et al: Immortalized murine osteoblasts derived from BMP 2-T-antigen expressing transgenic mice. Endocrinology 137:331-339, 1996.
18. Mundy G, Garrett R, Harris S, et al: Stimulation of bone formation in vitro and in rodents by statins. Science 286:1946-1949, 1999.
19. Sugiyama M, Kodama T, Konishi K, et al: Compactin and simvastatin, but not pravastatin, induce bone morphogenetic protein-2 in human osteosarcoma cells. Biochem Biophys Res Commun 271:688-692, 2000.
20. Maeda T, Matsunuma A, Kawane T, et al: Simvastatin promotes osteoblast differentiation and mineralization in MC3T3-E1 cells. Biochem Biophys Res Commun 280:874-877, 2001.
21. Emmanuele L, Ortmann J, Doerflinger T, et al: Lovastatin stimulates human vascular smooth muscle cell expression of bone morphogenetic protein-2, a potent inhibitor of low-density lipoprotein-stimulated cell growth. Biochem Biophys Res Commun 302:67-72, 2003.
22. Nakai D, Nakagomi R, Furuta Y, et al: Human liver-specific organic anion transporter, LST-1, mediates uptake of pravastatin by human hepatocytes. J Pharmacol Exp Ther 297:861-867, 2001.
23. Yamazaki M, Tokui T, Ishigami M, et al: Tissue-selective uptake of pravastatin in rats: Contribution of a specific carrier-mediated uptake system. Biopharm Drug Dispos 17:775-789, 1996.
24. Ziegler K, Blumrich M, Hummelsiep S: The transporter for the HMG-CoA reductase inhibitor pravastatin is not present in Hep G2 cells: Evidence for the nonidentity of the carrier for pravastatin and certain transport systems for BSP. Biochim Biophys Acta 1223:195-201, 1994.
25. Rao S, Porter DC, Chen X, et al: Lovastatin-mediated G1 arrest is through inhibition of the proteasome, independent of hydroxymethyl glutaryl-CoA reductase. Proc Natl Acad Sci U S A 96:7797-7802, 1999.
26. Luckman SP, Hughes DE, Coxon FP, et al: Nitrogen-containing bisphosphonates inhibit the mevalonate pathway and prevent post-translational prenylation of GTP-binding proteins, including Ras. J Bone Miner Res 13:581-589, 1998.
27. Woo JT, Kasai S, Stern PH, et al: Compactin suppresses bone resorption by inhibiting the fusion of prefusion osteoclasts and disrupting the actin ring in osteoclasts. J Bone Miner Res 15:650-662, 2000.
28. Schilephake H: Bone growth factors in maxillofacial skeletal reconstruction. Int J Oral Maxillofac Surg 31:469-484, 2002.
29. Meraw SJ, Reeve CM: Qualitative analysis of peripheral peri-implant bone and influence of alendronate sodium on early bone regeneration. J Periodontol 70:1228-1233, 1999.

30. Binderman I, Adut M, Yaffe A: Effectiveness of local delivery of alendronate in reducing alveolar bone loss following periodontal surgery in rats. J Periodontol 71:1236-1240, 2000.
31. Kaynak D, Meffert R, Gunhan M, et al: A histopathological investigation on the effects of the bisphosphonate alendronate on resorptive phase following mucoperiosteal flap surgery in the mandible of rats. J Periodontol 71:790-796, 2000.
32. Whang K, Zhao M, Qiao M: Administration of lovastatin locally in low doses in a novel delivery system induces prolonged bone formation. J Bone Miner Res 15:S225, 2000.
33. Thylin MR, McConnell JC, Schmid MJ, et al: Effects of simvastatin gels on murine calvarial bone. J Periodontol 73:1141-1148, 2002.
34. Dunstan CR, Boyce R, Boyce BF, et al: Systemic administration of acidic fibroblast growth factor (FGF-1) prevents bone loss and increases new bone formation in ovariectomized rats. J Bone Miner Res 14:953-959, 1999.
35. Garrett IR, Escobedo A, Esparza J, et al: Cerivastatin increases BMP-2 expression in vivo and bone formation in concentrations of two orders of magnitude lower than other statins. J Bone Miner Res 14:S180, 1999.
36. Wilkie D, Bowman B, Lyga A, et al: Cerivastatin increases cortical bone formation in OVX rats. J Bone Miner Res 15:S549, 2000.
37. Oxlund H, Dalstra M, Andreassen TT: Statin given perorally to adult rats increases cancellous bone mass and compressive strength. Calcif Tissue Int 69:299-304, 2001.
38. Crawford DT, Qi H, Chidsey-Frink KL: Statin increases cortical bone in young male rats by single, local administration but fails to restore bone to ovariectomized (OVX) rats by daily systemic administration. J Bone Miner Res 16:S307, 2001.
39. Skoglund B, Forslund C, Aspenberg P: Simvastatin improves fracture healing in mice. J Bone Miner Res 17:2004-2008, 2002.
40. Gutierrez G, Garrett IR, Rossini G: Dermal application of lovastatin to rats causes greater increases in bone formation and plasma concentrations than when administered by oral gavage. J Bone Miner Res 15:S427, 2000.
41. Ming XF, Viswambharan H, Barandier C, et al: Rho GTPase/Rho kinase negatively regulates endothelial nitric oxide synthase phosphorylation through the inhibition of protein kinase B/Akt in human endothelial cells. Mol Cell Biol 22:8467-8477, 2002.
42. Laufs U, Fata VL, Liao JK: Inhibition of 3-hydroxy-3-methylglutaryl (HMG)-CoA reductase blocks hypoxia-mediated down-regulation of endothelial nitric oxide synthase. J Biol Chem 272:31725-1729, 1997.
43. Feron O, Dessy C, Desager JP, et al: Hydroxy-methylglutaryl-coenzyme A reductase inhibition promotes endothelial nitric oxide synthase activation through a decrease in caveolin abundance. Circulation 103:113-118, 2001.
44. Armour KE, Armour KJ, Gallagher ME, et al: Defective bone formation and anabolic response to exogenous estrogen in mice with targeted disruption of endothelial nitric oxide synthase. Endocrinology 142:760-766, 2001.
45. Garrett IR, Gutierrez G, Chen D, et al: Statins stimulate bone formation by enhancing eNOS expression. J Bone Miner Res 16:S141, 2001.
46. Laufs U, Liao JK: Post-transcriptional regulation of endothelial nitric oxide synthase mRNA stability by Rho GTPase. J Biol Chem 273:24266-24271, 1998.

16

47. Garrett IR, Esparza J, Chen D, et al: Statins mediate their effects on osteoblasts by inhibition of HMG-CoA reductase and ultimately BMP2. J Bone Miner Res 15:S225, 2000.

48. Bauer DC, Mundy GR, Jamal SA, et al: Statin use, bone mass and fracture: An analysis of two prospective studies. J Bone Miner Res 14:S179, 1999.

49. Edwards CJ, Hart DJ, Spector TD: Oral statins and increased bone-mineral density in postmenopausal women. Lancet 355:2218-2219, 2000.

50. Chan KA, Andrade SE, Boles M, et al: Inhibitors of hydroxymethylglutaryl-coenzyme A reductase and risk of fracture among older women. Lancet 355:2185-2188, 2000.

51. Wang PS, Solomon DH, Mogun H, et al: HMG-CoA reductase inhibitors and the risk of hip fractures in elderly patients. JAMA 283:3211-3216, 2000.

52. Meier CR, Schlienger RG, Kraenzlin ME, et al: HMG-CoA reductase inhibitors and the risk of fractures. JAMA 283:3205-3210, 2000.

53. Meier CR, Schlienger RG, Kraenzlin ME, et al: Statin drugs and the risk of fracture. JAMA 284:1921-1922, 2000.

54. Pasco JA, Kotowicz MA, Henry MJ, et al: Statin use, bone mineral density, and fracture risk: Geelong Osteoporosis Study. Arch Intern Med 162:537-540, 2002.

55. Funkhouser HL, Adera T, Adler RA: Effect of HMG-CoA reductase inhibitors (statins) on bone mineral density. J Clin Densitom 5:151-158, 2002.

56. Chung YS, Lee MD, Lee SK, et al: HMG-CoA reductase inhibitors increase BMD in type 2 diabetes mellitus patients. J Clin Endocrinol Metab 85:1137-1142, 2000.

57. Montagnani A, Gonnelli S, Cepollaro C, et al: Effect of simvastatin treatment on bone mineral density and bone turnover in hypercholesterolemic postmenopausal women: A 1-year longitudinal study. Bone 32:427-433, 2003.

58. Chan MH, Mak TW, Chiu RW, et al: Simvastatin increases serum osteocalcin concentration in patients treated for hypercholesterolaemia. J Clin Endocrinol Metab 86:4556-4559, 2001.

59. Lacroix AZ, Cauley JA, Jackson R, et al: Does statin use reduce risk of fracture in postmenopausal women? Results from the Women's Health Initiative Observational Study. J Bone Miner Res 15:1066, 2000.

60. Van Staa TP, Wegman SLJ, De Vries F, et al: Use of statins and risk of fractures. J Bone Miner Res 15:1067, 2000.

61. Cauley JA, Jackson R, Pettinger M, et al: Statin use and bone mineral density (BMD) in older women: The Women's Health Initiative Observational Study (WH I-OS). J Bone Miner Res 15:S155, 2000.

62. Rejnmark L, Buus NH, Vestergaard P, et al: Statins decrease bone turnover in postmenopausal women: A cross-sectional study. Eur J Clin Invest 32:581-589, 2002.

Index

Note: Page numbers followed by "f" indicate illustrations; those followed by "t" indicate tables.